Narrative Exposure Therapy (NET)
for Survivors of Traumatic Stress
3rd edition

AF766523

About the Authors

Maggie Schauer is a psychotraumatologist, PD Dr., at the University of Konstanz, Germany. Together with Frank Neuner and Thomas Elbert, she has developed Narrative Exposure Therapy (NET). She is a founding member of the NGO *vivo international,* of the NGO *babyforum* (counteracting neglect and maltreatment in early childhood*)* and of *NET The Institute.* Maggie has researched multiple and complex traumatization after family and organized violence, childhood trauma, torture, and human rights violations, especially the transgenerational consequences of violence and neglect. In her pursuit of a deeper understanding of human nature as a philosopher and psychologist, she is dedicated to synthesizing insights from a diverse spectrum of disciplines and to alleviate suffering and inspire and support survivors and therapists in trauma work in both clinical and humanitarian contexts. In 2015, Maggie, together with her colleague Michael Odenwald, was awarded the August-Forel Prize, Ellikon, Switzerland, for her research on the relationship between war, trauma, and drug intake. She was also honored with the Jaap Christoffels Visiting Professorship of the University of Amsterdam for her contributions as a scientist and clinician in the field of childhood trauma. In 2016, together with Thomas Elbert, she received the Carl Friedrich von Weizsäcker Prize of the German National Academy of Sciences for her life's work. Among many other achievements, she has recently been appointed to the board of directors of the Italian Society for Traumatic Stress Studies SISST. Maggie is based in Germany and Italy. E-mail: maggie.schauer@uni-konstanz.de

Frank Neuner is Professor and Chair of Clinical Psychology and Psychotherapy at Bielefeld University, Germany, including the university's outpatient clinic for mental disorders. He has gained an international reputation for the co-development of NET. Frank published the first randomized treatment trial for posttraumatic stress disorder with refugees living in a war region, which was followed by a series of highly cited published randomized controlled trials of his working group. He is interested and has expertise in epidemiology, etiology, and treatment of severe trauma-associated psychological disorders following repeated intense adversities such as war and child abuse. Currently he is developing low-threshold measures to improve access to psychotherapy for refugees. E-mail: frank.neuner@uni-bielefeld.de

Thomas Elbert is Professor Emeritus of Clinical Psychology and Behavioural Neuroscience at the University of Konstanz, specializing in research on the consequences of social and traumatic stress. He has conducted laboratory and clinical studies as well as field studies and care projects directly in conflict areas. Moreover, he has asked what motivates people to perpetrate acts of violence, whether domestic or in organized groups. Thomas is a member of the German Academy of Sciences Leopoldina, the Berlin–Brandenburg Academy of Sciences, and the Academia Europaea. He has received the Hector Science Prize; the German Psychology Prize, which honors outstanding achievements in psychological research; and, together with Maggie Schauer, the prestigious Carl Friedrich von Weizsäcker Prize awarded by the German Academy of Sciences. As founding member of the non-profit organisation *vivo international*, Thomas is committed to overcoming the psychological and physical consequences of traumatic stress and preventing violence. The International Society for Research on Aggression honoured him with the Scott Award in 2024. E-mail: thomas.elbert@uni-konstanz.de

Narrative Exposure Therapy (NET) for Survivors of Traumatic Stress

3rd edition

Maggie Schauer

Frank Neuner

Thomas Elbert

hogrefe

Library of Congress of Congress Cataloging in Publication information for the print version of this book is available via the Library of Congress Marc Database under the Library of Congress Control Number 2024951775

Library and Archives Canada Cataloguing in Publication
Title: Narrative exposure therapy (NET) for survivors of traumatic stress / Maggie Schauer, Frank Neuner, Thomas Elbert.
Names: Schauer, Maggie, author | Neuner, Frank, author | Elbert, Thomas, author
Description: 3rd edition. | Includes bibliographical references.
Identifiers: Canadiana (print) 20240530802 | Canadiana (ebook) 20240530810 | ISBN 9780889375956 (softcover) | ISBN 9781616765958 (PDF) | ISBN 9781613345955 (EPUB)
Subjects: LCSH: Post-traumatic stress disorder—Treatment. | LCSH: Narrative therapy. | LCSH: Victims of violent crimes—Rehabilitation. | LCSH: Narrative medicine.
Classification: LCC RC552.P67 S33 2025 | 616.85/210651—dc23

© 2025 by Hogrefe Publishing. All rights, including for text and data mining (TDM), Artificial Intelligence (AI) training, and similar technologies, are reserved.

www.hogrefe.com

The authors and publisher have made every effort to ensure that the information contained in this text is in accord with the current state of scientific knowledge, recommendations, and practice at the time of publication. In spite of this diligence, errors cannot be completely excluded. Also, due to changing regulations and continuing research, information may become outdated at any point. The authors and publisher disclaim any responsibility for any consequences which may follow from the use of information presented in this book.

Registered trademarks are not noted specifically as such in this publication. The use of descriptive names, registered names, and trademarks does not imply, even in the absence of a specific statement, that such names are exempt from the relevant protective laws and regulations and therefore free for general use.

Cover image: The cover photo shows a Lifeline and was taken by photographer Claudia Gori at the Eremo dei Frati Bianchi in Cupramontana, Italy.

This is the 3rd edition of *Narrative Exposure Therapy: A Short-Term Treatment for Traumatic Stress Disorders* (ISBN 978-0-88937-388-4).

Figures 11, 16, 17, 26, 28, 30, 31, 35, 37, 38, 40, 41, and 42 as well as parts of Figures 7, 22, 23, and 27 were designed by MUSCLEBEAVER Animation & Illustration Studio Munich.

The authors are the proprietors of the word/figurative mark (logo) for NET Narrative Exposure Therapy, which is protected by the German Patent Office (Az.: 30 2021 018782.9).

PUBLISHING OFFICES

USA:	Hogrefe Publishing Corporation, 44 Merrimac St., Newburyport, MA 01950 Phone 978 255 3700; E-mail customersupport@hogrefe.com
EUROPE:	Hogrefe Publishing GmbH, Merkelstr. 3, 37085 Göttingen, Germany Phone +49 551 99950 0, Fax +49 551 99950 111; E-mail publishing@hogrefe.com

SALES & DISTRIBUTION

USA:	Hogrefe Publishing, Customer Services Department, 30 Amberwood Parkway, Ashland, OH 44805 Phone 800 228 3749, Fax 419 281 6883; E-mail customersupport@hogrefe.com
UK:	Hogrefe Ltd, Hogrefe House, Albion Place, Oxford, OX1 1QZ Phone +44 186 579 7920; E-Mail customersupport@hogrefe.co.uk
EUROPE:	Hogrefe Publishing, Merkelstr. 3, 37085 Göttingen, Germany Phone +49 551 99950 0, Fax +49 551 99950 111; E-mail publishing@hogrefe.com

OTHER OFFICES

CANADA:	Hogrefe Publishing Corporation, 82 Laird Drive, East York, Ontario, M4G 3V1
SWITZERLAND:	Hogrefe Publishing, Länggass-Strasse 76, 3012 Bern

No part of this book may be reproduced, stored in a retrieval system or transmitted, in any form or by any means, electronic, mechanical, photocopying, microfilming, recording or otherwise, without written permission from the publisher.

Printed and bound in the Czech Republic

ISBN 978-0-88937-595-6 (print) • ISBN 978-1-61676-595-8 (PDF) • ISBN 978-1-61334-595-5 (EPUB)
http://doi.org/10.1027/00595-000

Acknowledgments

We express our gratitude to the many outstanding clinicians and researchers who have contributed to furthering the development of NET. Specifically, Elisabeth Kaiser, Claudia Catani, and Katy Robjant deserve our appreciation for their valuable discussions and essential clinical experience contributions. The NGO *vivo* has enlisted brilliant and talented minds to assist and shape clinical trials in culturally diverse settings, including war and crisis zones. Their continued support is greatly appreciated.

We are affiliated with the NGO *vivo international* (https://www.vivo.org) and *NET The Institute* (https://www.net-institute.org). The organizations can be reached by e-mail at info@vivo.org and info@net-institute.org.

Contents

Preface

We dedicate this book to those who risk their life to achieve a world without violence.

Trauma is contagious, causing suffering to loved ones, families, and communities, and placing an ever-increasing burden on our societies. Creating opportunities to process the stressful and meaningful biographical events through supported narrative in talking therapy is a remedy that is ideally suited to our innate and powerful need to share and belong, and can serve to prevent and even reverse the consequences of trauma. We humans are storytellers. Narrative Exposure Therapy (NET) is a straightforward, accessible therapeutic foundation that aims to integrate scientific evidence with the experiential knowledge of survivors in a joint approach to healing and testimony, while safeguarding the rights and dignity of people affected by violence, crisis, and conflict.

We are grateful to have been able to build these interventions on good science, on respect for the integrity of individuals and communities, on compassion, knowledge, collegiality, honesty, and openness, according to our vision statement "for a world without violence."

If adverse interpersonal childhood experiences can be prevented, the (involuntary) spread of the consequences of trauma can be halted. This will end the transgenerational cycle of violence that reverberates through the generations, causing untold suffering and destruction.

Maggie Schauer, Frank Neuner, & Thomas Elbert
(November 2024)

1 Introduction: Voices of Victims

Experiencing or witnessing a threat to one's life and integrity is considered a traumatic event because it has a lasting impact on the survivor's body and mind. Survivors are often overwhelmed by traumatic memories with frequent exposure to traumatizing experiences, resulting in pervasive fear and distress long after the danger has passed. Individuals who have experienced psychological trauma may feel as though their body and mind are under constant threat, leading to confusion between past and present dangers. Intrusive memories of traumatic events can create a distorted perception of reality, making it difficult for survivors to feel safe in the present moment. This detachment from the present and future can result in feelings of alienation and a disconnection from one's body and soul.

Natural disasters and life-threatening accidents are events that can happen to anyone. Therefore, scientists have long believed that survivors do not perceive disasters as a personal attack. However, humans tend to interpret even natural coincidences as personal, trying to link them to some reason or cause as a form of punishment for their actions.

Intentionally inflicting severe pain and harm violates humanity. Trauma destroys the essence of human interaction within a social setting, including communication, speech, autobiographical memory, dignity, peace, and freedom. It also isolates survivors and halts the natural flow of their personal narrative. In this introduction, we want the voices of those who have survived violent acts and childhood abuse and neglect, as well as torture, terror, and suffering, to be heard. Primo Levi, an Italian Jew born in Turin in 1919, who was deported to the concentration camp Auschwitz in 1943, wrote one of the most significant documents about the horrors of the concentration camp. In *If This Is A Man*, he demonstrated that the dehumanization and degradation of the victims that precedes physical murder is even more terrible than the murder itself.

> *A dream full of horror has not stopped visiting me, at sometimes frequent, sometimes longer, intervals: I am sitting in a peaceful relaxed environment, apparently without tension or affliction; yet I feel a deep and subtle anguish, the definite sensation of an impending threat. And, in fact, as the dream proceeds, slowly and brutally, each time in a different way, everything collapses and disintegrates around me, the scenery, the walls, the people, while the anguish becomes more intense and more precise. Now everything has changed into chaos; I am alone in the center of a grey and turbid nothing, and now I know what this thing means, and I also know that I have always known it; I am in the Lager once more, and nothing is true outside the Lager. All the rest was a brief pause, a deception of the senses, a dream.... I have fallen into a rather serious depression. I ask you as a "proper doctor," what should I do? I feel the need for help but I do not know what sort.*
>
> Primo Levi (February 7, 1963, p. 25; Auschwitz survivor in a letter to his friend and doctor David Mendel.)

Primo Levi had experienced even more trauma. As a child, he suffered from frequent chest infections. His father, Cesare, was often away working abroad in Hungary, leaving Primo and his mother alone. Primo was described as thin and shy, and he was severely bullied at school for many years, which he believed was due to his perceived "ugliness" (Thomson, 2019). Undoubtedly, the time spent in concentration camps was a traumatic and inhumane experience of unnameable proportions for victims and witnesses. However, it is important to recognize that other factors, such as experiences of marginalization, lack of attachment figures, physical illness, and more, occurring in contexts of persecution and human rights violations, contribute to the deterioration of mental health amidst organized violence and wars. Levi's death in 1987 came as a terrible shock to his friends and admirers around the world – his death certificate cites "suicide." Natalia Ginzburg, a Jewish writer, wrote, "Of those years [in Auschwitz] he must have had terrible memories: a wound he always carried with great fortitude, but which must have been nonetheless atrocious. I think it was the memory of those years which lead him towards his death." (quote in Gambetta, 1999).

The memory of trauma should never be erased. Many survivors believe that denying their experiences is more harmful than the trauma itself. In his account of life as a Moroccan political prisoner, inspired by his own 18 months detainment in an army camp in the late 1960s, Ben Jelloun puts this sentiment into words:

Oh, I see, (you) want to destroy the evidence of the horror suffered ... tear down, lie, mask, dance on the ashes of the people. ... Even if the soldiers succeed in erasing the traces of the dungeon, they will never erase the memory of what we have suffered from our memory. Oh, my memory ... You must persevere. Oh, you, my memory, my child, who will carry these words beyond life, beyond the visible. ... Worse than the horror suffered is its denial.

Tahar Ben Jelloun (translated from the original by the author, 2001, p. 220)

Treatments that help to organize memories of fear and horror are of central importance: They can induce a permanent anchoring of implicit memories in the past, thus preventing the unwanted frequent threat of reactivation of trauma-associated memories by triggers. This integration of traumatic events is particularly important because unresolved trauma memories can influence emotions and actions throughout a person's life and can be transmitted to the social environment as well as transgenerationally. Equally essential, however, is the testimony so that past violations remain acknowleged.

Bearing witness, however, is often prevented by the inherent dynamics of the trauma itself. Inexplicable fear and speechlessness silence survivors. Trauma agents persist due to incomplete memory encoding, preventing conscious recollection of the past. Fleeting traces manage to slip through the gates of attention and trigger vivid and realistic memories of the distressing events, causing immediacy for fear and horror. "As-if" reenactments of the past become a part of the present, but are too terrifying to express vocally. Consequently, terror induces an inability to speak.

When I think of this time, fear is rising. In the past, we had to suppress it because of the permanent danger, but today I feel strange, because I only remember fragments. Why is that so? I feel as if a part of me is still hiding. I am staring into the darkness and only now and then something flashes up and lays open, a memory of my previous life.

Ervin Staub (1998), child survivor of the Holocaust, whose history of persecution unfolds in multiple events beginning when he was just 6 years old.

Survivors of continuous or complex trauma have often endured frequent interpersonal abuse from early childhood. It can take decades for the first clear sensory intrusive memories to surface, despite a lifetime of experiencing symptoms of unknown origin and untold misery.

One day I looked in the mirror. On my arms and legs there was hardly any place where I had not cut or burned myself.... I was 30 years old. This time I was hospitalized for 14 weeks. It was my 57th stay as an inpatient in a psychiatric ward. I had suffered from eating disorders, bodily pains, and drug abuse since 16 years old by then. During the 2nd week, I suddenly experienced my first flashback of sexual abuse through my grandfather. I saw him raping me. After this stay, I had panic attacks and nightmares. More and more memories appeared. I realized that my father had done the same thing to me. I felt immense disgust. I slit my wrists; another attempt to die. After that, I stayed again for 5 months on a locked ward. Terrible fractions of memory of a time when I was sold to men in child-prostitution were haunting me. I wished I had succeeded to starve myself to death....

Excerpt from a diagnostic interview at University of Konstanz, held at the Center for Psychiatry Reichenau, Germany (2010) with a person suffering from borderline personality disorder.

The memories of past horrors can consume the body and mind, even in the present moment. Listen to the voice of one woman describing the overwhelming nature of these recollections:

When I remember this body, so close to me, so ugly, so intimate, it is still as if a dark, evil, black thing entered me at the level of my stomach. It is a thing with arms, like an animal, like a snake, a writhing thing that enters me and twists and turns inside me. Ugh... It shakes me. I know it wants to spread, it wants my whole body, it wants to take me over completely. It wants me to lose control. It has an evil, dark intention.... There is such desperation in me, such total loss of control, such helplessness. I have to hide, I go far, far away in my mind, I cannot bear this.... I feel like I want to explode, I feel like a bomb inside. But I never told anyone.... Now that I am almost 50 years old, who will understand the memory of a little girl? People will think I am crazy...

Excerpt from a vivo-documented NET testimony (2003) during therapy with a 49-year-old female survivor of childhood sexual abuse.

Loneliness and social isolation are common experiences for survivors. They are often unable to talk about the traumatic experiences of the past or to understand their altered personalities. Instead, survivors feel controlled by the emotions that have become a part of their existence. One woman describes how this experience has affected her:

Even now many years later the pictures of this day keep coming back to my mind. I look at normal people, like a teacher or a friend, and suddenly the face of the perpetrator appears. Then I get angry and aggressive and try to hurt the person. I throw things and get violent. Sometimes I find myself sitting in strange places, like on top of the roof crying and I have no idea how I got there. It is as if there are two personalities living inside me. One is smart and kind and normal, the other one is crazy and violent. I try so hard to control this other side of me. But I fail. Sometimes I feel tears running down my cheek and I wonder why. ... I have never told anybody what had happened to me during that day and even my father does not know what goes on in my mind and body when I get out of control. This is why I always feel a distance to everybody around me. People don't understand why I act strange sometimes, and I cannot tell them.... When I saw children playing and being happy, I had to cry because I thought I could never do something like that again.

Excerpt from a vivo-documented NET testimony (2003) during therapy with a 13-year-old Somali child survivor.

Trauma and narrative may seem like opposing forces that cannot be reconciled, because those who experience such violations are often in too much pain to recount their stories. However, these two aspects are closely related and form the foundation of this approach and work: Victims must speak out for the betterment of their own mental health and their social surroundings. And violence cannot remain hidden indefinitely, as they can transmit and spread trauma in numerous ways, resonating down generations.

After the war, for ten years I didn't speak, I was not a witness, for ten years ... and I was waiting for ten years, really.... I was afraid of language. Oh, I knew for ten years I would do something: I had to tell the story. One day, I visited an old Jew.... He sat down in his chair, and I in mine, and he began weeping. I have rarely seen an old man weep like that. I didn't know what to do. We stayed there like that, he weeping and I closed in my own pain. And then, at the end, he simply said, "You know, maybe you should talk about it...." In that year, the tenth year, I began my narrative.

Elie Wiesel (1996); excerpt from an interview in 1996 with the Nobel Peace Prize laureate and survivor of the Auschwitz Concentration Camp.

The main conflict of psychological trauma is the struggle between being unable to speak about the experience and the desire or fear to reveal what happened. This conflict arises from the desire to deny the horrific events and the urge to disclose the extent of the atrocities. Regaining one's dignity and finding the truth by implicating the perpetrator are both essential to the internal healing process.

Some victims face the additional obstacle of not feeling understood in this drama of the unspeakable. Elie Wiesel once testified to the belief that their experiences cannot be fully shared by others.

It is not because I cannot explain that you won't understand, it is because you won't understand that I can't explain.

Elie Wiesel (1996)

If the core issue of feeling misunderstood due to communication barriers is not recognized, therapeutic interventions will be ineffective. The process of disclosing a traumatic experience begins with acknowledging the difficulty in expressing it. By providing a safe space for victims to articulate their trauma without pressure, they can regain their ability to communicate and overcome their sense of silence and memory loss. Clinical intervention techniques alone are insufficient to address the societal and political dimensions of trauma, including the experiences of terror, torture, and abuse. Victims may feel silenced due to the potential implications of speaking out about their abuse. Mental health professionals may also feel overwhelmed when listening to stories that demonstrate a gross violation of human rights.

The ordinary response to atrocities is to banish them from consciousness. Denial, repression, and dissociation operate on a social as well as an individual level.... Far too often secrecy prevails, and the story of the traumatic event surfaces not as a verbal narrative but as a symptom. Remembering and telling the truth about terrible events are prerequisites both for the restoration of the social order and for the healing of individual victims.

Judith Herman (1992), from the introduction to *Trauma and Recovery*.

Explicitly addressing the sociopolitical aspects of healing is crucial for achieving true healing. Externalizing feelings of abuse and distrust is necessary. Postconflict peace and reconciliation depend on society's willingness to acknowledge abuse and on individuals' mental health. *Narrative Exposure Therapy* (NET) aims to improve the health of individuals and society by recognizing their inherent interrelatedness. The *NETfacts health system* supports communities affected by violence, based on individual narrations (see Chapter 4).

Based on this theoretical foundation, NET is a treatment for individuals who have experienced multiple and complex traumas. It is a comprehensive approach that addresses both the testimony and healing aspects (Schauer et al., 2005). NET weaves the *hot implicit* memories into the story that is unfolded by the *cool declarative* memories (see Elbert & Schauer, 2002; Schauer, Elbert, & Neuner, 2007; Metcalfe & Jacobs, 1996). In this way, intrusive memories are integrated into their original context, and a coherent autobiographical narrative develops. Because narrative and oral tradition are an integral part of every culture, NET is a culturally universal intervention for reducing the suffering of traumatic stress in survivors of severe and repeated life-threatening events, such as domestic or organized violence, including torture (see Amnesty International and UN General Assembly, 1984; for a definition for "torture"; Pérez-Sales, 2017), war, rape, civil trauma, and childhood abuse. NET encourages traumatized survivors to tell their detailed life story chronologically to a trained therapist who listens carefully, writes it down, reads it back, and assists the survivor in the task of integrating fragmented traumatic memories into a coherent narrative. The detailed description of personal experiences facilitates a sensory, emotional, physical, and meaningful recollection, and thus exposure, of traumatic memories. Originally developed for survivors of multiple and complex forms of trauma who come from diverse backgrounds and live in insecure situations, often under conditions of ongoing trauma, *Narrative Exposure* serves not only therapeutic purposes but also a social and political agenda. Part of the process is similar to creating a legal testimony. The logic of this component follows, to some extent, the testimony therapy procedure that Lira and Weinstein developed in Chile during the Pinochet regime (Cienfuegos & Monelli, 1983). NET documents child and human rights violations while treating survivors through the narrative process.

Overall, this present manual has been written with the goal of integrating the psychological rehabilitation of trauma survivors – victims and perpetrators – with issues of human rights and dignity at the social, academic, and political levels. This work bridges the gap between academia and practice. It is aimed at mental health practitioners working in the field (i.e., in crisis regions and post-conflict settings) as well as those working in clinics, human rights organizations, public health institutions, and academic settings. At the same time, this manual is written in a way that makes it accessible to committed members of the general public. Because storytelling, oral tradition, and verbal expression are concepts shared by all of humanity, NET can be tailored to any culture, group, or context.

A key strength of NET is its great potential for dissemination, including to counselors in low-income countries and war and crisis regions (Neuner et al., 2008; Ertl et al., 2011; Jacob et al., 2014; Köbach et al., 2017). Thus, NET can be implemented in health care in low-income countries just as it can be useful in high-income regions. For example, Stenmark et al. (2013) showed for central Norway that traumatized survivors can be successfully treated for posttraumatic stress disorder (PTSD) and depression in the general psychiatric health care system. Whatever the cultural setting, dropout rates are generally low. The manual has been translated into Arabic, Dutch, English, Farsi, French, German, Italian, Japanese, Korean, Portuguese, and Slovak.

Based on scientific evidence from a variety of disciplines (clinical psychology, psychotherapy, neuroscience, public health, and refugee studies), NET has been compiled and successfully tested in the field. In their systematic review and meta-analysis, Siehl et al. (2021) analyzed 56 clinical trials from 30 countries and found large between-group effect sizes for PTSD symptom reduction in favor of NET, with the most pronounced improvements seen at 6- to 12-month follow-up, with sustained changes in psychopathological symptoms, physical health, psychological functioning, and overall quality of life. Early studies have suggested that NET can effectively be applied in insecure situations such as war zones in East Africa (Neuner, Schauer, Klaschik, et al., 2004; Schaal, Elbert, & Neuner 2009). This has been further supported by numerous controlled trials whereby local counselors, who underwent thorough training, successfully provided treatment (Neuner et al., 2008; Jacob et al., 2014; Köbach et al., 2017; Köbach et al., 2021; Robjant et al., 2019).

NET has the potential to alleviate the suffering of individuals experiencing domestic violence, even during ongoing intimate partner violence (Orang et al., 2018). Research by Stevens et al. (2020) suggests that NET can be successfully implemented during pregnancy among impoverished and distressed populations. A modified version of NET, called KIDNET, has also been developed for children who have experienced trauma. Further information is available in Chapter 4, and in Schauer et al.,2024. NET has been utilized across all age groups, including older persons experiencing traumatic stress (Bichescu et al., 2007; Lely, De la Rie, et al., 2019; Lely, Knipscheer, et al., 2019; Lely et al., 2022). The adaptation for older adults is referred to as ElderNET (see Chapter 4, below).

Following the NET approach of advocacy, NET has been adapted for the needs of populations that are at increased risk for traumatization and discrimination, including transgender and gender diverse adolescents (Julian et al., 2023) and adults (Lange, 2020), parenting and pregnant adolescents (Volpe et al., 2017), and members of tribal communities in the US (Bedard-Gilligan et al., 2022).

Neurophysiological markers confirm objectively sustained changes in response to NET: In Schauer et al. (2006), we reported changes in magnetic brain activity: Over a 6-month period, oscillatory neural activity in the NET group, but not in the control group, became more similar to that of healthy controls. Adenauer et al. (2011) observed NET-induced neurophysiological changes in response to aversive pictures, that improved reappraisal of the actual danger of the current situation, thereby reducing PTSD symptoms in those treated with NET.

In addition, molecular biological measures suggest that NET leads to permanent physiological changes: Morath, Moreno-Villanueva, et al. (2014) observed that NET is able to reverse elevated levels of damaged DNA to normal levels in individuals with PTSD, findings that may have implications for physical health, including carcinogenesis. The reversibility of pathophysiological processes in individuals with PTSD through psychotherapy suggests that there is a therapeutic window to not only reverse the psychological burden of PTSD, but also to reduce the long-term and potentially lethal somatic effects of traumatic stress. This effect may be particularly pronounced in vulnerable populations, as suggested by our findings in a Ugandan refugee camp (Neuner et al., 2008).

In this process, witnesses and survivors of child abuse and serious human rights violations are invited to work through their traumatic memories while narrating and testifying to the details. This practice allows for the processing of painful emotions and the reconstruction of clear contingencies of dangerous and safe conditions, which usually leads to significant emotional recovery. With the survivor's consent, the documents (testimonies) resulting from this therapy can also be used directly for the prosecution of human rights violations or for awareness-raising purposes to counteract societal forgetting and denial.

Look, you must speak.
As poorly as we can express our feelings, our memories,
but we must try.
We have to tell the story as best as we can.
We cannot guarantee success, but we must guarantee effort.
In truth, I have learned something:
Silence never helps the victim. It only helps the victimizer....
If I remain silent, I poison my soul.

Elie Wiesel (1996)

Traditional ways of assessing and narrating human experiences have failed to incorporate and explain traumatic events, yet it is crucial to discuss them to heal the damage they have caused in personal lives and history. However, how can we communicate these stories? What are the consequences of sharing that nightmare? What is the impact of acknowledging and supporting such a testimony?

Now we recognize our duty to tell the full story, however painful ... the survivors need to come forward after all these years of silence... the silence that had been both a trap and a sanctuary for many survivors.

Dori Laub, child survivor of the Holocaust and clinical professor of psychiatry at Yale University and the Fortunoff Video Archive for Holocaust Testimonies at Yale (personal communication, 2001)

Survivors of violence are given the opportunity to seek justice through documentation, resulting in a meaningful step forward. The previously iniquitous violence they have suffered is given a new purpose, and the process of preventing future violence is strengthened by NET's explicit societal and political mission to uphold the UN Declaration of Child Rights and Human Rights, proving to be a valuable asset in numerous ways. Human rights groups, international criminal tribunals, and courts that rely on survivors' data can benefit from the comprehensive nature of a victim's and witness's report. Advocacy efforts on behalf of one's community may also draw upon testimonial evidence offered by NET. But, above all, it serves as a record of an individual's life, a lasting memory that can be passed down to future generations, resulting in a sense of agency.

Based on scientific evidence, our personal experiences, and practical observations, it is possible that trauma-focused biography therapy, when combined with testimony work, may have empowering effects on both individual and societal levels. Ensuring suitable mental health services for trauma victims is essential, particularly in resource-poor and conflict-ridden countries (Schauer & Schauer, 2010). Many survivors experiencing extreme stress disorders lack the ability to carry out essential survival activities, such as establishing feasible economic and social living arrangements for themselves and their families. Victims may experience intrusive thoughts and nightmares, deteriorating physical health, and increased feelings of worthlessness and suicidal thoughts. The lives of trauma survivors are often marked by hopelessness, poverty, and an inability to fulfill their social roles, but studies have shown that survivors are able to return to work, tend to their fields, and reengage in social and intimate relationships, after treatment. The process of individual and communal recovery can commence through trauma treatment. It serves as an essential connection between an individual's mental well-being and community and economic development.

Healing deep-seated antagonism or changing ideologies of antagonism through various types of interactive conflict resolution procedures can contribute to [reconciliation].... Members of each group can describe the pain and suffering of their group at the hands of the other.... They can grieve for themselves.... They can begin to grieve for the other as well. Members of each group can acknowledge the role of their own group in harming the other. Mutual acknowledgement of responsibility can lead to mutual forgiving. Healing from trauma, which reduces pain, enables people to live constructive lives, and reduces the likelihood of violence by victims and thus a continuing cycle of violence.

Ervin Staub (1998, p. 232)

If it is indeed true that recalling and truthfully recounting traumatic events are necessary for both the recovery of the individual victim and the restoration of social order, reconciliation, postconflict peace, and economic development (Herman, 1992), why would we ever participate in a "conspiracy of silence"?

There are important issues that arise as we engage in this work. For example, it is necessary to consider whether exposing survivors to traumatic memories is beneficial or harmful to their healing process. Additionally, we need to ask ourselves if we are willing to listen to these stories and how to address our own fears and discomfort as we do so. Throughout our search for answers, it is crucial that we respect and honor the voices of the victims.

If you had seen such things that I went through, you'll never forget. Before I had told my story, the horrible experiences felt like wounds in my body that didn't want to heal. I was always sad. I didn't know what could help. The pictures were always there and I was shaking with fear, so I wasn't able to dig in the fields. Because of the pain I couldn't find the words. Only pieces of speech. Then you came and were not afraid to listen to me. To hear all of it. I never thought anybody could bear hearing this. Now I hold the story in my heart and on the paper in my hands. I cannot read, but my children will finally know what has happened, what enables them to fight for peace. Because I went through the pain, I got my past back. Now my heart is free ....

Excerpt from a vivo-documented NET testimony with a 35-year-old female survivor of the Sudan Genocide, 2000.

Documenting and examining an individual's complete life history offers numerous benefits, as demonstrated by the practice of NET. This method enables the individual to reflect on their entire life, facilitating their comprehension of complex connections between explicit and implicit emotional aspects of significant experiences. Additionally, it initiates an inner process by which one can understand and realize the origin and perception of their feelings, thoughts, and behavioral patterns. Through this exploration, individuals may develop a new sense of self-awareness, considering both their current identity and the person they were during the traumatic experience. Aligning with their younger self during storytelling can foster growing self-compassion and self-acceptance. With the assistance of a committed listener, experiencing corrective relationships and having one's life stories read by the therapist can support mentalization.

Personal strengths and resources that individuals accumulate over the course of their lives, in NET referred to as "flowers," can be identified and validated. A secure and thorough process of interaction and emotional exploration can reveal the importance of interconnected events and lead to an understanding of related patterns and schemes. As linked events are brought to attention, a perception of an individual's "destined" path in life can emerge. Insights about the past fall into place, so that implications and desires for the future begin to emerge. The role of the therapist, mental health professional, or trauma counselor is to provide a safe and personal connection while being fully present as a listener, bearing witness, honoring, and respecting the survivor and every part of their life as it happened and as it continued to unfold moment by moment.

2 Theoretical Base

Traumatic Stress

Traumatic Events

The term "trauma," as defined within the fields of clinical psychology and psychiatry, differs significantly from its colloquial usage. It is not a mere breakdown in coping strategies in response to challenging life events. Rather, trauma entails a profound wound to the soul, resulting in a shift in our perception and fundamental assumptions about the world, following horrifying experiences (see Elbert & Schauer, 2002, for a brief outline of the concept). Its core symptoms, including intrusions, insomnia, hyperarousal, andnegative thoughts and feelings , are conceptualized as posttraumatic stress disorder (PTSD). Psychological trauma means a "wound of the mind" and an injury to humanity. Consequently, the objective behavior, perception, and self-report of a specific symptom pattern and the examination of survivors' regulatory systems – neural, hormonal, and immunological – became tools for observing mental injury. Naturally, efforts are made to avoid reminders and suppress fear and negative emotions. This is analogous to someone who has experienced physical harm and now refrains from moving or touching the injured area to prevent further pain. In the next chapter, we will explore how trauma survivors who still experience the effects of past events may also endure severe emotional distress when reminded of their fearful experiences (Elbert et al., 2022).

Traumatic events are characterized by danger and elicit specific physiological responses of alarm and defense in the brain, endocrine, immune, gastrointestinal, and reproductive systems (Tseng et al., 2023). These adaptations play an important role in modulating victims' responses to threat. These events impact significantly on individuals. Life- and integrity-threatening events can be truly horrifying, whether one has directly experienced them or had to witness them. Witnessing can be equally traumatic as being a victim, due to humans' social nature and tendency to reflect others. This is especially true when the injury is to a loved one or family member, or when the witness identifies closely with the injured person.

Traumatic experiences are often classified as either man-made or caused by natural disasters. The former includes exposure to childhood abuse, sexual violence, combat, torture, witnessing killings, being held as a prisoner of war, or experiencing catastrophes such as airplane crashes or severe car accidents. Natural disasters classified as traumatic may include floods, earthquakes, hurricanes, or volcanic eruptions. In contrast, experiences of loss, such as losing a business, or of bereavement may not cause an immediate alarm response or activate any other psychophysiological defense, and are then not considered *traumatic* in a clinical sense. However, losing a loved one in a traumatic event can result in severe trauma reactions. Viewing a disturbing film or reading a violent book does not constitute a traumatic experience for adults. But that is only true if the viewer is aware that the content is fictional and therefore does not react in a state of panic or alarm.

Only stressful events that trigger a state of physiological alarm or fright, or a shutdown response (refer to details in the section Stress and Defense Cascade, below), and result in the victim or eyewitness feeling terrified or helpless, are considered traumatic. The body and mind undergo a cascade of responses due to this experience, which, when consistently re-experienced, can cause damage to both. This cascade causes rapid changes in the body and brain through a combination of neural activity, hormonal reactions, and changes in immune function. These changes have an impact on all organs, resulting in extensive alterations to heart rate, muscle tone, blood flow, and metabolism. Additionally, digestion is temporarily halted while the immune system adapts to counter the potential danger.

What is psychological trauma?

It refers to the experience and effects of events that threaten one's life, integrity or safety, causing the person to feel horrified, powerless, and physically and psychologically overwhelmed, reacting with alarm or shutting down (such as dissociation or even fainting) during and after the experience. These responses can have long-lasting effects on an individual's mental, emotional, and physical well-being.

Stress and the Defense Cascade

The body, including the brain, possesses the capacity to respond to threats in a supple and adaptable manner. In contrast to homeostasis, which refers to an organism's ability to maintain a stable internal state, the adjustment to stressors exhibits significant flexibility. These stressors can be physical, such as exposure to cold, noise, or sleep and food deprivation. They can also come in the form of fear-provoking situations, whether they are real or imagined, that trigger an alarm response or shutdown process, potentially leading to trauma-related disorders. Mammals, including humans, select from an array of attack and defense mechanisms to mitigate negative effects (McEwen, 2002; Schauer & Elbert, 2010). Even with minor cues, the brain can activate any appropriate alternative from the behavioral predispositions shaped by genetic and epigenetic factors (Elbert & Schauer, 2014). A coherent sequence of six defense responses that escalate as a function of proximity to danger and threat has been established by evolutionary biology and psychophysiology alike: *freeze* (orienting), *flight*, *fight*, *fright*, *flag*, and *faint* (Schauer & Elbert, 2010).

First, the freezing (orienting response) facilitates a "stop-look-listen" perception and evaluation of the threat. Pavlov (1927) described the reflex as "Shto Eta" (what is it?), a response that directs the sensory systems toward the source of stimulation. It can be perceived as a set of bodily reactions that aid in processing the stimulus, including posture adjustments, dilation of the pupils, orientation toward potentially meaningful stimuli, reduction in motor activity, and a momentary decrease in heart rate. If the stimulus is perceived as a threat, an alarm response is initiated, with instant sympathetic arousal and adrenal release that enable the organism to counter danger (strong heart rate acceleration, blood pressure elevation, and vasoconstriction in hands and feet, but vasodilation in the muscles) – to prepare for a flight-or-fight response, the body shifts blood to the muscles that require it and reduces blood flow to the skin to prevent blood loss in case of injury. Additionally, sweating on the palms and feet helps to prevent harm and improves grip.

Highly aversive stimuli that appear proximate to the organism do not elicit an orienting response but rather a defensive reflex. For instance, a very intense sound with a short rise time, such as a noise at 100 dB, is likely to be from a nearby threat and elicits a startle response – this includes pupils constricting and an increase in heart rate. Such a defensive reflex blocks out the event. The peritraumatic panic reaches its maximum in the fright response (tonic immobility with high dual autonomic tone), which may enhance survival when there is no current possibility of escaping or winning a fight (direct physical contact with the perpetrator).

However, pushing a car's "gas pedal" (sympathetic arousal) and brake (vagal activity) at the same time is costly and may lead to heart failure. Therefore, finally, parasympathetic dominance (bradycardia, drop in blood pressure, and vasodilation) takes over, which, in extreme cases, may result in a vasovagal fainting (-like) response (absence of efferent motor commands and functional deafferentation; Figure 1).

The actual sequence of trauma-related response dispositions carried out in an extremely dangerous situation depends on the appraisal of the threat by the organism in relation to its own power to act (e.g., age, sex), as well as the perceived characteristics of the threat or perpetrator.

The cascade of these responses to stress is directed by four bodily systems (see overview in Elbert & Rockstroh, 2003; McEwen, 2002; Teicher et al., 2002). The *hippocampus* is primarily responsible for functions associated with orchestrating the construction of explicit memory. The *hypothalamic-pituitary-adrenal* (HPA) axis is the elite force of the defense cascade and is involved in the feedback regulation of cortisol, a stress hormone secreted by the cortex of the adrenal gland. It helps us to maintain and regulate the response to stress over time. A second axis that produces a rapid, short-lived response involves the *amygdala* (related to the development and processing of emotions), the *locus coeruleus*, *adrenaline* secreted by the adrenal gland, and the *sympathetic nervous system*, all of which are critical for directing blood flow, heightening awareness, and mobilizing the appropriate immediate defense response. A third, less-explored axis involves the *vasopressin-oxytocin peptides* and arguably the *ventral vagal complex*. It increases social bonding, enhances the ability to relate, and thus dampens defensive responses. Finally, in addition to these three axes, the *immune system* is involved in adaptive and maladaptive responses (see Segerstrom & Miller, 2004, for an overview): Short-lasting acute and naturalistic stressors are associated with adaptive up-regulation of some, but down-regulation of other, parameters of immunity, while

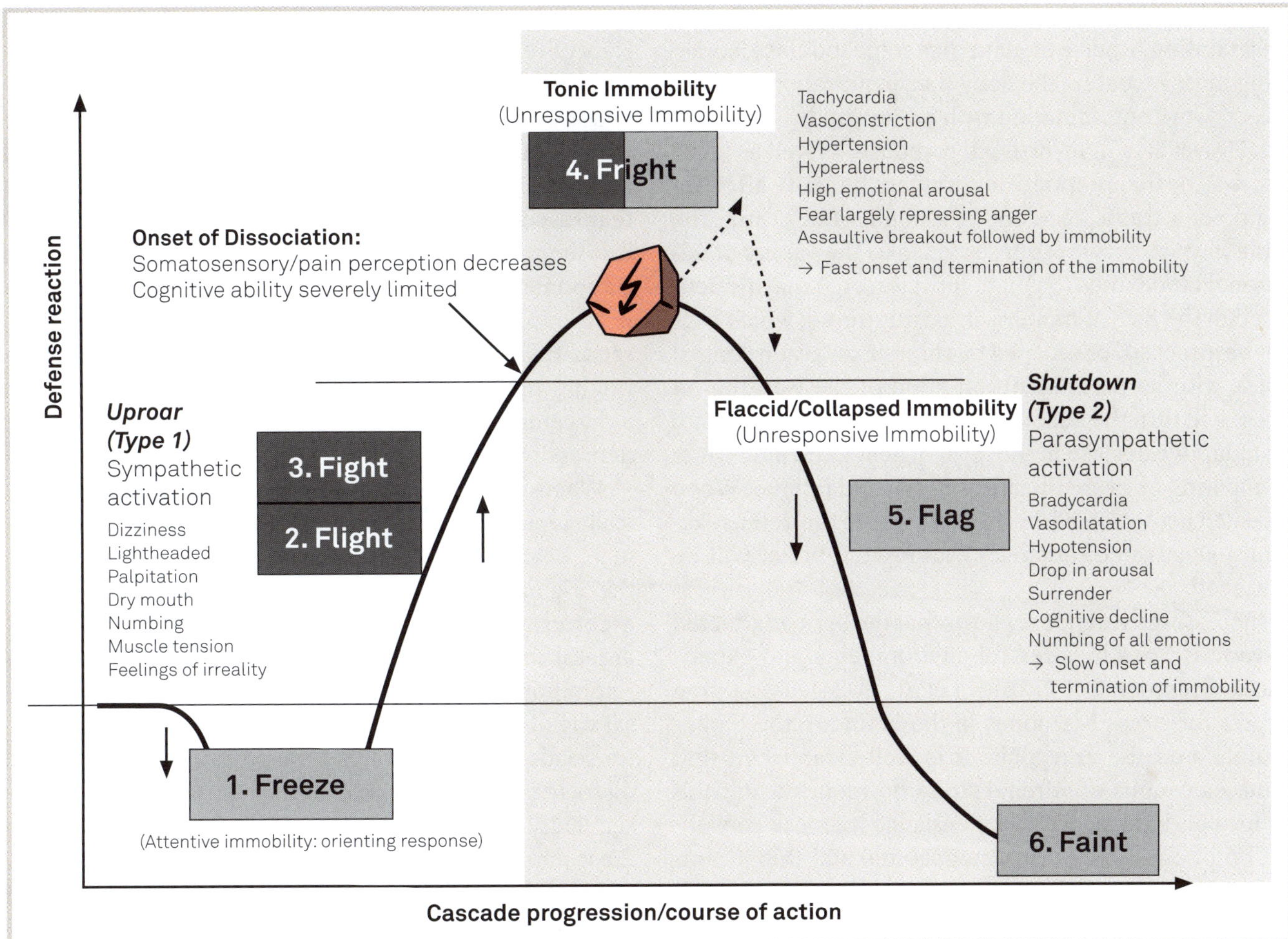

Figure 1. The defense cascade progression along different actions. *Uproar* results in a maximum of sympathetic arousal at the fright stage, eventually overtaken by the dominance of dissociative *shutdown*. It is important to note that during life-threatening situations, individuals may not necessarily experience every stage of the defense cascade. The sequence of trauma-related response dispositions in an extremely dangerous situation is influenced by various factors. The defense response is structured to assess an individual's ability to defend themselves and secure their integrity and social bonds in response to a threat. This includes the evaluation of the threat in relation to the organism's own capabilities to counteract, such as age, sex, physical condition, and defensive abilities, as well as the specifics of the threat, such as the type, speed of approach, context, potential for injuries, blood loss, invasion into the body, etc. In addition, a particular response may be classically conditioned and thus depend on previous experiences with threatening events. Adapted with permission from "Dissociation Following Traumatic Stress: Etiology and Treatment," by Maggie Schauer and Thomas Elbert, *Zeitschrift für Psychologie/Journal of Psychology, 218*, 109–127 (https://doi.org/10.1027/0044-3409/a000018). © 2010 Hogrefe Publishing.

chronic stressors lead to immune suppression. All of these biological systems aid in crisis management and are also involved in the stress-protective effects of positive social interactions. Furthermore, disrupted metabolism of specific biological systems may be associated with clinical disorders.

When unremitting stress forces the axes of stress response to tilt in one direction, the result can be anything from a long-lasting head cold to depression. When tilted the other way, toward a flattening of the rhythm of stress hormones, undesirable consequences may be abdominal fat, loss of muscle mass, and mental ailing (McEwen, 2002). When the danger is over, the stress response should shut down. However, ongoing perceived stress, be it real or supposed, can send the HPA axis on a roller-coaster ride, until it eventually becomes exhausted and unresponsive. The stress hormones ultimately make their way back to the brain, affecting both behavior and health.

The various stages of the defense cascade have evolved to allow adequate responding, such as running for escaping acute danger; or dissociative responding or even fainting, when a predator has come too close, something invasive enters the body (i.e., penetration of sharp objects), or contamination with bodily fluids is impending. However, a fight-or-flight response, as well as fainting, may be inappropriate in a modern human – after, for example, a traffic accident or a bomb attack. Still, the same physiological responses (such as the supply of additional blood and oxygen to muscles, etc.) may be activated in the face of modern stressful stimuli, which cannot be attacked, or escaped by running away. Prolonged stress with its permanent initiation of the warding off stress will turn the adaptive physiological responses into maladaptive disease in the form of aches and pains, loss of appetite, or overeating, insomnia, and fatigue. When repeated activation of the memories keep the defense responses activated, organs, including the brain, will be damaged.

Increasing evidence suggests that the brain is affected in various ways by stressful environments and experiences (Bremner, 2002; Vaidya et al., 2024). Two prime targets for stress hormones in the brain are the hippocampus and the amygdala. It is well-established that acute elevations of adrenal stress hormones (catecholamines and glucocorticoids) enhance memory consolidation of emotionally arousing, contextual (hippocampus-dependent) information in a dose-dependent manner in animals (Roozendaal et al., 2001) and humans (Buchanan & Lovallo, 2001; Cahill et al., 1994). These enhancing effects of stress hormones are mediated by structures within (the basolateral nucleus of) the amygdala (Cahill et al., 1995; McGaugh, 2002). Whereas the support of stress hormones might be adaptive, whenever lasting memories of vital information (e.g., dangerous situations) have to be established, this mechanism may become maladaptive in conditions of extreme stress, when persistent and intrusive memories of a traumatic event promote the development of trauma-related disorders. However, acute elevations of glucocorticoids not only have enhancing effects on memory consolidation, but also impairing effects on memory retrieval (de Quervain et al., 1998, 2000; Roozendaal et al., 2003). Furthermore, chronic glucocorticoid excess can lead to disruption of brain synaptic plasticity, atrophy of dendritic processes, and reduced neuronal ability to survive a variety of coincident insults (Sapolsky, 1999). Moreover, perinatal stress changes the HPA axis, delays cognitive and emotional development, and may impair avoidance learning for the rest of a person's life (Bock et al., 2003; Meaney et al., 1988; Teicher et al., 2002).

Thus, stressful experiences differentially activate a variety of responses designed by evolution to counter danger. The different chemical messengers may cause deficits in hippocampus-based learning and memory, and their effects on the amygdala and the medial prefrontal and cingulate cortex may lead to impaired inhibition of fear responses. As a result, emotional and autobiographical memory may become fragmented (see the section Rationale for NET). In addition, repeated or chronic exposure to traumatic stress may result in long-term dysregulation of these systems, leading to impaired functioning and to symptoms of stress-related disorders such as hyperarousal, dissociation, flashbacks, avoidance, and depression.

When confronted with trauma reminders, survivors typically replay their original response of the traumatic event (e.g., Keane et al., 1985; Schauer & Elbert, 2010). When the original threat has triggered a fight-or-flight response, a corresponding alarm response with high emotional arousal and sympathetic responding may be elicited by the reminding cues. However, if a parasympathetically (dorsal vagal) dominated shutdown was the prominent peritraumatic response to the traumatic incident, comparable dissociative responses may dominate responding to subsequently experienced threat and may also reappear when the traumatic memory is reactivated during therapy. The current concept of PTSD does not distinguish whether the reminder of the traumatic experiences results in a fight-or-flight alarm, an "uproar," or in a dissociative block, a shutdown with a subsequent excessive vagal tone. For the therapist, however, it is mandatory to note if the physiological responding during treatment is dominated by high emotional arousal or by a dissociative responding. To understand responding during trauma-focused treatment, it is thus necessary to understand the response repertoire humans have when confronted with various forms of threat to their lives (Figure 1).

Individuals who respond to trauma with numbing, freezing, dissociation, or even fainting would be predicted to produce a muted or reduced psychophysiological response when recalling the event. Intrusions can be understood as repetitive displays of fragments of the event, which then elicit a corresponding combination of hyperarousal and dissociation, depending on the dominant physiological response during the threat.

An evolutionary perspective suggests that shutdown enables survival in the following situations:

- When the organism is in direct and close encounter with a dangerous perpetrator for example, when there is skin contact;

- in the presence of body fluids with danger of contamination – for example, blood or sperm;
- when bodily integrity is already injured, or in the face of impending or enforced invasion – for example, sexual penetration, sharp objects (e.g., teeth or knife) at the skin, or medical procedures.

These situations require physiological adaptations, including immobility and analgesia for pain (in order to "play possum," avoid tearing of tissue, pretend entire submission). Switches in consciousness, information processing, and behavior also occur, which are perceived as strange because they are outside the range of ordinary experiences. The Schauer & Elbert (2010) neurobiological model, as well as its applicability to diverse human populations, has gained widespread acceptance (see, e.g., McKinnon et al., 2016; Lanius et al., 2018; Schalinski et al., 2011; Bichescu-Burian, 2012; Chessell et al., 2019; Jongedijk et al., 2014; Kecala et al., 2022; Terpou et al., 2019).

Violence: The Major Source of Traumatic Stress

Forms of Violence

Violence appears in different forms. Prominent classifications of violence are defined according to context (Derriennic, 1971). A major dimension for qualifying types of violence rests on the degree of organization. Examples of unorganized types of violence include assaults, domestic violence, sexual abuse, and other violent crimes against individuals. Organized violence includes wars, armed conflict, political persecution, and any other systematic violation of human rights. Political motives provide the context for a more systematic order of organized or state-sponsored violence, which include torture, massacres, hand-to-hand combat, crimes against humanity, and bombardments. It is crucial to recognize the political context of war and torture and understand how organized violence impacts both the individual and society at large. Equally significant is acknowledging the consequences of domestic violence and abuse on a survivor's life.

Survivors of Organized Violence

An obvious consequence of organized violence is that many people have to flee from their region of origin because of war, persecution, or other forms of continuous threats (Davies et al., 2022).

There is ample evidence that war and the social environment interact, and that childhood abuse and neglect, together with social exclusion, drive poverty and transgenerational cycles of trauma and violence leading to a *mental health crisis* of unprecedented dimensions (Schauer, 2016) These adversities have reached a critical point of hopelessness and intolerability that has set a mass migration movement in motion, to "flee a miserable life without a future in the home country, hoping to grant a better life for our children" (personal statement of a refugee in an EU shelter). The perilous journey, often over many months, adds trauma exposure, which contributes to psychological and physical health problems. Uprooted people from different backgrounds show high prevalence rates for psychological problems (Cooper et al., 2019). Aggression and deprivation have destructive impacts on mental health, resulting in a psychiatric emergency of pandemic proportions. We argue that the psychological impact of this is not only devastating for the individual, but also is a factor in perpetuating both conflicts and mental ill health. This in turn fuels aggression and conflicts and leads to the uprooting of people trying to leave social disadvantage and "failed states," reaching out for more desirable living environments and creating a market for human traffickers and people smugglers; again a source of severe traumatization adding to a challenged capacity for integration in a new context. Exposure to traumatic stressors, especially early in life, are the building blocks for psychopathology and substance misuse, with consequences extending beyond the individual, to the family, society, and the next generation: essentially, individual traumas multiply into ever-larger traumas within society (Schauer & Robjant, 2018).

The United Nations High Commissioner For Refugees (UNHCR) most recently estimated that, for the first time in recorded history, the number of people forcibly displaced is now over 110 million (UNHCR, 2023). No matter where refugees or internally displaced people flee to after war and persecution, most exiled people are not safe or accommodated (Karunakara et al., 2004). Many reports indicate that initial receptions by host government authorities and humanitarian agencies are impersonal and threatening, and that refugees assume roles of dependency and helplessness (Doná & Berry, 1999), while at the same time they are perceived as threatening by their hosts (Landmann et al., 2019; Müller-Bamouh et al., 2016; Augsburger et al., 2017). While development of social networks, family reunions, and permanent settlements do occur (Castles & Miller, 1993), harsh living conditions, continued anxiety about forced repatriation, and uncertainties regarding resettlement can cause considerable stress for the refugees (Cunningham & Cunningham, 1997). Host country refugee policies are often dictated by domestic concerns, usually of a foreign policy nature, and not necessarily determined by security and protection concerns or by the wishes of host communities in receiving countries (Tandon, 1984). There are many reports that refugee camps and internal displacement camps breed violence, and people are often victims of violent acts perpetrated by the army, militias, humanitarian workers, and by their hosts (Malkki, 1995; Turner, 1999; UNHCR, 2002). In countries throughout the world, people are being detained and imprisoned arbitrarily without a fair trial. Many face torture or other forms of ill-treatment, as has been continuously documented by Amnesty International. They may be held in inhumane conditions that are cruel and degrading. Cumulative exposure to these stressors piles up and eventually results in PTSD, depression, and related disorders (see next section). Among the public health impacts of climate change, environmentally induced forced migration is a severe and adverse outcome that regularly results in a multitude of significant social and resource losses. Displaced populations are frequently exposed to trauma and violence, highlighting the significant impact of this issue. Specifically, the effects of population displacement on mental health and psychosocial functioning require dedicated focus (Shultz et al., 2019).

> **What is organized violence?**
>
> Organized violence is violence with a systematic strategy. It is put into operation by members of groups with a centrally guided structure or political orientation (police units, rebel organizations, terror organizations, paramilitary, and military formations). It is targeted for continuous use against individuals and groups who have different political attitudes or nationalities, or who come from specific racial, cultural, and ethnic backgrounds. It is characterized by the violation of human rights including disregard of women's and children's rights. The consequences reach far into the future of the targeted society. Taking the Uppsala Conflict Data Program (https://ucdp.uu.se) as trustworthy, and considering the number of armed conflicts during the period from 1946 to 2018, the volume of organized violence conflicts has more than doubled. Especially intrastate and internationalized intrastate conflicts have increased.

Survivors of Family Violence

The quality of parent-child interactions predicts the risk for psychopathology over the lifespan.

Michael J. Meaney (2008)

Family violence, also known as domestic abuse, spousal abuse, child abuse, or intimate partner violence, has many forms including physical aggression (hitting, kicking, biting, shoving, restraining, slapping, throwing objects), emotional abuse (insulting, scolding, nagging, humiliating) sexual violence, or threats thereof (see Box 1). Unemployment, poverty, substance abuse (e.g., excessive alcohol consumption), and mental illness of spouse or parent are important risk factors for family violence (Orang et al., 2018; Serpeloni et al., 2023; Volpe et al., 2016, 2017; De Bellis, 2002; Dube et al., 2003; Jaffee, 2005; Margolin & Gordis, 2000). Childhood trauma has psychopathological and developmental consequences including adverse emotional, behavioral, and cognitive consequences (Schauer et al., 2020; De Bellis, 2002). High levels of stress, fear, and anxiety are commonly reported by victims of domestic violence. Maltreatment of children, defined as neglect, physical abuse, sexual abuse, and emotional abuse (which includes witnessing domestic violence), has always been the most common cause of interpersonal trauma and PTSD in children and adolescents (Teicher et al., 2022; Felitti et al., 2019; De Bellis et al., 1999; Widom, 1999). In clinically referred samples, the reported incidence rates of PTSD resulting from sexual abuse range from 42% to 90% (McLeer et al., 1994; McLeer et al., 1998) and are above 50% when arising from just witnessing domestic violence (Pynoos & Nader, 1989).

Children who grow up in an environment of violence and maltreatment later show severe forms of disorders of the trauma spectrum. Pathological levels of stress are thought to disrupt the normally integrative functions of mental activity, leading some aspects of experience to be segregated from conscious awareness. A number of studies have demonstrated significant associations between childhood physical or sexual abuse and dissociation (Dutra et al., 2009). Meta-analyses have confirmed the associations among infant disorganized attachment behavior, parental maltreatment, parental psychopathology, disturbed parent–infant interaction, and childhood behavior problems (Madigan et al., 2006). When intense and persistent stress occurs while the brain is undergoing enormous change, the impact may leave an indelible imprint on its structure and function (Matz et al., 2010; Teicher et al., 2002).

Box 1. Some of the possible consequences of child maltreatment in certain areas of development and functioning

Emotion

More mental health problems
- Trauma-related disorders (PTSD, dissociation, anxiety)
- Externalizing problems, including conduct disorder, aggressive and antisocial behaviour
- Internalising problems up to depression
- Little response to first-line treatments
- Frequent relapses

Suicidal attempts (only in people with adverse childhood experiences)

Lower self-esteem

Less secure attachment to caregiver

Lower quality of caregiver–child relationship

Cognition

Lower cognitive abilities

Lower working memory capacity

Lower attention capacity

Lower school achievement

Childhood sexual abuse (CSA) is a complex constellation of experiences that involve an adult or older child using a child for sexual gratification and can include, but is not limited to, rape, unwanted touching, threatened sexual violence, exhibitionism, and use of children in pornography or sex work (World Health Organization [WHO], 2017). CSA is especially a risk factor for the emergence of adult psychopathology (Hailes et al., 2019), such as depression (Andersen & Teicher, 2008), borderline personality disorder (Lieb et al., 2004; McLean, & Gallop, 2003), eating disorders (Schaaf & McCanne, 1994; Smolak & Murnen, 2002), somatization disorder (Farley & Keaney, 1997; Kinzl et al., 1995; Morrison, 1989; Walker et al., 1992), and negative effects on physical health (Anda et al., 2006; Felitti et al., 1998).

A prospective study (Widom et al., 2009) found that significantly more abused and neglected children overall met the criteria for borderline personality disorder (BPD) as adults, compared with controls, than did physically abused and neglected children (Porter et al., 2020).

Early stress or maltreatment is an important risk factor for the later development of substance abuse (Shin et al., 2018; Kiburi et al., 2018; Scheidell et al., 2018). As an adult, the survivor will maintain a state of vigilance, hyperarousal, readiness for sympathetic hyperactivation, and suspiciousness to swiftly detect danger, and the potential to mobilize immediate aggression when threatened with danger or loss. Early childhood abuse and neglect lead individuals into social isolation, hostility, and depression and substance abuse, and foster the emergence of disease processes.

Based on a meta-analysis that included 37 studies with a total of 253,719 participants, Hughes et al. (2017) reported increased risk of all examined health outcomes for individuals with substantial adverse childhood experiences, compared with individuals with no such stressful experiences. Associations were moderate for somatic diseases such as cancer or cardiovascular problems, and strong for mental ill health. For problematic drug use and interpersonal and self-directed violence odds ratios (ORs) reached above a substantial 7.

In war zones, children are often victims of both organized and family violence. The combination of these two forms of adversities potentiates their vulnerability for trauma-spectrum disorders (Catani et al., 2009, 2010).

The range of familial violence

Familial and domestic violence take many forms, including physical aggression, sexual abuse, emotional neglect, verbal abuse, intimidation, and various forms of deprivation. Domestic and familial violence are common and thus often aggravate effects of other stressful experiences. Hence therapists should assess every client for these forms of violence (using a checklist). Survivors of early maltreatment and abuse often show a range of problems and severe symptoms of complex trauma. Compared with traumatic stressors experienced during adulthood, continuous and developmental trauma during development has even more serious consequences on the brain (see the section Neurobiological Basis of Memory and Trauma Disorders) and mind, and thus on the mental and physical well-being of the survivor.

The Concept of PTSD

The lasting pathological reactions to traumatic, stressful experiences are called posttraumatic symptoms. The prefix "post" means after or later – so "posttraumatic" meaning, in this case, injury of the soul. The study of the psychological consequences of traumatic events has a long tradition in psychotherapy research. In the 1970s, investigations studying the consequences of traumatic stress were stimulated by the finding that a large proportion of Vietnam veterans had major difficulties reintegrating into their prewar roles. Scientists influenced by the women's movement responded to the observed severe psychological problems in rape victims by conducting research in this area.

A trauma spectrum disorder like PTSD requires that symptoms result from experienced or witnessed threatening experiences to the survivor's life, physical and psychological integrity, or biological fitness. Additionally, according to the definition, the victim's immediate response must involve fear, terror, or helplessness, thus triggering a defensive reaction. If the therapist is uncertain about whether to classify an event as "traumatic," during the assessment, in a clinical sense, it may be helpful to ask for the survivor's peritraumatic reaction. For example, the therapist might ask, "Mike, you mentioned witnessing an explosion. Were you in close proximity to the site and did you experience fear in that moment, or did you see the explosion from a far distance without significant emotional responses?" Objective assessment can aid in identifying events and treating trauma-related disorders.

Repeated exposure to traumatic stressors will always result in various symptoms. For instance, insomnia or headache are common adverse consequences. However, other causes may lead to such symptoms. Therefore, the diagnostic manuals focus on rather specific symptoms and these include:

Intrusive symptoms – that is, unwanted intense memories up to a seemingly literal reliving of the threatening event. This may also come in the form of nightmares while one is sleeping, or flashbacks that occur during waking hours. These are accompanied by multiple sensory experiences (e.g., hearing threats approaching, feeling the weight of the perpetrator on the body, seeing the soldiers over and over again, smelling the alcohol, tasting blood in the mouth, etc.) as well as the sense of being stuck in the traumatic situation. Intense flashbacks seem to be unique to PTSD (Brewin, 2001, 2016; Malaktaris & Lynn, 2019).

Avoidance behavior – that is, attempting to avoid the fear and pain caused by any memories of the trauma is consistently associated with trauma reactions. *Active avoidance* means avoiding any stimuli related to the trauma that may trigger the memories thereof. For instance, one might avoid people, news reports, or places that are associated with the event, or avoid talking or thinking about the event. *Passive avoidance* or *numbing,* also related to dissociation phenomena, includes general emotional numbing as well as detachment from other people including negative alterations in cognitions, emotions, and personality.

High general distress (Marshall et al., 2019) and *emotional arousal* is easily triggered by the feeling of being back in a life-threatening situation that creates a persistent sense of threat. The reaction can be anything from an exaggerated startle response, to irritability, to an explosion of anger and rage. It also leads to difficulty focusing on present tasks – that is, concentration problems – and contributes to insomnia. The frequent tensions are also a source of headaches.

The *Diagnostic and Statistical Manual of Mental Disorders,* 4th edition (DSM-IV; American Psychiatric Association [APA], 1994) triad of diagnostic criteria has been modified in the 5th edition (DSM-5; APA, 2013), splitting avoidance into its more active form and "negative cognitions and mood" as a separate category, and proposing four rather than three symptom clusters (Friedman et al., 2011). This category encompasses dysphoric mood states and social, self-conscious emotional stress associated with PTSD, such as guilt, shame, and disgust. It also covers negative cognitions such as self-blame and persistent negative expectations about oneself and the future. Complex PTSD (CPTSD), which has been adopted as a new diagnosis in the *International Classification of Diseases,* 11th edition (ICD-11; Maercker et al., 2022), is characterized by three core posttraumatic symptom clusters, along with chronic and pervasive disturbances in emotion regulation, identity, and relationships.

How does a traumatized person feel?

Traumatization involves experiencing the lingering effects of a past traumatic event. Re-experiencing the traumatic event occurs when the survivor involuntarily relives (features of) the situation either during waking hours through flashbacks or at night through nightmares. Both are accompanied by intense feelings of fear and helplessness, similar to those experienced during the traumatic event. The body responds with a stress reaction during the experience. The individual experiences, for example, accelerated heart rate, profuse sweating, and excruciating physical discomfort. The recollection of the event can be persistent, despite the individual's attempts to suppress it. The flashbacks can manifest in various ways, from a momentary perception of the event taking place in the present, to profound emotions of terror and insecurity. The individual may even have the belief that the traumatic event is taking place in real time. Survivors report the memories pulling them back to their past and being trapped in those moments of intense despair. Nightmares frequently lead to the survivor waking up feeling afraid and unable to return to sleep. Re-experiencing episodes are observed to occur due to internal reactualizations (body posture, somatosensory, visceral, thermoception, vestibular, nociception, etc.) or environmental cues that resemble the ones encountered during the traumatic event, usually specific sounds, smells, or similar emotional cues. Future avoidance of such stimulus configurations and situations are common, though the exact factor triggering the memories may remain unclear to the survivor. For example, they may stop seeing certain people, doing certain activities, and may avoid emotional excitement, among others, all in an attempt to avoid reminders of the past experiences. The traumatized individual may learn to become numb or detach from their feelings and the reality, which can lead to a loss of loving emotions and the ability to feel close to people, even one's spouse or children.

The survivor may lose hope or feel that the future holds nothing for them. Meanwhile, the sustained or repeatedly triggered fear leads to heightened arousal and distress, resulting in increased alertness and preparedness to confront danger at any given moment. Individuals may develop mistrust and regard danger as ever-present, or they may face difficulties in focusing on everyday tasks or attentively listening to others. Frequent activation of stress responses can impose significant costs on the body and potentially lead to a variety of physical complications.

The PTSD concept, with its dominant features of intrusive re-experiencing and hypervigilance, reflects the *arousal* side of the defense cascade (see the section Stress and the Defense Cascade): During sympathetic dominance, sensory function and physiological arousal are heightened. However, some types of trauma (e.g., sexual abuse) result in a conditioned parasympathetic *shut down* response with functional sensory deafferentation. These trauma survivors will not readily exhibit the intrusions required for a diagnosis of PTSD (Schauer & Elbert, 2010). Sometimes it may take years, if not decades, after a period of continuous trauma, for the first explicit intrusive memories to emerge. Nevertheless, these survivors are severely traumatized and exhibit many other symptoms of trauma spectrum disorders. This more complex set of symptoms has led to the suggestion that CPTSD be regarded as a distinct condition, one which has now been introduced in ICD-11. Again, symptoms can be diverse and may include the following:

1. Intrusions or other forms of supposed threat perceptions may trigger intense and fluctuating emotions which are difficult to understand by the social environment. Feelings of emptiness or emotional numbness are common.
2. Those intrusions, together with the adverse interpersonal experiences, cause problems in forming and maintaining healthy relationships. Distrust, fear of intimacy, or difficulties with boundaries are not uncommon.
3. Low self-esteem, a distorted self-image, feelings of guilt or shame, self-blame, or a sense of being fundamentally flawed or worthless are characteristic symptoms.
4. The victim has distorted perceptions of the perpetrator, a preoccupation with the abuser, an intense need for validation or approval, or an irrational belief that the abuser is all-powerful.
5. Dissociation involves a sense of disconnection from oneself, others, or the world, leading to an inability to express aggression or resistance. Ultimately, the closure of the thalamic gates (reduction of sensory sharpness) may result in the feeling of being an outside observer of one's own self. This experience can lead to gaps in memory consolidation.
6. Being under perceived threat changes the bodily systems. This causes chronic physical symptoms such as headaches, gastrointestinal issues, neuroinflammation, autoimmune responses, unexplained pains, etc.
7. Some survivors are constantly on edge, easily startled, or hyperaware of potential threats.
8. Impulsive or self-destructive behaviors, self-harm, substance abuse, or eating disorders may be utilized to alleviate tension and stress reactions, while also initiating endogenous opioid release.

The symptoms have been listed here, as it is important to acknowledge the wide range of suffering involved.

Psychosocial Problems and Comorbid Disorders in Adults and Children

Epidemiological studies have found that one or more comorbid psychiatric disorders, especially depression or dysfunctional anxiety, diagnosed in addition to PTSD, occur in 80% of cases (Kessler et al., 1995). Usually, these disorders are trauma-related, but not scored for a PTSD diagnosis. For instance, a survivor who is experiencing vivid flashback episodes might experience a panic attack, indicative of panic disorder. Or, if someone feels detached and isolated from others, this person might abandon previous interests and hopes, start drinking, or become clinically depressed. An increasing exposure to traumatic stressors is a main driver of many additional symptoms, watering down the borders with other psychiatric disorders. It should be remembered that disorder categories constitute heterogeneous syndromes rather than specific nosological entities causing distinct diseases. As causes remain mostly unknown, the disorder categories have been defined by sets of presenting signs and symptoms. Therefore, it is not surprising that diagnostic manuals differ – for example, CPTSD has been introduced in ICD-11 but not DSM-5. Trauma-related disorders range from personality disorders, prolonged grief disorder, depressive episodes, panic disorder, and dissociative disorders, and may even increase the likelihood of psychotic disorders. Trauma is also a frequent driver of substance use disorder and promotes violent behavior, and suicidality, which does not occur without repeated adverse experiences during childhood. The validity of psychiatric disorder classes has not been established, and thus psychotherapy may move toward transdiagnostic treatments, if it is not hampered by administrative restrictions and the need for conceptual paradigms.

Trauma consequences may occur at all ages, but may be particularly devastating in children, as they may impair the child's developmental trajectory from a very early age (see diagnostic criteria for children 6 years and younger: DSM-5 PTSD<6Y; De Young & Landolt, 2018), throughout childhood (e.g., Haag et al., 2019; McLaughlin & Lambert, 2017; Sayed et al., 2015; Choi et al., 2019), and transgenerationally (e.g., Conradt et al., 2020; Ullmann et al., 2017). Factors such as altered memory function, frequent severe headaches, sleep disturbance, or loss of ability to concentrate lead to a decline in school performance or difficulties in forming interpersonal relationships. In a survey of adolescents, Somasundaram (1993) found psychosocial problems and comorbid disorders as a consequence of these children being exposed to traumatic experiences during the civil war in Sri Lanka (that lasted from 1983 to 2009; see Table 1).

Table 1. Psychosocial problems in Tamil adolescents (*N* = 625; adapted from Somasundaram, 1993)

Psychosocial problem	%
PTSD	31
Somatization	32
Anxiety	34
Depression	29
Hostility	45
Relationship problems	34
Alcohol and drug misuse	7
Functional disability	35
Loss of memory	44
Loss of concentration	48
Loss of motivation	33

In an international, epidemiological survey among Tamil children during the war in Sri Lanka (Elbert et al., 2009), we found that 57% of the children reported that traumatizing war experiences and the symptoms resulting from it interfered with their life. Social withdrawal, difficulties in leading a normal family life, and problems in school performance were most common. The greater the number of traumatic events reported, the greater the number of difficulties in social and emotional functioning reported by the child. Neuropsychological testing and school grades validated the outcome further and demonstrated the problem associated with this mental disorder. A psychological test of memory (the Rey-Osterrieth Complex Figure) revealed that nearly all children without PTSD scored adequately for their age and were able to copy a figure from memory. However, interaction of PTSD diagnosis with recall shows that traumatized children are less able to perform well on this test and are unable to recall the different elements of the Rey Figure correctly. The recall score (% correctly recalled elements) dropped from 73% in the children without a trauma-related disorder, to 55% in those suffering from PTSD (Figure 2).

Clinical interviews in this study further revealed that depressive symptoms were frequent in traumatized children. In response to questions relating to affective disorders, only 12% of the children without PTSD reported symptoms of a mood disorder, in comparison with 68% of those with PTSD, and more than 40% of the latter fulfilled the diagnosis for an affective disorder. The risk of suicide was 26% in the children who presented with PTSD versus 7% in children without PTSD. Somatic symptoms (physical illness–related symptoms) were also more frequently reported in children with PTSD than in those without PTSD. For instance, 81% of children with PTSD reported suffering from headaches during the last 4 weeks. In addition, children with the disorder had significantly lower school performance rates in key subjects compared with non-PTSD children (Elbert et al., 2009).

Often, children are also indirectly affected by trauma. Their parents' and caretakers' symptoms of PTSD, such

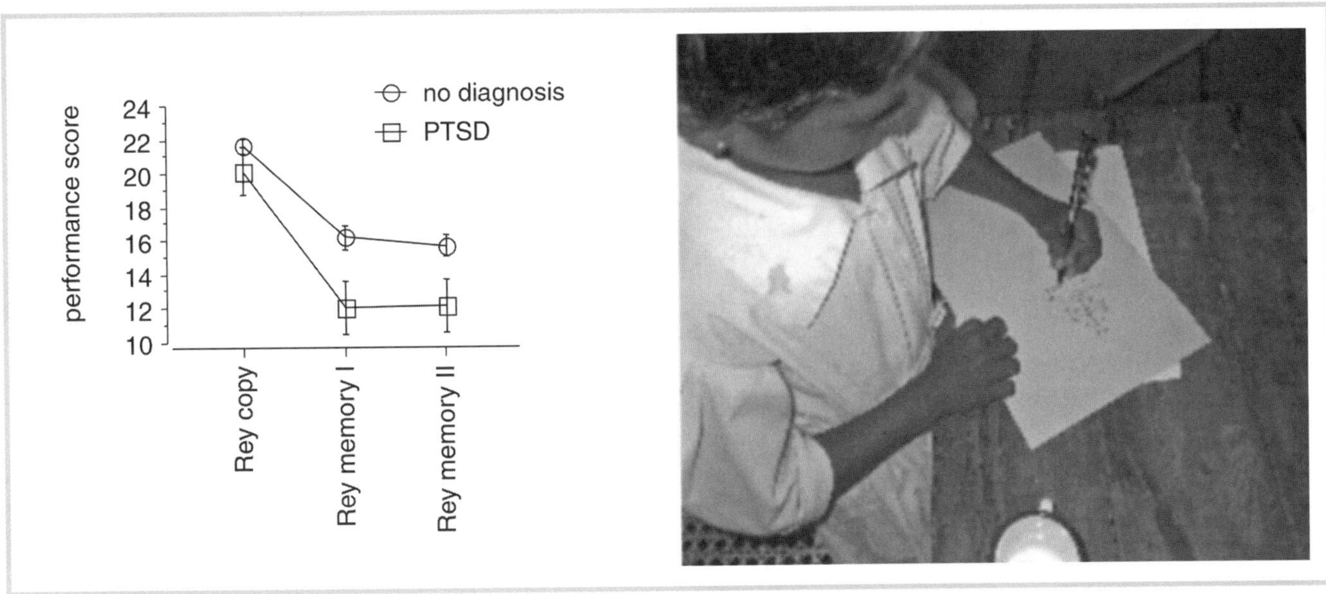

Figure 2. Children with and without PTSD could copy a Rey Figure equally well, but memory performance (right side: recall of the figure from memory) was better in children without PTSD (circles) than in those who presented with PTSD (squares). Adapted from "Trauma-Related Impairment in Children – A Survey in Sri Lankan Provinces Affected by Armed Conflict," by T. Elbert et al., 2009, *Child Abuse & Neglect, 33*, pp. 238–246, © 2009, with permission from Elsevier.

as emotional numbing and avoidance, prevent normal emotional feelings and loving behavior toward their children. As a result, family members of a traumatized person are forced to operate within a domestic context in which intimacy is severely impaired. In many cases, tension, domestic violence, and substance abuse increase. Children are more likely to be abused or neglected as a consequence. Furthermore, severe traumatic experiences have multigenerational effects. Some evidence suggests there are higher rates of anxiety and depression in children of survivors compared with nontraumatized comparison groups. However, more rigorous scientific studies are needed to uncover the psychopathological consequences in the offspring of survivors.

In elementary school children, PTSD may manifest as repetitive reenactments or drawings of frightening experiences. This can be used to gain access to the most distressing events. For example, a child may be asked to draw what comes to mind (see Step 0 in the section General Advice: Utilizing Creative Media With Children, in Chapter 3).

PTSD and Drug Abuse

PTSD and substance use disorders (SUDs) frequently co-occur, with often complex relationships. Substance use – for example, use of alcohol, cigarettes, marihuana, cocaine, heroin, amphetamines, khat, or banji seeds – can be attempts to cope with trauma memories. Individuals suffering from disorders of the trauma spectrum tend to consume more drugs in an effort to reduce the mental pain associated with their symptoms. While substance use may temporarily alleviate the distress, the long-term use of substances will worsen PTSD symptoms, leading to a vicious cycle of dependence, substance intoxication, trauma symptoms, and retraumatization (see, e.g., Narvaez et al., 2019)

The co-occurrence of both trauma spectrum disorders and SUDs presents substantial treatment challenges. Integrated approaches that address both conditions simultaneously are often more effective than treating them in isolation. It is crucial to address the underlying trauma and provide coping strategies for the mental health problems, while also addressing the substance use and implementing relapse prevention techniques. NET has been used in individuals who consume substances, but only to an extend that allowed adherence to treatment. Drug consumption in these cases gets reduced and frequently controlled (e.g., Köbach et al., 2017; Hinsberger et al., 2020; Robjant et al., 2019). However, if possible, detoxication must precede treatment.

If drug abuse is found in children and adolescents, it is always a cry for help and as such should not be punished. It is of key importance to emphatically explore the reasons for such behavior, together with the troubled youngster. Traumatic events, but also suffering related to neglect or abuse during childhood years, are likely causes. A number of treatment programs exist that can reach substance abusers and their families. Successful trauma treatment, however, is necessary for these programs to work.

PTSD and Physical Health

Given that the reminders of trauma can be so intense that they trigger physical responses, including the activation of stress hormones that affect many somatic systems, it is not surprising that the frequent activations come at a cost not only to mental but also to physical health. In fact, individuals with trauma spectrum disorders have a higher risk of developing chronic problems such as cardiovascular disease, respiratory disease, gastrointestinal problems, and autoimmune disorders. Trauma consequences may be associated with metabolic changes, including alterations in hormone levels and the regulation of appetite and metabolism. These changes can contribute to weight gain or loss, metabolic syndrome, and an increased risk of developing conditions such as diabetes.

The chronic stress response associated with PTSD can contribute to inflammation and other physiological changes that increase the risk of these conditions. The relationship between stress and physical illnesses, in particular infectious diseases, has been well-established and there are several models about the immunological mechanisms that may be responsible for this effect (e.g., Kiecolt-Glaser et al., 2003). For instance, experiencing traumatic events leads to severe reductions in naïve cytotoxic and regulatory T cells, which can explain the increased risk for infections and autoimmune diseases, respectively (Sommershof et al., 2009). Morath, Gola, et al. (2014) showed that symptom improvements in response to NET were mirrored in an increase in the originally reduced proportion of regulatory T cells in the NET group at the 1-year follow-up. These cells are critical for maintaining balance in the immune system, regulating the immune response, and preventing autoimmune diseases.

As mentioned above, individuals with PTSD typically suffer from insomnia and nightmares. Sleep problems can have a significant impact on physical health, as adequate sleep is critical for the body's restorative processes. In turn, this results in a number of physical health problems, including increased susceptibility to illness, impaired cognitive function, and cardiovascular problems. Park et al. (2020; see also Weinhold et al., 2017) have shown that NET improves insomnia.

Individuals with trauma disorders frequently report chronic pain and repeated pain perceptions. Symptoms may include headaches, muscle tension, stomachaches, and general bodily pain. It appears that PTSD exacerbates these symptoms if they were already present before the posttraumatic stress.

Not all individuals with PTSD will experience the same physical health outcomes, suggesting integrated treatment approaches that address both the mental and physical health aspect. However, in resource-poor regions where many health treatments are not available, studies have shown that NET can also improve such symptoms as cough, diarrhea, and fever (Neuner et al., 2008).

Finally, it should be mentioned that NET is able to reverse, in individuals with PTSD, increased levels of damaged DNA back to a normal level (Morath, Moreno-Villanueva, et al., 2014). The reversibility of pathophysiological processes in individuals with PTSD via psychotherapy indicates that there is a therapeutic window not only to address the psychological burden of the disease PTSD but also to reduce the long-term somatic effects of this mental condition.

Vulnerability for PTSD

Not everyone who is exposed to traumatic stressors develops mental health issues. Two key factors contribute to the vulnerability for developing PTSD:

- Cumulative exposure to traumatic stressors: The frequency and severity of traumatic events, especially when prolonged or repetitive in nature, explains most of the variance of the risk, whereby childhood maltreatment is particularly toxic (e.g., Nandi et al., 2015; Behnke et al., 2020). The best prediction of PTSD is the assessment of the number of traumatic events experienced (Neuner, Schauer, Karunakara, et al., 2004; Wilker et al., 2015; see Figure 3), including childhood adversities (Figure 4).
- Lack of social support: The availability of social support following a traumatic event is crucial. Individuals with limited or inadequate social support networks have found to be more vulnerable to developing PTSD For instance, Sommer et al. (2016) have demonstrated that supportive relationships, such as those with family, friends, or community groups, can help mitigate the impact of trauma to an extend as cognitive behavioral treatments do.

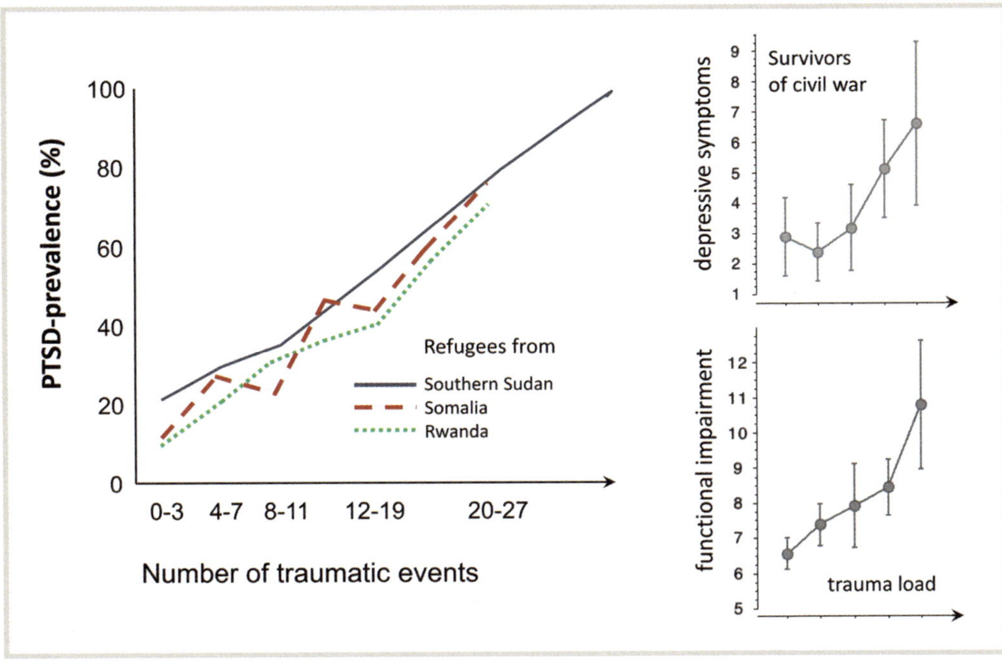

Figure 3. The likelihood of developing trauma-related distress increases with the cumulative experience of the types of traumatic events experienced, which we also refer to as "building blocks" of trauma-related disorders. The greater the number of traumatic events experienced, the greater the likelihood of PTSD, depressive symptoms and functional impairment. Left panel: based on data from studies of refugees in Uganda by Neuner et al. (2004) and Onyut et al. (2009); right panel: based on data from war zones in Sri Lanka, Elbert et al. (2009).

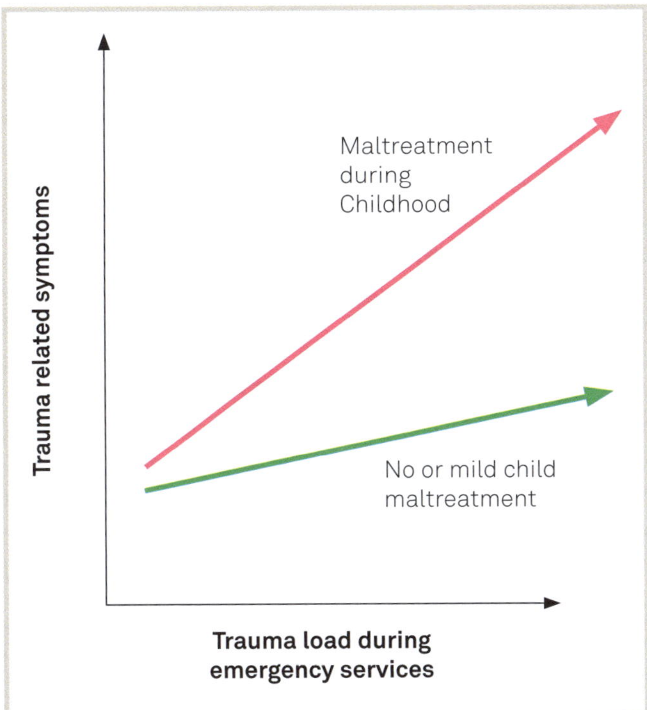

Figure 4. Differential building block. This graph illustrates how child maltreatment massively aggravates the effects of later occupational trauma exposure in emergency service personnel. This has been well demonstrated in studies by Behnke et al. (2020).

Other factors that may affect the likelihood of developing PTSD include the individual's sense of control and safety following the traumatic event, as well as their coping strategies. For example, social withdrawal and persistent feelings of helplessness can increase the risk of PTSD. In contrast, a sense of empowerment and desire for retaliation against the group responsible for the trauma can contribute to resilience (Weierstall et al., 2012; Elbert et al., 2017b; Sommer et al., 2017).

While the role of single traumatic events in causing chronic PTSD can be uncertain, numerous studies have consistently found that experiencing previous traumatic events increases the likelihood of developing PTSD after subsequent trauma (Brewin et al., 2000). Our studies indicated that the cumulative number of traumatic events experienced was the primary predictor of PTSD among the populations in Sudan and Uganda's West Nile region affected by war. It is crucial to consider the impact of multiple traumatic events on PTSD onset and development. In the population studied, it was discovered that individuals who reported experiencing over two dozen traumatic events in their lifetime met the criteria for PTSD. Resilience is lacking at this level of repeated threat (Neuner, Schauer, Karunakara, et al., 2004; Schauer et al., 2003). This suggests that the development of PTSD is cumulative or additive, as trauma and exposure to violence contribute over time with a sufficiently high "dose" in each instance (Schauer et al., 2003). This building block effect has been observed in a variety of cultural and contextual settings. For example, Schaal and Elbert (2006) studied samples of Rwandan genocide survivors, while Onyut et al. (2009) studied Rwandan and Somali refugees. Elbert et al. (2009) and Catani et al. (2010) conducted similar research on Tamil children. Moreover, this effect has been observed among Congolese refugees by Ainamani et al. (2020; see also Figure 3 and Figure 4). The study by Ainamani et al. indicated a higher prevalence among women, but once the traumatic load is factored in, the effect decreased. This can be attributed to the fact that women are more commonly victimized by sexual violence, a traumatic experience that becomes apparent during the NET procedure, yet frequently goes unreported to the examiner.

Given that the regulatory systems, especially the neural structures, are particularly plastic during development, it comes as no surprise that childhood maltreatment moderates this building block effect. A highly illustrative example has been provided in an excellent study of emergency service personnel by Behnke and colleagues (2020). The occupational trauma exposure had a much more devastating effect in those who also reported childhood maltreatment (as assessed by the MACE, available at https://doi.org/10.1371/journal.pone.0117423; see also Figure 4).

A proportion of trauma-related sufferers remit over time, even in the absence of treatment. Our data have consistently shown that higher trauma exposure is associated not only with a higher prevalence of current and lifetime PTSD, but also with a lower likelihood of spontaneous remission from PTSD, as a clear dose–response effect (Kolassa et al., 2010). Several studies have examined the factors that influence remission from PTSD after a single traumatic event. Unfortunately, previous traumatic stressors and exposure to violence, including domestic violence, have often not been assessed, or at least not adequately. After motor vehicle accidents, higher initial symptom severity scores, new trauma to family members, more severe physical injuries, and persistent physical injuries 4 months after initial diagnosis were associated with lower rates of remission from PTSD 6 months after initial diagnosis (Blanchard et al., 1997). A study of patients in primary care with PTSD found that remission during a 2-year follow-up was associated with lower comorbid anxiety disorders and higher psychosocial functioning at intake (Zlotnick et al., 2004). In a population of physical and sexual assault victims, maintenance of PTSD was higher if the victim held negative trauma-sensitive beliefs before the assault, if the victim experienced psychological defeat or confusion during the trauma, or if the survivor had a negative appraisal of initial posttrauma symptoms or used avoidance or safety seeking as a maladaptive control strategy after the trauma (Dunmore et al., 2001; Wilker et al., 2017).

Culture and Symptoms of the Trauma Spectrum

Culture undoubtedly influences how individuals experience and interpret trauma reactions. For instance, in certain cultures, physical symptoms may be more commonly reported than emotional distress stemming from PTSD. Nonetheless, when questioned directly, individuals from any cultural background describe the entire range of symptoms. Consequently, there is no indication supporting the notion that cultural factors impact the prevalence and authenticity of trauma-related symptoms. Contrary to claims that there is no universal response to trauma, recent research into posttraumatic reactions and the neurobiological mechanisms underlying them provide compelling evidence that PTSD is a disabling and pathological outcome of traumatic events which occurs across cultures.

Recognition of trauma and human rights violations can decrease suffering related to trauma, particularly if an individual receives support from others already during the acute aftermath of trauma (McGuire et al., 2018) and later (Gottvall et al., 2019; Pugh, 2022). Hence, cultural norms that raise stigma and limit help-seeking behavior will augment suffering and need to be acknowledged by mental health experts – but not accepted (Harandi et al., 2017).

Scientific research has led to the development of effective treatment methods and the discovery of less successful or harmful approaches in various areas of medicine and healing. Withholding this knowledge from resource-limited nations under the guise of "cultural sensitivity" is unjust and unethical (refer to Neuner & Elbert, 2007, for further analysis). The practice of implementing large-scale psychosocial projects with nonevaluated treatment approaches is unacceptable. What is necessary are empirically valid guiding principles for public mental health interventions for which evidence has been gathered. Such research is intended to bring awareness and action into a nearly neglected field of public health, human rights implementation, humanitarian intervention, development aid, policy making, and funding; which will substantiate the thesis that a programmatic innovation is needed, rendering a paradigm shift in this field inevitable (see Schauer & Schauer, 2010).

Social Trauma

The current concept of PTSD is based on the assumption that some types of experiences can be classified as traumatic, because they differ from other types of stressful events, causing more exceptional pain and lasting damage. The idea is that traumatic events that threaten the *physical integrity* of a person, which involve a threat to life and limb or sexual violence, are, per se, more harmful than other stressors. Both the DSM and the ICD criteria of PTSD and CPTSD include a gate criterion, which restricts this diagnosis to the consequences of traumatic events that involve a physical threat. However, this concept of PTSD has been increasingly challenged by clinical researchers (Weisman et al., 2011; Azoulay et al., 2023; Bjornsson et al., 2020; Neuner, 2023).

Many individuals report experiencing highly stressful events and conditions that do not meet the clinical criteria for trauma. For instance, some individuals report being verbally abused by their parents, told they were unwanted, or that their attachment figures had desired their death. Others have experienced ridicule and systematic exclusion from their peers in school. Some have reported discrimination based on their ethnicity or refugee status. It is clear that emotional maltreatment, verbal abuse during childhood, peer bullying, and social exclusion can all have harmful effects, even if they do not result in physical harm. Studies have shown that emotional maltreatment can have a more severe impact than physical and sexual abuse on social anxiety (Iffland et al., 2012), substance abuse (Potthast et al., 2014), dissociative symptoms (Haferkamp et al., 2015), symptoms of BPD (Gratz et al., 2011), and other personality disorders ((Johnson et al., 2000). What is common to all of these events is not primarily physical, but concerns the social integrity of the person. There is reason to assume that, from an evolutionary perspective, injuries to social integrity in the form of a reduction in status and belonging can be perceived as equal to, or even more dangerous than, a direct threat to bodily integrity and health. This perspective sheds light not only on the traumatic nature of emotional abuse, but also on the fact that traumatic events often carry social messages and therefore threaten both a person's physical and social integrity. A rape victim, for instance, may perceive humiliation as the worst aspect of the event, and even victims of natural disasters have reasons to perceive social injustice, as it is often the least privileged in a society who suffer most after disasters. As a result, the emotional impact of an extremely stressful event, whether classified as traumatic or not, is not limited to fear, helplessness, and dissociation, but often includes social emotions such as shame, guilt, and humiliation. We (see Neuner, 2023 and the Threats to Human Life [THL] checklist in Appendix 1) have postulated that an intense threat to social integrity elicits a defensive response of the organism that resembles the reaction to physical threat, in that it is not a single, unitary reaction but a cascade of distinct types of affective states. While the initial stage may trigger basic emotions such as fear and anger, increasing threats that limit the individual's range of responses lead to shutdown reactions ranging from shame and humiliation to social defeat (see Chapter 5 and the sections on guilt and shame). Shame, a form of perceived devaluation by others, involves the experience and the signaling back of a social status degradation (Schauer, 2018). Downward cast eyes, slack posture, and lowered head are obvious signs of it. For NET, shame can be a sever obstacle, as it promotes silence, leads to speechlessness, and increases the avoidance of talking. Ultimately, the fear of exclusion and rejection becomes dominant, as someone is convinced that deep down they are lower ranking, sometimes even perceived as being defect or worthless in the eyes of the other(s). The affect of humiliation involves the appraisal that the experience is painful, and the individual feels unable to defend themselves in the situation. It is typically accompanied by helpless (and suppressed feelings of) anger, and rumination about how the person would have wanted to react in that moment (Fernández et al., 2015). As the threat to status becomes repetitive or more intense, the person will no longer feel anger and injustice, but will attribute the loss of status to the self. The common response to such intense social injury has been called social devaluation, as the common denominator of social emotions involving a self-concept dominated by inferiority, submissiveness, and sometimes even self-hatred. Ultimately, the affective response, like shutdown dissociation, means mentally giving up. It includes demobilization, a feeling of paralysis, low muscle tension, and a desire to disappear. This affect has also been characterized as a *defeat reaction*, which has been linked to depressive disorders in both animals and humans (Sloman & Gilbert, 2000). Peritraumatic defeat seems to be an important predictor for PTSD development and also treatment response (e.g., Kleim et al., 2007; Wilker et al., 2017). It can however result in violent responding (Gilligan, 2020). It is helpful for the therapist to understand the biological meaning and function of shame within the social structure (Schauer, 2024).

Rationale for NET

For the development of effective treatment methods, it is essential to understand the psychological and biological processes that underlie disorders of the trauma spectrum, including PTSD. Key features of memories of traumatic events emphasize the relevance of memory processes for the explanation of PTSD symptoms.

Nature of Traumatic Memory

A distinct symptom of PTSD is the re-experiencing of the traumatic event in the form of flashbacks. These involuntary intrusions can be triggered by any cues that remind a person of the traumatic situation. The reliving can include all kinds of sensory information, such as pictures, sounds, smells, and bodily sensations (Terr, 1993; van der Kolk, 1995). A feature of flashbacks is the feeling that this event is happening again right at that very moment. This means that during a flashback, victims are not fully aware that what they are experiencing is active memory arising from past experiences; on the contrary, they feel they are back in the traumatic situation. The memory of the traumatic event does not seem to be fixed in the context of the time and space in which it actually occurred (Ehlers & Clark, 2000).

The person may see, feel, or hear the sensory elements of the traumatic experience, yet they may be prevented from being able to translate this experience into communicable language. Despite frequent episodes of reliving the experience through flashbacks or nightmares, it is difficult if not impossible for them to narrate the event in a detailed, consistent, and chronological manner. Survivors report that they can remember the event all too well, as they suffer from painful involuntary recollections. However, if asked to report the event, their narration may be disorganized, fragmented, and incoherent (van der Kolk, 1995). In a remarkable series of studies, Breithaupt and colleagues (e.g., Breithaupt et al., 2022) showed that emotional experiences form the core of narrations guiding the selection and ordering of the story elements, hence they "operate as anchors for remembering and retelling stories" (Breithaupt et al., 2022, p. 581). It is interesting to note that AI (e.g., ChatGPT) may also prioritize emotional situations, but basically keeps mentioning the identical sensory elements, while humans experience the emotions, regardless of emphasis on certain sensory elements and even during retelling experiences from others. Consequently, as Herman (1992) puts it, humans who have survived atrocities often tell their stories in a highly emotional, potentially contradictory, and fragmented manner, which undermines their credibility and is thereby an attempt to serve contradictory twin imperatives of truth telling and secrecy. Survivors can begin their recovery only when the truth is finally acknowledged and words have been given to the full emotional realm of the experiences. Otherwise, "secrecy prevails, and the story of the traumatic event surfaces not as a verbal narrative but as a symptom" (Herman, 1992, from the introduction).

Harvey and Bryant (1999) showed that narrative disorganization correlates with symptoms of acute stress disorder. Their systematic observations found evidence of a breakdown in the ability to put into words the most emotional part of the traumatic event, over a period of time that could have lasted anywhere from a few seconds to hours or even days. Physiologically, they might react as if they had been exposed to the threatening situation again, but this might be dissociated from semantic knowledge – not part of explicit memory. When the victim experiences derealization, they cannot "own" what is happening and therefore cannot take steps to do anything about it.

For survivors of longer-lasting events, and for those who were exposed to a series of traumatic events, as is often the case for victims of organized or family violence (especially childhood abuse), this problem in narrating one's history can persist for extended periods of time (Cloitre et al., 2020). This effect was described by Rosenthal (1997), who documented the life stories of Holocaust survivors:

> *It is difficult to establish a relationship between the different stages of life – this means the time before the persecution, the time of persecution and the time after having survived. Within these stages, the relationship of the different events can be substantially broken into pieces. Whole stages can sink into the sphere of speechlessness and are accessible for the biographer only in single fragments, pictures and moods.*
>
> Rosenthal (1997, p. 40)

Thus, the characteristic of the memory of a traumatic event is twofold: On the one hand, a person has very vivid recollections of the event, including many sensory details; on the other hand, it is very difficult for the victim to face the memories and to learn to put the details into coherent speech and chronological order. This is because traumatic events are stored differently from memories of everyday events. This pathological representation of traumatic memories is what leads to the core symptoms of PTSD (Brewin, 2001; Brewin et al., 1996; Ehlers & Clark, 2000; Metcalfe & Jacobs, 1996; van der Kolk, 1996). Hence, this difference in storage of memories will be addressed next.

To understand the pathological characteristics of traumatic memories, it is first necessary to understand how normal past events are stored in memory. Based on neuropsychological research, Squire (1994) differentiated two types of memory: *declarative* (explicit) and *nondeclarative* (implicit). Declarative memory consists of memory of personal events, as well as memory of facts and knowledge of the world. For instance, declarative memory represents significant events such as a marriage or a graduation, as well as knowledge about the history or geography of the world. In contrast, nondeclarative memory covers skills, habits, emotional associations, and conditioned responses. Based on this taxonomy of memory, Squire (1994) determined that declarative or explicit memories can be deliberately retrieved, whereas nondeclarative or implicit memories are not deliberately retrieved and do not require conscious recollection. Nondeclarative memories do have an impact on a person's behavior and experiences, but are activated through other processes, such as environmental or internal cues, similar to the memories of trauma survivors.

Using the example of declarative memory, we know that the memory of a wedding or the story of the French Revolution can be deliberately retrieved or activated when desired (assuming one was paying attention in history class!). However, nondeclarative memories do not involve a deliberate recall. For example, for most people, opening a door is a highly practiced skill that is automatically activated without ever remembering how and when that skill was learned. The memory of a traumatic event can be triggered by an external cue such as a smell or a sound. Putting these two types of memory together, we can see that a single event can be stored as two different types of memory. For instance, a person learns to ride a bike. The day the rider learned to ride the bike is stored in that person's memory as a historical, autobiographical event in their life. This is an example of declarative memory. However, as the person becomes more adept at bike riding, it is no longer necessary to remember each step of riding the bike. Riding a bike thus becomes a skill that is easily activated without deliberate recall. It is coded as a nondeclarative memory.

Tulving (2001) further distinguished between *episodic* and *semantic* memory. As the name implies, episodic memories are stored as episodes – that is, happenings in particular places at particular times – and they cover information about what, where, and when. Tied to episodic memory is the recollective experience. Episodic memory allows people to consciously re-experience previous events and to activate their sensory-perceptual experience. In contrast, semantic memory is our knowledge base – for instance, it might include knowing that 5 times 12 equals 60 or that Greenland has been covered with ice. This type of memory is not necessarily related to experience in the sense that a visit to Greenland had to be made to build up the respective semantic representation.

Sensory-Perceptual Representation

If you think about past life events, you may not only retrieve abstract knowledge about what has happened (e.g., "On September 21st, I went to Jaffna by boat"), but also sometimes imagine the event in the form of a *recollective experience* (Tulving, 2001), as in "I feel the breeze over the water, the swinging of the boat". In the case of recalling the event as a recollective experience, you directly access visual and other sensory information about past events previously stored in your mind, in addition to being aware of the sequence of events that happened.

Obviously, this form of vivid and detailed recollection is not possible for all events experienced in life. For everyday events, which have less significance to a person, these representations usually only last minutes or hours (Conway, 2001). They can only become more stable if they are integrated with other memory structures. In this case, detailed images of this event can be retrieved years later. This enduring storage of sensory-perceptual representations only happens for events stored in a highly emotional state, as this means they are significant for the achievement or failure of individual goals (Conway & Pleydell-Pearce, 2000).

Lang's *bioinformational theory of emotion* (Lang, 1979) offers a good framework within which to understand the nature of sensory-perceptual representations and their embedding emotions. In this view, emotions are considered *response propositions* or more general action dispositions – that is, modes in neural networks (neuronal connections within the brain and body) that favor distinct sets of actions.

These representations consist of sensory-perceptual information about the stimuli present in the past situation in different modalities (visual, auditory, olfactory, etc.). In other words, a single traumatic memory can be

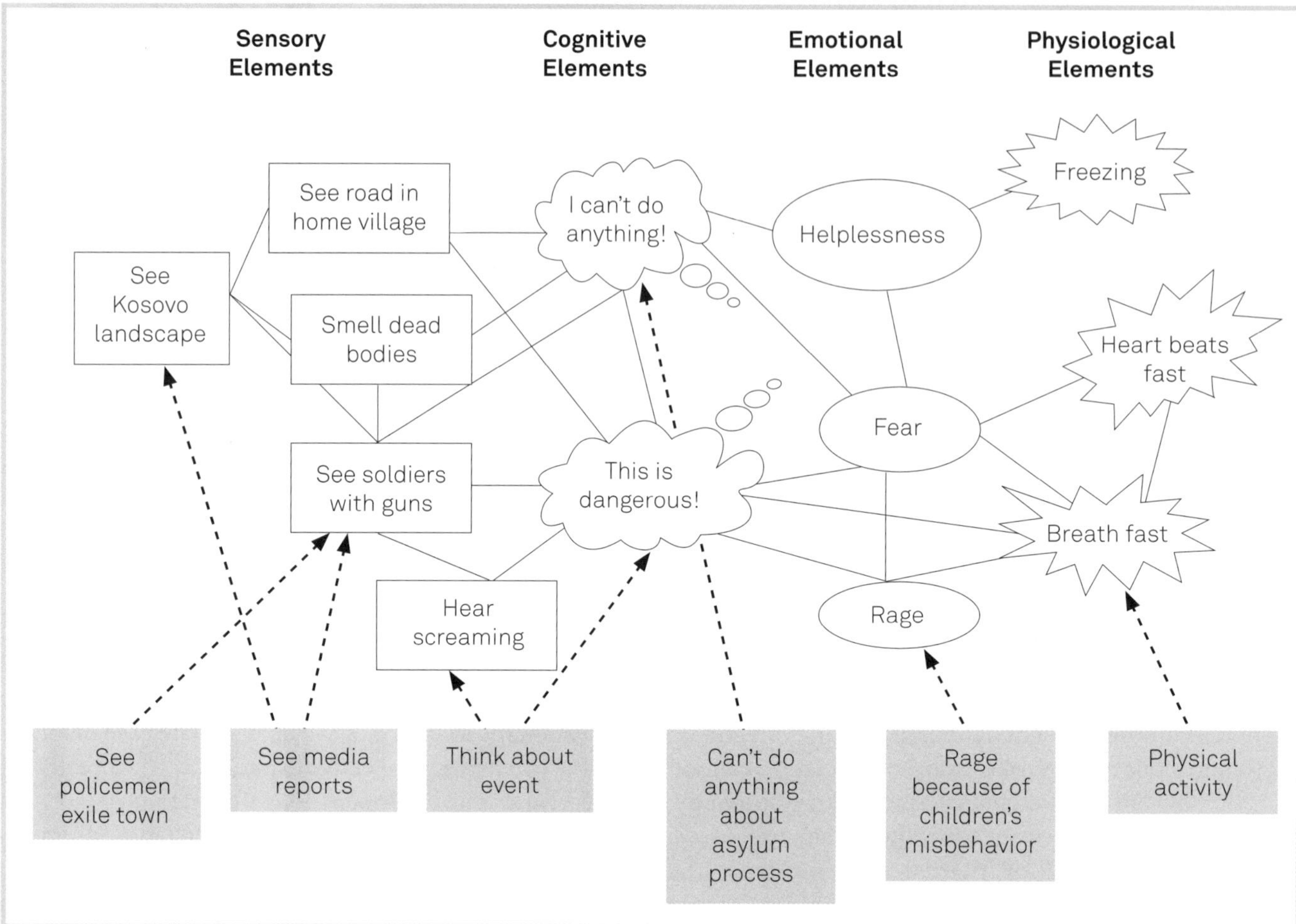

Figure 5. Schematic presentation of a hypothetical sensory-perceptual representation, including sensory, cognitive, emotional, and physiological elements. The network represents a Kosovar refugee's memory of the attack on his home village. The boxes below indicate environmental stimuli with the potential to activate the representation.

experienced by a victim in many different ways, all simultaneously. At the same time as a person is experiencing the sensory aspects of the memory, for instance, other parts of this network or system within the brain are processing cognitive or emotional information in response to the stimuli. Additionally, the body is also responding with a set of corresponding physiological reactions. Another set of response propositions include the motor and physiological responses to the stimulus or memory. All elements of this network of brain activity are connected such that the activation of a single item (such as a sensory experience) lowers the threshold for activation of other elements (see Figure 5 for an example).

The sensory-perceptual representations of traumatic events have also been called *fear structures*. Lang (1979, 1984, 1993) concluded that fear structures or fear networks operate in anxiety disorders. This theory explains the ability to remember and relive past events in the form of *recollective experiences* (in which the subjective, sensory components of memory are experienced; as conceptualized by Tulving, 2001). In addition, this model predicts that these recollections of the event will occur simultaneously with physiological and emotional responses similar to those that occurred when the event happened. For instance, if someone experienced great levels of fear and terror accompanied by heart palpitations while watching a horrible event, this fear and terror and the heart palpitations will be relived upon remembering the event. These predictions have been confirmed by Lang (1979, 1984, 1993) and coworkers using subjective, behavioral, and physiological measurements during mental imagery.

Conway (2001) stated that the retrieval of a sensory-perceptual representation, a memory with sensory information, is the final step in recalling a memory of a past event. He asserts that this process of recovering sensory information takes some effort on the part of the individual and that the process lasts for several seconds of time, rather than occurring instantaneously. However, the impact of emotional structures on behavior is not limited to the deliberate retrieval of memories of past events, as for instance during voluntary mental imagery. Elements of the structure can also be automatically retrieved by a cue, and lead to emotional behavior. For instance, the smell of dead bodies may activate pictures of a road in the home village in the network depicted in Figure 5, without the person choosing to bring these pictures back to mind. Edna Foa and Mike Kozak, a Lang scholar, have related the network theory to PTSD (Foa & Kozak, 1986), whereby a PTSD network would differ from representations (the coding of memories) of normal events in several ways:

- Fear structures encoded during a traumatic event are unusually large (including many nodes or neural elements within the brain) and cover a wide variety of single elements being coded, such as sight, sound, different emotions, and physical sensations. This means that nodes in the fear structures can be easily activated, as many stimuli in the environment have similarities to one or the other element and thus can act as cues (see also Figure 6).
- Interconnections between single elements, such as sight and sound, are unusually powerful. Consequently, the ignition of only a single element, such as a firecracker exploding, may be sufficient to activate the whole structure, causing all of the related memories to return. This explains why traumatized people can have sudden flashbacks when reminded of the traumatic event. According to this theory, an environmental stimulus or internal cue, such as thinking about the event or an intense heartbeat that resembles one part of the stimulus configuration of the traumatic situation can cause the full firing of the sensory information. In turn, the associated emotional, physiological, and motor responses stored in the fear structure will also be triggered. According to this theory, a flashback is the activation of the fear network (which may also be referred to as the "trauma network").

In addition to phenomena of intrusive recollections, this theory can also explain the typical PTSD symptom of avoidance. The activation of a fear structure is experienced as a fearful and painful recollection, and consequently many survivors of traumatic stressors learn to prevent this by avoiding those cues that remind them of the traumatic event. A survivor of war, for instance, walks uphill (higher heartbeat), passes by the fire station (fire, man in uniform), while hearing an airplane from the distance. All these are cues that together form a powerful activation of the fear network. Hence traumatized individuals will learn to avoid both internal and external cues, so they try not to think about it, not to talk about it, and to keep away from persons and places that remind them of the event. In addition, running away or other types of motoric flight behavior (feeling the need to flee a specific situation) can be part of the fear structure. The potential of physiological arousal to trigger the fear network can be so strong that any affective arousal, even positive emotions, are avoided. The victim seems to have become emotionally numb. It is important to notice that the sensory-perceptual representations of extremely stressful and traumatic events are not restricted to emotions such as fear, helplessness, and dissociation, but often encode also reactions to social threats, in particular humiliation, social devaluation, or social defeat.

Autobiographical Contextual Memory

The sensory-perceptual representation is only one type of memory about past experiences. When a person retrieves a memory about a past event, the type of memory that is generally retrieved first is called *autobiographical memory* (see Figure 7; Conway & Pleydell-Pearce, 2000). At the top of the hierarchy of autobiographical memory organization is the memory of *lifetime periods.* Lifetime periods represent general knowledge of persons, places, actions, activities, plans, or goals that characterize a special period. They cover distinct time periods with identifiable beginnings and endings. An example of a lifetime period is "the time when I lived with John." Lifetime periods are typically organized along major themes of persons or places related to goals in life. Typical themes include relationships, occupations, and places one lived. Lifetime periods related to different themes can overlap with respect to the time period to which they refer. For example, the time covered by "when I was working at the farm" may overlap with the time span of "when I lived with John."

A type of knowledge base, or classification of memories, one step down from lifetime periods is the memory of *general events.* A general event refers to a relatively broad or common happening. It typically describes a broader category or type of occurrence such as "having lunch at the cafeteria" or "riding my bike to school." A *specific event*, on the other hand, refers to a particular

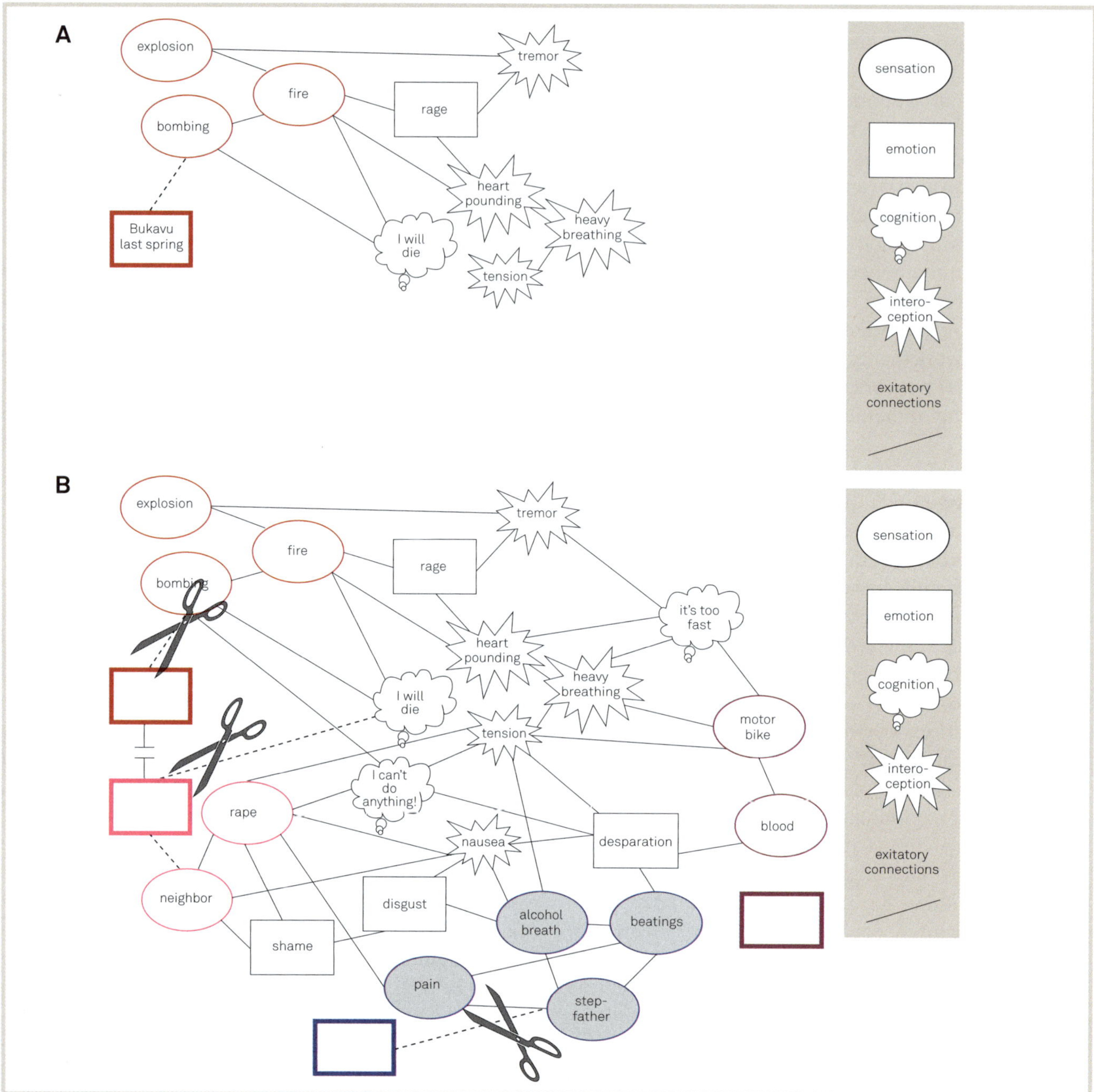

Figure 6. Schematic presentation of a fear network resulting from multiple traumatic experiences. Panel A: The experience of a single traumatic event – such as in this case, the experience of a bombing in the city of Bukavu, Democratic Republic of the Congo (DRC), last spring – is well connected to autobiographical memory. Panel B: If, however, the same experience is integrated into an already existing network of traumatic memories (experiences of domestic violence, earlier accidents, etc.), the connection to the "cold" autobiography gets lost. The sensory, cognitive, emotional, and physiological elements interconnect with increasingly mutual excitatory power. The elements of the cold memory, the codes for the where and when, however, inhibit each other, as the brain's architecture does not allow the activation of representations of two different places or two different periods at the very same time. The memory for the where – the location, for instance – is coded with the help of "place cells" in the hippocampus and the adjacent structures in the temporal lobe. Place cells are neurons that exhibit a high rate of firing whenever the person is actually at the specific location or imagines themselves to be in an environment corresponding to the cells' "place field." As only one set of cells can remain active at any given time, the fear network gets disconnected (symbolized by the scissors) from time and place, and the fear generalizes, giving rise to a permanent feeling of impending threat. Adapted with permission from "Dissociation Following Traumatic Stress: Etiology and Treatment," by Maggie Schauer and Thomas Elbert, *Zeitschrift für Psychologie/Journal of Psychology, 218*, 109–127 (https://doi.org/10.1027/0044-3409/a000018). © 2010 Hogrefe Publishing.

occurrence with unique characteristics, details, or context that distinguish it from other events within the same category. It has a defined scope, time, and location. Examples of specific events could include "I had a bike accident at the intersection in front of my aunt's home."

Conway and Pleydell-Pearce (2000) define *event-specific knowledge* as corresponding to the sensory-perceptual representations described above, such as "when my mother was taking me to school" (on my first day at school). Event-specific knowledge (mother was taking me to school) is usually linked to more general event structures ("my first day at school"), and the activation of the sensory-perceptual details of an event (e.g., the picture of the classroom) is accompanied by the activation of knowledge about the sequence of the event ("first we went to school, and then I saw the classroom") and the location of the event in lifetime periods ("we still lived in our homeland then"). As an exercise, the reader may mark the following as either lifetime periods, general or specific events, or emotional-sensory network:

I remember this warm day in spring, some 20 years ago. It was near my parents' house. I was still going to kindergarten; it was my last year before primary school. My father had bought me a purple bike the day before. He was pushing me, and I can remember well the exciting feeling I had when I started rolling on my own. I was tense but very happy at the same time! I had the feeling "yes I can!"

Taking this concept of memory, we can now examine how memory is affected by traumatic experiences (Figure 7). First, we will take a closer look at how autobiographical memory, general memory, and lifetime periods are all affected in survivors of traumatic stress. The first assumption is that PTSD symptoms develop as a consequence of *generalization and with it distortion of autobiographical memory*. In contrast to those who remember major events as general events, there is evidence to suggest that in persons with PTSD, the traumatic experiences are *not* clearly represented as a series of specific events. Hence, the events often cannot be clearly positioned in a lifetime period. Even though one's memories and the sensory-perceptual representations of traumatic events are very strong and long lasting, there does not seem to be a reliable autobiographical structure to which the memory can be assigned (Figure 6). Trauma survivors suffering from a manifest disorder are often unable to narrate their traumatic experiences. The result is a disorganization and distortion of the sequence of autobiographical memories. In this passage, Metcalfe and Jacobs (1996) describe the typical characteristics of isolated activation of a sensory-perceptual representation in patients with PTSD:

Memories and reactions that are attributable to the isolated hot-system encoding may seem irrational both to the individual him-

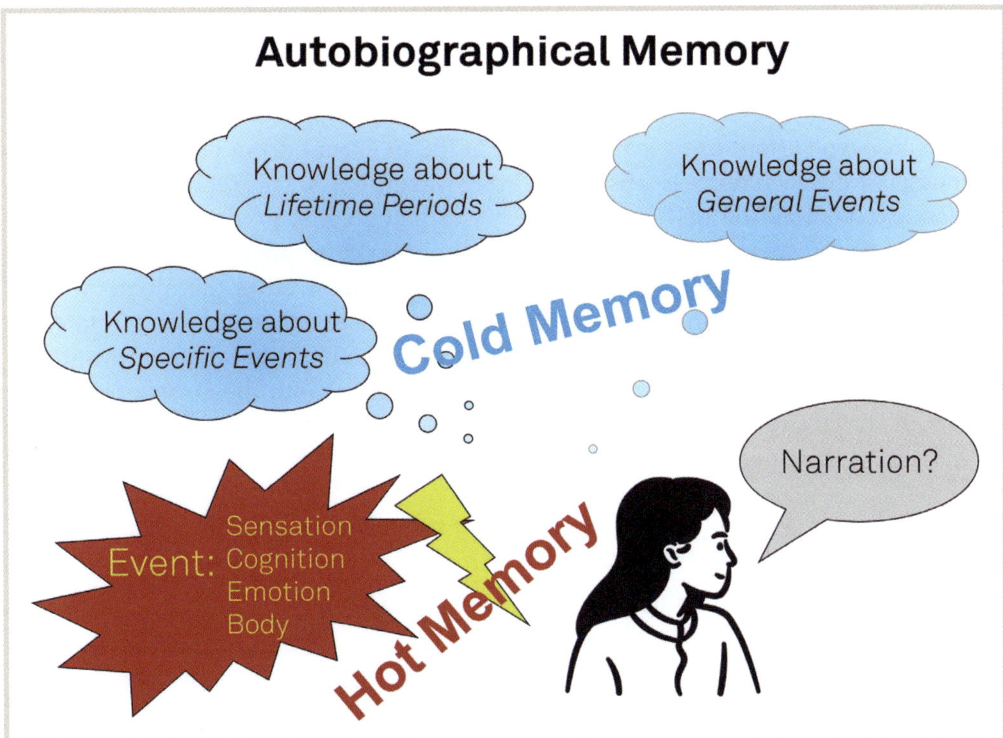

Figure 7.
Structure of autobiographical memory.

or herself, and to the therapist, since such fragments are ungrounded by the kind of narrative and spatio-temporal contextual anchors that tie our ordinary experience to reality. Such memories are disturbing, not only because of the direct fear they evoke, but also because of their strangeness.

Metcalfe & Jacobs (1996, p. 2)

The sensory-perceptual-emotional representations of the traumatic event have also been called *hot memory* (Metcalfe & Jacobs, 1996; Elbert & Schauer, 2002) or *situationally accessible memory* (Brewin et al., 2010), whereas the autobiographical context memory has been called *cold memory* or *verbally accessible memory*.

Figure 6 illustrates the model that exposure to severe stressors increases the probability of developing mental health problems: Each stressor incrementally enlarges a neural representational network, whereby it is common to all sensory elements that they get connected to an emotional-cognitive core of fear and helplessness. Given a high enough level of cumulative exposure to threatening stressors that elicit alarm responses in the mind and body of a survivor, it will eventually wipe out all protective factors that might initially help to counter the onset of a psychiatric illness, notably PTSD and depression. Thereby the brain's networks will integrate experiences of abuse (emotional or physical) and neglect during childhood with those experiences later in life that relate to fear and depression. This may explain the somewhat surprising observation that stressors may make a survivor more vulnerable when they are experienced in quite different contexts rather than in the same environment.

Some events, such as emotional abuse, and often sexual abuse, are not single experiences, but the accumulation of many single events over an extended period of time. In this case, the sensory-perceptual representation will change fundamentally (Neuner, 2023). First, the repetitive experience of events will lead to a generalization of stimulus features. It is not the specific face of a person that is associated with a defensive reaction, but the commonality of different events – that is, the facial and bodily expression of a person that indicates disrespect or devaluation.

The second difference is that the repeated activation of certain response elements – that is, a state of dissociation or defeat – causes a preferential priming of these responses. This means that even minor tangential reminders of the abuse can cause the organism to short-circuit other defensive responses (such as fear or anger) and to react with immediate shutdown or defeat.

The *place cells* in the hippocampal region encode the specific locations or places. They fire when an individual is in a particular location, referred to as its *place field*. Place cells also play a significant role in memory formation and retrieval, particularly in relation to spatial memories as the firing patterns of place cells create a spatial representation of the environment, forming a cognitive map. This spatial representation forms a critical component of episodic memory – that is, remembering specific events within their associated spatial context. This mechanism not only encodes the current location but also contributes to the formation of memories of past experiences in those locations. The firing patterns of place cells during an experience become associated with the memory of that experience. Consequently, when an individual is in a location that was previously encoded by place cells, the activation of those cells can trigger the retrieval of hot memories associated with that place. The reverse process – that is, the possibility that hot memories activate the related place and context – however, becomes impaired when there is not just one place connected to fear and helpless. The more traumatic stressors are experienced in a greater spatial context, the less likely the enlarged hot memory associations will activate a specific place. The hot memories become assigned to the "here and now," and the threats from the past are perceived as real in the present. The more so, the greater the number and variety of traumatic experiences, a phenomenon that we have referred to as *building block effect* (Schauer et al., 2003).

Furthermore, place cells participate in the consolidation of memories during sleep. During sleep, the hippocampus replays the neuronal firing patterns that were observed during wakefulness. This replay, including the firing patterns of place cells, is thought to facilitate memory consolidation by strengthening the connections between neurons involved in the memory trace. However, when the fear or other emotions related to these experiences lead to high emotional arousal during the sleeping and dreaming, the survivor awakens screaming in terror, as if they were reenacting the trauma in sleep.

Disorders of the trauma spectrum and memory

During a traumatic event, mainly sensory and perceptual information (e.g., the sound of gun shots or the smell of blood) is stored in memory during a highly emotional state. The mind and body become extremely aroused (rapid heartbeat, sweating, and trembling) and are set for actions such as hiding, fighting, or running away. This emotional and sensory information is stored separately from the information related to the content. It is stored in an interconnected neural network which may establish a so-called fear network (Figure 6). This fear network includes sensory, cognitive, physiological, and emotional experiences, including the action disposition related to the experience (= hot memory, situationally accessible memory, sensory perceptual representation). Environmental stimuli (e.g., a smell or noise) and internal cues (e.g., a thought) can activate this fear structure later at any given time. The ignition of only a few elements in the network is sufficient to activate the whole structure. This is thought to be a flashback – that is, the feeling as if one were back in the traumatic situation with its sounds, smells, feelings of fear, response propositions, and thoughts. Since the activation of the fear network is a frightening and painful recollection, many survivors learn to avoid cues that act as reminders of the traumatic event. They try not to think about any part represented in the fear/trauma network, not to talk about it, and to keep away from persons and places that remind them of the frightening event. In contrast to the extensive fear memory, individuals who suffer from PTSD have difficulties with autobiographical memory – that is, they are unable to place the fear of the events appropriately in time and space and to clearly position them in a lifetime period (Figure 6). This, and the avoidance of activating the fear structure, makes it difficult for survivors to narrate their traumatic experience.

Neurobiological Basis of Memory and Trauma Disorders

A recognition of how memories are formed and coded within the brain may help us understanding the range of impairments that may occur in survivors of trauma-related suffering. There appear to be several regions of the brain that may be affected to an extent that it can be detected in brain-imaging studies, most notably the hippocampus, the amygdala, and the medial prefrontal cortex, which includes the anterior cingulate cortex (Kolassa & Elbert, 2007).

- The medial temporal lobe and the connected **hippocampus** are brain structures that play a major role in the transformation and construction of the (cold) memories that contain autobiographical information, including the temporal and spatial context of an event. Thus, these neuronal circuits are vital to episodic memory formation and emotional regulation by putting specific events into their proper context, binding together multiple events that co-occur during an experience, and converting short-term into long-term memories – that is, they play a central role in the encoding of context, also during fear conditioning. McClelland and colleagues (McClelland et al., 1995) suggested that the hippocampus is especially important for the coding of information that contradicts previously learned knowledge. This is especially important for survivors of traumatic experiences, as much of what they experience during times of trauma contradicts basic assumptions that have been learned in life about security, trust, and human nature.
- The **amygdala and cingulate cortex** are relevant for *hot* memories. The amygdala is involved in the assessment of threat-related stimuli and has been suggested to be at the center of the defense cascade involved in the acquisition and expression of conditioned fear. Two prominent nuclei of the amygdala are the basolateral complex (BLA) and the central nucleus (CeA). The BLA is involved in the acquisition and storage of fear memories. It receives sensory information from various sources, such as the thalamus and sensory cortices, and integrates this information to form associations between sensory stimuli and fear responses. For example, if a person encounters a dangerous situation and experiences fear, the BLA helps establish a memory linking the sensory cues associated with that situation to the emotional response of fear. This allows for the future recognition and response to similar threats. The CeA is primarily responsible for the expression of fear responses. It receives information from the BLA and other brain regions and sends output signals to regions involved in generating emotional and behavioral responses, such as the hypothalamus, brainstem, and autonomic nervous system. Activation of the CeA can lead to the activation of the body's stress response, triggering physiological changes associated with fear, such as increased heart rate, heightened arousal, and the fight-or-flight response. The amygdala thus plays a pivotal role in mediating stress-related effects on behavior and modulating hippocampal function.
- The **medial prefrontal cortex** inhibits activation of the amygdala and is involved in the extinction of conditioned fear. It includes the anterior cingulate cortex, which is implicated in evaluating the emotional significance of stimuli and in attentional function (Cardinal et al., 2002).

In people with PTSD, the amygdala appears to be hyperreactive, meaning that it shows increased responsiveness to trauma-related cues. This heightened activity can lead to exaggerated fear responses and hypervigilance. In turn, higher brain regions, such as the hippocampus and the medial frontal cortex, are affected, as they are unable to handle the overload of stimuli that results from symptoms such as an exaggerated startle response and flashbacks. Stress hormones that result from these experiences impair the ability of the brain to function properly and to create memories correctly. Based on research with rodents (for a review, see, e.g., McEwen, 2002), there is evidence that the stress hormones released during traumatic events affect both the function and (when happening during childhood) the structure of the hippocampus. Exposure to glucocorticoids (stress hormones that occur during traumatic events) normally increases the activity of the hippocampus; however, if a certain threshold is exceeded, its functioning begins to decline drastically. Under very high levels of stress, the functioning of the hippocampus becomes severely impaired, and the hippocampus, along with the medial frontal cortex, is unable to mediate the exaggerated symptoms of arousal and distress that occur in the amygdala in response to reminders of the traumatic event (Nutt & Malizia, 2004). In humans, a series of cross-sectional studies examined structural abnormalities of the hippocampus and other brain regions in subjects with various traumas. Originally, Bremner et al. (1997, 2003) reported that the hippocampus is smaller in individuals with PTSD than in comparison subjects. Subsequently, it became increasingly evident that this effect of a sizeable volumetric reduction depends on the developmental period when the traumatic stress has been experienced first (see Figure 8). When drug intake, such as excessive alcohol consumption, is controlled, traumatic stress in adults, even when severe, such as in torture survivors, will not result in a reduction of hippocampal volume (Eckart et al., 2010).

Several studies found changes in the limbic cortex, and particularly in the anterior cingulate cortex. Some authors have argued that the cause-effect relationship is preexisting - that is, that an individual with a smaller hippocampus may be more prone to develop PTSD when exposed to a traumatic event - and these researchers explored whether or not a reduction in the volume of the hippocampus occurs in survivors of a recent trauma who develop PTSD. Shalev and his group found that smaller hippocampal volume is not a preexisting risk factor for

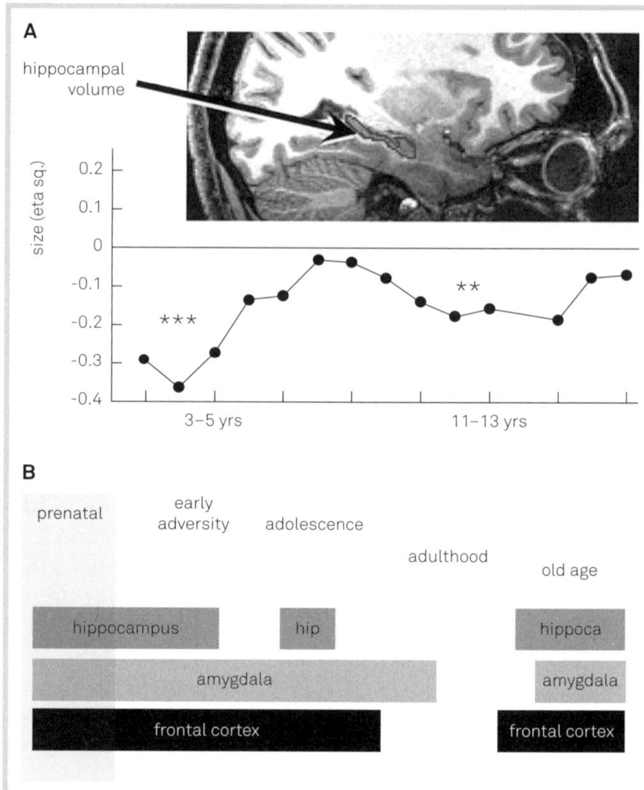

Figure 8. The impact of traumatic stress on memory. (A) Depending on the developmental period, chronic or repeated exposure to traumatic stressors may significantly reduce (negative values) hippocampal volume later in life (based on data from personal communication with Marty Teicher, 2008–2010). (B) The sensitivity of brain regions to alter their structure in response to stressors varies with developmental periods, depending on the type of the stressor (type × timing, see, e.g., Schalinski, Teicher et al., 2016).

the development of PTSD, but that it later occurs in individuals with chronic or complicated PTSD (Bonne et al., 2001).

In our own research, we have identified structural alterations of the cortex (Eckart et al., 2010): Survivors suffering from PTSD (and to a lesser extent, trauma-exposed controls) showed reduced gray matter volumes in the right inferior parietal cortex, the left rostral middle frontal cortex, the bilateral lateral orbitofrontal cortex, and the bilateral isthmus of the cingulate. An influence of cumulative exposure to traumatic stress on the isthmus of the cingulate and the lateral orbitofrontal cortex indicated that, at least in these regions, structural alterations might be associated with repeated stress experience. These results indicate that lateral prefrontal, parietal, and posterior midline structures become structurally remodeled by repeated traumatic stress experiences. As these regions are particularly involved in episodic memory, emotional processing, and executive control, these changes might be part of the physiological substrate of PTSD symptoms.

In addition to these massive structural changes, there are other brain regions that show functional alterations in survivors of organized violence: We observed massively changed oscillatory properties in left temporal brain regions, with peak activities in the region of the insula (Figure 9). Furthermore, we found altered slow wave activity in right frontal areas in individuals with PTSD compared with controls (Kolassa et al., 2007). The theory of the associative fear/trauma network would predict effective and widespread synchronized afferent inputs to a cortical area. Consequently, a representation will become unusually large. As a result, more and more neurons become coupled with each other and the resulting networks begin to oscillate (in the low frequency range; Kolassa et al., 2007; and Figure 9) and, through this reverberation, generate continuous organized response activity leading to a permanent pressure for activating these networks. In other words, it is the otherwise highly valued plasticity of the brain that leads to an ever-increasing pressure for intrusions as the number of traumatic experiences increases. In summary, magnetic brain-imaging studies provide neurophysiological support for the theory of a fear/trauma network (Figure 9).

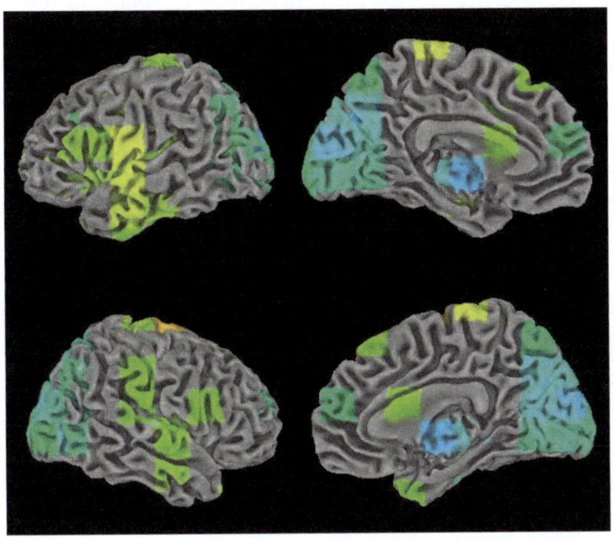

Figure 9. The reorganization of brain functions under traumatic stress. Abnormal slow brain waves were recorded and localized in brains of a torture victim, using magnetic source imaging. Volume elements (voxels) where abnormal brain waves are generated have been marked with darker shades of gray. Examples of abnormal oscillatory activity as shown here include frontotemporal regions, notably the insula (a site of multimodal convergence) and the region around Broca's area in the left hemisphere. Abnormality in these regions may be related to the "speechlessness" of the terror. (Based on data from the authors' clinic; see also Kolassa et al., 2007)

PTSD and the brain

The functioning of brain structures important for memory coding, such as the medial temporal lobe including the adjacent hippocampus, is strongly affected by traumatic stress via stress hormones. Under very high levels of traumatic stress, the function of the hippocampus and related neural networks becomes impaired. With cumulative exposure to traumatic stressors multiple but incompatible sets of place cells become activated. Their parallel activation produces noise in the spatial coding, and the mutual inhibition of sets of place cells tend to suppress the coding. During times of severe stress, this adds to an incomplete and distorted storage in autobiographical memory. Many other brain areas are affected in turn. On the other hand, the more arousing a stressor is emotionally, the more active those areas of the brain become which encode emotional content, including nuclei of the amygdala – the structure in the brain that prepares the body for danger. During a traumatic event and later in response to a reminder of the trauma, the amygdala and the interconnected frontal lobe regions respond ever more vigorously to the stimuli of the event. The individual then is "overconditioned" to respond to fear. This may explain the exaggerated emotional responses to threat situations in trauma survivors.

Processing of Affective Experiences

Regulation of Emotions

Whereas most people react with intensive emotional upheaval or a massive dissociative response immediately following a traumatic experience – including symptoms of acute stress and PTSD symptoms – only a minority develop chronic trauma-related symptoms. Recovery from acute stress symptoms seems to be the usual process in human beings who have been exposed to isolated events.

In order for the victim to recover from the debilitating effects of trauma-related suffering, the mind and brain must begin to *control or inhibit the fear response,* leading to a modification or extinction of the fear network. One theory is that by activating the fear structure in a safe context – for example, by allowing the memories to be triggered with another person present – this process can begin to take place. Triggering the memories in a momentarily safe and socially accepting environment allows for the possibility of introducing new elements, ones that are incompatible with the original fear-based connections, into the existing fear structure. For example, the newly introduced thought or cognition "I am safe" contradicts the main cognitive elements of the fear structure that have been resulting in a permanent state of impending threat. By allowing the individual to experience the current fear structure in conjunction with the current incompatible information, the fear structure can be modified such that maladaptive associations between the stimulus (fearful memories) and response (symptoms of PTSD) decrease over time. In other words, by exposing the individual to both the cues that may trigger fearful memories of the trauma, along with new contradictory information, the fear will begin to lessen over time as the new information is integrated. Normally, this process of integration occurs naturally after an emotional event without any specific intervention, but in the case of repeated traumatic stress, it may be inhibited due to an avoidance of the fear structure or because the individual prematurely terminates the process out of fear of the stimuli. Moreover, repeated stress will enlarge and reinforce the fear structure while disconnecting its elements more and more from the contextual cues (when and where the traumatic stressor has been experienced) at the same time. This will lead to the development of chronic PTSD.

Research on *fear conditioning* has challenged this view. Several investigators have shown that an *extinction or elimination of fear responses* will not necessarily change the original stimulus–fear associations, as the original fear response can easily be reinstated in a context different from the context of extinction learning. For example, just because an individual has become accustomed or desensitized to hearing fireworks does not mean that a repeated traumatic event will not reinstate the original fear structure. Instead, extinction probably occurs through the inhibition of the fear response by a *regulative process* (LeDoux, 2000). This regulative process is based on a more thorough evaluation of the current situation than the automatic evaluation by the fear structure – that is, the brain is able to process the information about the event more slowly and thoroughly rather than just reacting emotionally to the information (Figure 10). Brewin (2001) suggested that this cortical evaluation depends on the availability of declarative memory of the stimulus. By using the information from declarative memory about the past event, the individual is better able to evaluate whether the current stimulus indicates a threat.

As noted in the box "PTSD and the brain", after a traumatic event, declarative knowledge, and especially autobiographical knowledge, which offers information about the context of the feared stimulus, is fragmented and noisy. This can lead to a lack of capability for the *cortical inhibitory control of the fear response.* The process of cortical inhibition of the conditioned fear response occurs as the person learns to distinguish between past and present threats. In other words, the person who experienced a traumatic event in the past learns that the same or similar stimuli in the present are not currently a threat. In normal emotional processing, the intrusive memories provide an opportunity for the individual to build up declarative memory about the event. As the person thinks and talks about this event, utilizing and integrating the memories and the stimuli presented by intrusive memories, cortical regulation begins to take place, and more functional and accurate autobiographical knowledge can be constructed about the traumatic episode. The construction of autobiographical knowledge about the traumatic event is no easy task, as the organization of autobiographical knowledge is connected to personal goals and to basic beliefs about the self. This means that active emotional processing takes time and effort. Secondary emotions such as anger and guilt may indicate problems in the cognitive processing of the event and the adaptive placement of the traumatic experience in the context of preexisting beliefs about the self, which also interferes with the construction of a coherent autobiographical representation. Because thinking about the traumatic event automatically causes painful emotions, many people avoid this process and try to eliminate intrusive memories as soon as possible. The fact that victims with poor social support following a traumatic event are at an increased risk for developing PTSD (Ozer et al., 2003; Sommer et al., 2016) might be explained by the lack of opportunity or encouragement to talk about the event. Persons who do not have strong support networks may be less likely to talk about the event, which would allow for emotional processing and the chronological reconstruction of autobiographical memory.

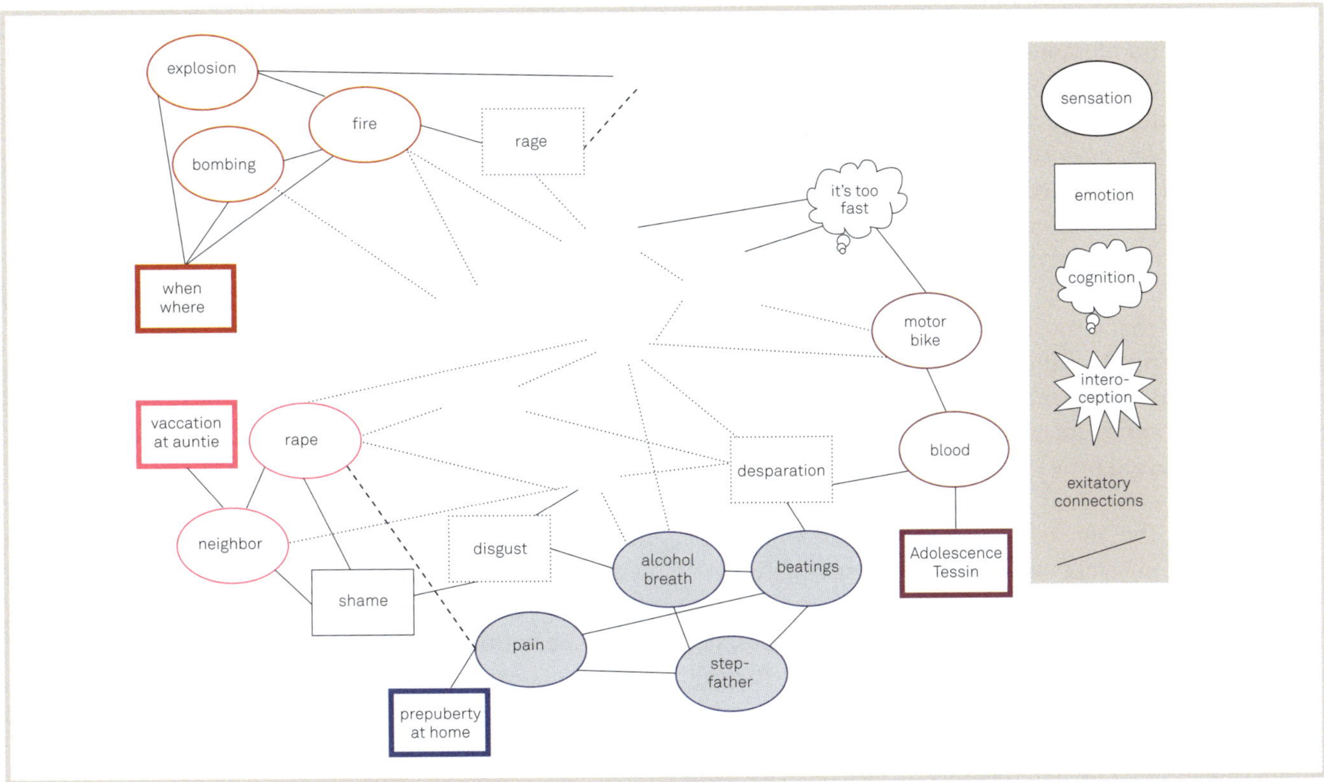

Figure 10. Connecting the cold, declarative elements to the hot memories will fractionize the fear/trauma network into its original elements. Cues are less likely to trigger neural representations of all the traumatic memories, but will activate a subset of representations, related to a particular traumatic event. The survivor will realize that the activated cognitions, emotions, and sensory elements relate to the past and no longer to the present.

Processing of the emotions connected with the fear structure

The explicit (declarative) autobiographical representation is needed to regulate the activation of the original fear structure and with it, the interconnected cognitions and emotions (= response dispositions). This will modify the connections within the fear structure (Figure 10). People naturally seem to try to control their fear structure by narrating their experiences. In many cases this is helpful, because this process naturally helps building up cool memory context information. However, because thinking about the traumatic event causes pain and fear, people avoid this process (despite the fact that it may prove helpful) and interrupt their recollections and storytelling. By avoiding that recall, they are inhibiting the habituating processing of the experience, and as a result the fear/ structure seems to consolidate itself, and chronic PTSD lingers. When, however, a survivor thinks and talks about the event, ideally in chronological order, and includes the stimuli presented by intrusive memories, autobiographical knowledge about the traumatic episode can be reconstructed, and the victim can learn to distinguish between cues of past and current threats. The construction of a narration enforces the activation and consequently the habituation of the fear. This exposure is the most powerful means to tearing down the fear network. In this process, a survivor is learning that sensory and emotional memory can be activated without fear.

Implications for Treatment

Basically, all evidence-based treatment approaches intend to relieve trauma symptoms by purposeful, controlled revisiting the traumatic events. Foa and colleagues (Foa & Rothbaum, 1998) were among the first to systematically develop (prolonged) *exposure therapy* as PTSD treatment, work which encouraged the development of NET. When implementing exposure therapy for PTSD, the participant is instructed to repeatedly talk about the traumatic experience, thus exposing the individual to the event and its related memories. Likewise, controlled, randomized studies have shown the superiority of exposure elements in cognitive behavior treatment in children and adolescents compared with other approaches (Saigh, 1992; Saigh et al., 1996). In particular, Foa and colleagues (Foa, Molnar et al., 1995) demonstrated that those participants who manage to construct a coherent narrative of the event during exposure therapy profit most from treatment.

The main focus of this therapy should be on the part of the memory that is most fragmented in autobiography and most intensively represented in sensory-perceptual representations. These moments of intense recollection of memories, complete with physical sensations, have often been referred to as "hot spots." In order for the victim to form a consistent autobiographical narration of this moment, the sensory-perceptual representations (memories of physical sensations) are inevitably activated, as they provide detailed knowledge about the event that is not yet available in declarative (autobiographical) structures. When recovering or reconstructing the autobiographical memories of the event, the individual should be encouraged to recount those moments within specific events that are most likely to cause intrusive symptoms such as flashbacks, physical sensations, or appear in nightmares. Because the sensory-perceptual representations of the memories in the brain evoke intense emotional reactions, successful therapy cannot proceed without a high level of emotional involvement.

Consistent with this view, Jaycox et al. (1998) showed that treatment success in exposure therapy is positively correlated with the level of fear initially experienced in treatment – that is, the higher the level of fear experienced initially, the greater the success of the treatment. The therapist should aid the survivor in organizing the declarative or autobiographical memories connected to the traumatic event and placing it in time and space. There is a decrease in emotional spectrum and response intensity as the memories become incapable of eliciting the core fear network (Figure 6). Ultimately, narrating the memories will no longer produce strong emotional reactions, confusion, and fear in the person (Figure 10).

Associations between stimuli and fear responses cannot always be erased in therapy with trauma survivors. For some individuals, there may always be some fear that is evoked when the event is recalled. Rather than trying to eliminate all fear, it may be necessary to make new associations. In this case, the new association would be the declarative or factual knowledge that is constructed and linked to the stimuli that evoke intrusive symptoms. For example, a goal for a victim whose fear is activated by the sight of fire might be to associate some declarative knowledge with the sight of fire, such as the time of day or season, rather than the emotional content of the memory. It may take several repetitions of the new associations before the declarative knowledge becomes the preferred representation that is activated when the event is recalled. Only when these associations are firmly established are the intense emotional reactions and associated intrusive symptoms inhibited by the new knowledge base and a modification of the fear structure initiated.

Moreover, even under difficult circumstances, most therapists evaluate the NET procedure as enriching and expressed their motivation to accept traumatized clients in the future (Potter et al., 2023). Although, participants symptom trajectories differ, and NET leads to clinically and behaviorally relevant reductions in PTSD symptoms both throughout and following treatment (Kaltenbach et al., 2018). Concerns about imaginal exposure have not been substantiated. While new and additional stressful life events contributed to transient symptom increases, they were not found to prevent the overall effectiveness of NET (Kaltenbach et al., 2020).

Speechlessness of Trauma: Sociopolitical Implications

In addition to the known fact that psychological trauma is a consequence or outcome of violence, there is also increasing discussion as to whether this psychological trauma can contribute to the number of violent conflicts – family or state-sponsored violence – in the world. Organizations that provide psychosocial interventions in war-affected societies have justified their interventions not only as a means of improving mental health care for individuals, but also by making the case that these interventions are relevant to society and on a political scale. One common assertion is that the treatment of traumatized societies is necessary to break the *cycle of trauma and violence* (UNICEF, 2001, 2022). The cycle-of-trauma argument implies that victims of violence are more likely to become perpetrators later on. At the same time, treatment of traumatized survivors is considered to facilitate forgivingness and reconciliation within the society.

Whereas it is unclear to what extent and how political processes affect the mental health of victims, it is very likely that the psychological status of victims has an effect on social and political processes beyond the assumed cycle of trauma. In every society there are individuals who want to speak out about what has happened and to pass their experiences on to their children as well as to the public. Some of them will be able to do so on their own, and various local human rights groups have evolved to give these people a forum. Many survivors of the Holocaust, for example, have chosen to document their own experiences as a means of educating subsequent generations (Bettelheim, 1986; Frankl, 1946/1959).

A considerable number of people, especially those who suffer from PTSD, are unable to narrate their personal histories because of the pathological effects of the traumatic events on their memory. This puts the victims at a disadvantage in comparison with the perpetrators and bystanders, who usually have no difficulties explaining their position. Offering victims a means of processing their traumatic events and documenting their history can help to give them a voice within their society. During the Pinochet regime in Chile, Lira and Weinstein (published under the pseudonyms Cienfuegos & Monelli, 1983) developed *testimony therapy* as a specialized treatment approach for torture victims, which directly addressed this issue.

Testimony therapy combines political as well as psychological goals. The biography of the survivor of human rights violations is documented in detail with an emphasis on the persecution history and traumatic events experienced. The resulting documents have been used to accuse the regime of human rights violations and, as a whole, became a powerful tool in the resistance to the Pinochet dictatorship. Thus, this treatment approach serves two distinct purposes: On the one hand, it serves as a method for facilitating the emotional processing of the victim's traumatic event, resulting in improved mental health, and at the same time, it acts as a document which can be directly used for political purposes. Other therapists have followed this example and used testimony therapy for different groups of survivors of wars and torture (Agger, 1994; Agger & Jensen, 1990; Weine et al., 1995; Weine & Laub, 1995; Weine et al., 1998). Despite these reports offering promising results for treatment, testimony therapy has not been widely used in mainstream psychosocial organizations, which primarily favor nonpolitical approaches.

Treatment of trauma-related suffering

The concept and theory of traumatic memory formation suggests that the goal of any trauma therapy must be to construct a coherent declarative (autobiographical) account of the sequence of events experienced by the survivor. The act of creating this coherent narrative allows the individual to become "ex-posed" (lat. "ex-position," positioned "outside") of the trauma while talking about it. This process allows for the control and reduction of stress reactions. The therapist's role is to facilitate engagement with specific memories of the traumatic experiences and to overcome the survivor's avoidance. At the same time, the therapist should assist the survivor in reorganizing the memories related to the traumatic event and connecting the events to time and space in the past. Visualizing or imagining the events is necessary for the traumatized individual to reconstruct their life story and will stimulate learning that these active neural representations are memories and not a life-threatening presence. The client is empowered to integrate the events into their life story.

The Nature of NET as a Treatment and Its Ethical Position

There is no greater agony than bearing an untold story inside you.

Maya Angelou (*I Know Why the Caged Bird Sings*)

NET has been developed to be a robust, low-threshold, evidence-based, and disseminable treatment module for trauma survivors. It aims to restore psychosocial functioning and health, while counteracting human rights violations. In this endeavor, it is a joint approach of healing and testifying.

This section provides an overview of the identity of NET as a model and its ethical position. For those readers who are less interested in this topic and wish to proceed directly to the intervention, we kindly ask that you skip these descriptions and continue reading on page 112.

NET Characteristics and Principles

Lifespan Perspective of NET

Trauma may have its roots long before the narrator is born, as the effects of traumatic dynamics resonate across generations. Children suffer interpersonal adversity in childhood almost always because of the abuse and emotional stressors endured by their caregivers and their grandparents (second generation caregivers) who raised the caregiver. The effects of violence and neglect, emotional, physical, or sexual abuse continue long after the maltreatment and stressful interaction have ended, through pathways such as epigenetics, mental health problems, model learning in the area of aggression and impulsivity, negative emotions and violence-proneness in the communal social fabric, highly expressed emotions in inconsistent parenting, and much more.

This trajectory is characterized by an increased likelihood of failure and disruption in the successful resolution of developmental tasks, which in turn may open pathways to maladaptation and psychopathology. NET aims to provide the opportunity and space to understand and relate victimization to persistent anxiety, devaluation, and later impulsivity, to humiliation, adolescent depression, and aggression. NET illuminates the connection between traumatic events and subsequent mental and somatic illnesses, and identifies personal developmental patterns as well as overarching themes and issues that run through decades of life, sometimes even across generations.

NET does not require that an individual identifies one or two worst events – that is, an *index* trauma (Schauer et al., 2005; Neuner, 2016). To label a single event that "broke" a person would be an arbitrary and sometimes even unethical decision.

To remove a major pathogen in our midst and end the cycle of spreading trauma, NET takes a different approach to allow healing: creating the opportunity to review all major life stories in sequence, beginning in early childhood, while also making interpersonal schemas tangible, as a natural and empowering way to overcome trauma consequences. The lifespan perspective makes it possible to see interpersonal patterns, to delve into early biographical times, and to make corrective relationship experiences with the help of a caring testimony bearer trained in memory-exposure-conversation.

This natural, life-affirming work provides connection and guidance to see trauma in its biographical context and to deal not only with traumatic moments but with life as a whole, giving it a sense of purpose and meaning.

NET as Trauma-Memory Focused Intervention

The focus of NET is on allocating highly arousing, important, and meaningful experiences (*hot memories*) to a time and space, thus producing coherent narratives about these experiences. In this way, NET enables individuals to create an autobiographical narrative that includes the most significant and arousing experiences from birth to present. Such an individualized trauma-memory focused therapy has been shown to be highly effective for the majority of survivors of traumatic stress, including those with severe dissociation and other complex forms of PTSD symptom patterns.

NET Across Cultural, Social, and Political Identities

As much as people are unique, a basic assumption of NET is that trauma reactions, with some cultural differences in the expression of symptoms, are a universal phenomenon, resulting from psychophysiological processes involved in the response to threat and stress. Likewise, the sharing of personal stories is a human practice across all groups of people. Storytelling helps survivors cope with life events and promotes interpersonal closeness. This may be why the NET process has been successfully applied in various cultures, genders, social classes, racial, ethnic and political expressions, and intersecting identities. NET can be incorporated into multicomponent ecological approaches and indigenous critical models to assist individuals, families, and social groups.

While diagnostic tools need to be carefully adapted and validated for each language and culture, only minor modifications to the narrative process are required when implemented for quite different survivor groups. Rather than focusing on differences between cultures and identities, the NET approach recognizes that in any given situation, people hold a wide variety of values and attitudes, and experience different and similar discriminations, disadvantages, and violent stressors. Ultimately, the experience of trauma touches on existential issues, and we are all one in this. Victims come from different economic and educational backgrounds, and they experience a variety of oppressions and social rejections. Accordingly, any treatment approach must be tailored to the individual needs of each survivor, rather than to clichés and stereotypes commonly attributed to specific cultures or groups and to our implicit assumptions about their needs (Schnyder et al., 2016; Bryant-Davies, 2019; Neuner, 2016; Schauer et al., 2020; Robjant et al., 2021; Spoont et al., 2017). Narrations strengthen the survivor's ability to connect with and own their developmental trajectory, and to regain dignity and fulfill the need for recognition by being seen and validated.

Mental Health First! NET in Task-Shifting and Screen and Treat Models of Care

Most people will experience shocking and potentially traumatizing events during their lives, but few will develop a psychiatric disorder from a single, a *mono-trauma* alone (Elbert et al., 2022; Kilpatrick et al., 2013). There are several factors that may lead to a trauma syndrome. The greatest impact results from the sum and variety of several potentially traumatizing life events ("building block"). With an increasing number of adverse and traumatic life events, the clinical symptoms become more severe and more lasting (Kilpatrick et al., 2013; Ni et al., 2022; Herron & Venner, 2023; Frost et al., 2019; Hamby et al., 2021), while the likelihood for spontaneous remission decreases (Kolassa et al., 2010).

Moreover, countless individuals reside in environments of continuous trauma, unable to seek refuge and occasionally incapable of safeguarding themselves and their progeny. Furthermore, poverty, malnourishment, scarcity, and the hazards of a shifting environment, including the impacts of climate change, exacerbate daily strain. These stressors cultivate violent tendencies in peer relationships as adults subject themselves to repeat victimization, inflict harm on others, and sometimes develop a compulsion for aggression. (Elbert & Schauer, 2014, 2018; Neuner et al., 2011; Hinsberger et al., 2020; Schauer & Schauer, 2010).

Survivors of trauma are stuck in their dreadful experiences and thus have difficulties with mental and daily functioning, this prevents economic self-sufficiency, as well as social and economic reconstruction and development. Childhood trauma can lead to lifelong economic consequences resulting directly or indirectly from associated behavioral problems, mental and physical health conditions, increased risk for violent behaviors, disability from physical injury, reduced health-related quality of life, lower levels of educational achievement, and impaired capacity of adults to generate income (Fang et al., 2012; Letourneau et al., 2018; Assari, 2020). Healing PTSD, in contrast, empowers survivors to live self-determined lives. Only then may living in safety finally be possible. Thus, treatment should be at the top of list of possible measures and only then is safety possible.

Trauma also has a noticeable and damaging effect on social contacts in particular. Although traumatized people are more at risk than dangerous, social contact and living with severely stressed people creates stress. The duration of contact and proximity to a "carrier" are also crucial in this form of epidemic. Especially when children live with traumatized caregivers who show symptoms of PTSD and CPTSD. Some of those affected, especially if they themselves experienced massively unfavorable childhood conditions, could be described as "spreaders," as they spread violence and hostility to a high degree and are impulsive and emotionally unpredictable.

Despite a wealth of evidence, the devastating and lasting infectious consequences of severe and traumatic stress, including intergenerational effects still goes unrecognized as it is not given due attention. The pathology and danger of contagion by trauma is rarely systematically assessed, often ignored by professionals, policy makers, humanitarian assistance, and, due to the characteristic avoidance symptoms, denied by those affected. This neglect perpetuates the cycle of violence. Individuals suffering from trauma-induced disorders are more likely to abuse substances and develop depressed disengagement and inconsistent parenting. They may display impulsive behavior and rejection, aggressiveness, or anxious irritability. People who spend time with them, particularly those who are dependent on them, can develop mental and somatic health problems as well as stress-related behaviors. These effects can have a burdensome and disruptive impact on various aspects of society, including communities, workplaces, and neighborhoods (see, e.g., Scoglio et al., 2022; Davis et al., 2022). In this way, traumatized individuals communicate their disease. These previously victimized spreaders can and should be identified using task shifting (help from trained paraprofessionals), screen and treat (active outreach to identify and offer targeted assistance according to need), and stepped care (utilizing a cascade model of interventions) approaches (WHO, 2021; Elbert, Wilker et al., 2017), as is necessary for overwhelmed health care systems. Individuals and their communities may be offered support and, upon informed consent, trauma-memory focused treatment (Siehl et al., 2021; NETfacts; e.g., Robjant et al., 2021; Köbach et al., 2021; FORNET, e.g., Elbert et al., 2012; Crombach & Elbert, 2014; Hecker et al., 2015; Hinsberger et al., 2020). Evidence-based psychological rehabilitation that can break the cycle of trauma transmission builds on trauma memory-focused interventions within cascading models of care. Specifically, the most effective, yet least resource-intensive treatment is to be delivered first to strengthen the capacity of individuals, families, psychosocial service providers, and primary health care providers to address the basic mental health needs. Being a safe, feasible, and relatively short intervention, having the ability to address multiple traumas, taking into account the individual's entire life journey in the therapy, and requiring less professional training, are all factors that make NET suitable for task-shifting approaches that can be implemented by diverse facilitators – from academic professionals to trained lay health workers in countries with an insufficient health sector (Smaik et al., 2023). Cascade models of stepped care and screen and prevent or treatment interventions (Schauer & Schauer, 2010; Ruf & Schauer, 2012; Kaiser et al., 2025) provide care for the vulnerable, identify the spreaders, and separate out those who cope well. Early prevention requires the identification of pregnant women in need and under stress (Elbert & Schauer 2014; Spyridou et al. 2014, 2015, 2016; Koenig et al., 2016, Radtke et al., 2015, Ullmann et al., 2017; Leeners et al., 2014; Stevens et al., 2020) followed by the timely offering of trauma treatment to avoid significant pregnancy complications associated with the increased risk of adverse perinatal outcomes. NET treatment during pregnancy has been shown to be well accepted and successfully implemented, suggesting promising outcomes (Stevens et al., 2020). Identifying mental health risk factors to promote positive attachment and the parent–child relationship through early appropriate intervention is as important as identifying children in need and at-risk youth (Schauer et al., 2017; Ruf & Schauer, 2012; Peltonen & Kangaslampi, 2019; Fazel et al., 2020; Wilker et al., 2020).

Task-shifting instead of regulation in the application and dissemination of trauma approaches is the need of our time (see Neuner, 2016). In the context of high-demand and limited resources, as is the case of most health care systems, any evidence-based trauma-focused therapy must be pragmatic, brief, and teachable to paraprofessionals who have no or limited university training. A number of randomized controlled trials have demonstrated that NET can be successfully delivered by trained paraprofessional therapists who do not have a formal medical or psychological background (e.g., teachers and fellow refugees in a refugee camp; Neuner et al., 2008; Robjant & Fazel, 2010). Low-threshold, evidence-based, trauma-memory focused modules are well tolerated, effective, and to the point, and they can complement traditional care models in the psychosocial and mental health sector, especially for populations with high and very high trauma loads. These modules are robust and disseminable, making them a valuable resource even for overburdened aid structures. In task-shifting "screen and treat" intervention models, such as NET, or "screen and counsel" care models, such as NAT (Narrative Trauma Work; Kaiser et al., 2025), trauma-informed and trauma-memory-focused mental health care can be provided by expanding the use of more personal (e.g., social- and health workers, community members, paraprofessionals, or well-trained lay counselors) who fulfill a role and work within a stepped-care approach to befriend, identify, and assess potential individuals in need, direct them to tailored help, and facilitate couseling.

NET to Help Traumatized People Avoid Revictimization

The fact of having experienced trauma, especially during childhood, greatly increases the likelihood of experiencing traumatic stress again through the dynamics of reenactment. Whether it is the propensity for risk taking, sensation seeking, or aggressive behavior exhibited by some trauma survivors (Babad et al., 2021); or the lack of self-care, concurrent self-hatred, or unstable sense of self (Maercker et al., 2022); continuous self-blame and shame (Langer & Neuner, 2021) experienced by some victims of more complex trauma reactions; or the lack of self-control due to self-medication with substances life is a dangerous place for people who continue to live under the domain of trauma. It has long been known that previously traumatized individuals seek increased attachment in the face of external danger. Adults, as well as children, can develop strong emotional attachments to people who sometimes bully, beat, and threaten them, and who please them through appeasement (Bailey et al., 2023; Steel, 2021).

The percentage of women who were raped as children or adolescents and who were raped again as adults was more than twice as high as the percentage of women with no early history of rape.

NISVS (CDC, 2024)

Memory disturbances and arousal states may interfere with good judgment, allowing the longing for attachment to overcome realistic fears and lead to compulsion to repeat, i.e. involvement in unhealthy relationships (Laplanche & Pontalis, 2018; van der Kolk, 1989). Many traumatized people expose themselves to situations reminiscent of the original trauma (Narvaez et al., 2019). The phenomenon of revictimization is not restricted to sexual violence, but involves all types of abuse, including physical and emotional victimization (Langer & Neuner, 2021.)

NET as Trauma-Focused Intervention for Insecure Living Conditions

Studies have documented that NET can effectively help survivors, even in unstable and socioeconomic poor living conditions. (see, e.g., Neuner et al., 2008, 2010; Orang et al., 2018; Edgar et al., 2022; Aysazci-Cakar et al., 2023; Emmelkamp, 2023). In most circumstances, good mental health is required to cope with or escape from conditions of continuous trauma. This is also true for survivors of family violence or community trauma. Victims are often helpless for years, if not decades. They continue to experience severe abuse in their homes, while often being isolated and bullied by outsiders, including peers and teachers. They often do not have access to help and treatment because they are silenced and threatened by the abuser. In addition, victims' own feelings of guilt and shame prevent them from seeking help and safety (Heron & Eisma, 2021; Orang et al., 2018; Stotz et al., 2015)

Overcoming the consequences of trauma is vital for individuals, their families, and their communities, especially in situations of acute and chronic stress on a large scale and in regions without social welfare systems, as manifest trauma leads to severe functional impairment and social marginalization. Many people with these trauma spectrum disorders do not have access to trauma-focused treatment due to a lack of trained therapists, geographic location, or inability to attend due to poverty and/or ongoing threats (Schauer, 2016).

Trauma-Memory Rehabilitation Is Not a Luxury, But the Foundation

It is essential and indispensable to accept that low-threshold and disseminable trauma-memory focused interventions for individuals and groups should be given the highest priority. And for this to happen, trauma-memory focused therapies need to be scalable, uncomplicated and robust.

Maslow's model of needs (Maslow, 1954) is often displayed as a pyramid, with the most basic needs that must be met in order to achieve well-being at the bottom: physiological, safety, belonging and love, esteem, and self-actualization. All these points are valid, but the hierarchy must be turned upside down to get it right: mental health must be given the highest priority, as we now know how much trauma corrupts all levels of development, emotions, and social life. It even prevents physiological health and a state of safety. Therefore, mental health and trauma rehabilitation through trauma-focused therapy must be considered at the base, the foundation for subsequent levels. The same applies to guidelines that suggest that specialized treatment for psychological problems should be offered only at the top of the intervention pyramid. It has become increasingly evident that not only a "small percentage of the population whose suffering ... is intolerable and who may have significant difficulties in basic daily functioning" (Inter-Agency Standing Committee [IASC], 2007). "In most large emergencies this group amounts to thousands of individuals" (IASC, 2007, p 13), after having been exposed to trauma, and, for all of these people, trauma plays a detrimental role in every aspect of their lives and aspirations.

A substantial portion of humans would profit from trauma-memory focused psychotherapy, be it on the individual level or as a community and group approach like the NETfacts health system.

The NETfacts Health System: NET as Part of a Combined Therapy for the Individual and the Community

Collective avoidance resulting from trauma leads to a fragmented collective memory of the community's past human rights violations, making a shared account of the group's history impossible. The lack of collective memory fosters ambiguous truths and fears, enabling a reactive construction of security based on selective information that leads to the endorsement of extreme opinions. Continued insecurity, violence, and crime can lead to increased anxiety and fear. The self-interest of perpetrators and the charged behavior of survivors escalate stigmatization and social exclusion, preventing or limiting coming to terms with the past, i.e., reducing tensions and protecting the construction of security. The exposure and recognition of traumatic facts that are subject to avoidance is key to a coherent collective memory and sense of community, and the prevention of further cycles of violence. The narrations obtained from NET may be used to inform the community at large about what has and is happening to many of their members. This process is the core of the NETfacts health system which addresses the structure of memory at both the individual and the collective levels (Robjant et al., 2021; Köbach et al., 2021). In this way, not only members but traumatized communities as a whole can be supported in their struggle to overcome the injuries of organized violence and marginalization and harmful group dynamics may be prevented.

NET as a Low Threshold Intervention

Trauma survivors suffering from trauma-spectrum disorders struggle with social and occupational functioning.

Oftentimes their capacity for healthy self-management and capability is jeopardized. Nevertheless, interpersonal respect should prohibit a mental health professional or a psychosocial helper from deciding when survivors are "qualified" to own their life story. Preventing people from working on their traumatic past with the putative intention to protect the individual follows a patronizing attitude. NET is built as a rather simple but straightforward procedure that does not require a so-called stabilization phase of preparation and learning, since the only competence a participant needs to bring in is the willingness to overcome avoidance and tell one's life-story.

Taking a closer look, biographical storytelling is quite a task, but most individuals starting from a preschool age are able to do it. It requires an episodic memory, linguistic abilities, the basic cognitive capacity for mental time travel, i.e. to imagine past events, the ability to change position from egocentric to allocentric perspective as well as to mentalize. Narrating one's own life to a skilled therapist and hearing it read back, is a straightforward and robust psychotherapy.

The pooled rate of dropout from RCTs of all different psychological therapies for PTSD is around 16–18% (Lewis et al., 2020; Imel et al., 2013). A review article shows that NET studies report no dropouts at all or significantly lower than other exposure approaches, at around ca. 2–6% (Jacob et al., 2017). The invitaton to tell the story of one's life seems to build on human nature to overcome the barrier of avoiding. We trust the basic right to inclusion and self-governance claiming that every person who wants to tell their story is perfectly suitable to have a voice. Neither are special self-regulation skills a must for admission nor any school education or the formal ability of reading or writing. In NET, the entire treatment takes place in the presence of a therapist who carefully assists and moderates uncomfortable or challenging moments. The NET therapist listens to the narration and ensures the safe (self-)management of strong arousal states, supporting the growing tolerance towards emotions and inner processes. This leads the narrator to authority over their own decisions towards a subjectively interpreted meaningful life and increased positive self-regard.

Many participants showing up for treatment live in unsafe conditions, use substances or are under psychoactive medication. Trauma treatments must take on these realities and nevertheless warrant safe offers. In NET, we strive to make minimal demands on the person in order to remove barriers for survivors to process their traumatic experiences (Neuner et al., 2002). Simply through focused listening and committed attention to the narrator's life story(s), therapists are a safe, guiding testimony bearer to unlock the resilience of survivors, even when faced with difficult and painful situations. Trauma therapy should be accessible, affordable, and inclusive, while also breaking down stereotypes.

Advocacy, Agency, and Testimony Through NET

For survivors of trauma the sense of control they feel in their life, the capacity to influence own thoughts and behavior, and their faith in the ability to handle a wide range of tasks and situations are key. A strong sense of agency helps to become psychologically stable, yet flexible in the face of conflict or change; an ability often missing in post- or continuous trauma situations. Maintaining and improving human rights situations requires understanding and acknowledging the destructive power of human rights violations they had to endure. Due to fragmented autobiographical representations, avoidance behaviors, and feelings of shame, as well as trauma-related feelings of helplessness and inferiority, victims of violence often have difficulties expressing themselves and talking about their experiences. So, bearing witness, allowing to testify and publicly outreach are key for a trauma treatment method. This speechlessness of trauma is a double-sided phenomenon, as the society and public are also ignorant regarding the stories of trauma survivors (Schauer, Neuner, & Elbert, 2011; Neuner et al., 2018; Robjant et al., 2020). However, to avoid causing harm or retraumatizing the survivor, testimony should ideally be protected by an evidence-based protocol within a psychotherapeutic framework (Wyles et al., 2023).

From this perspective, NET can provide comprehensible documentations of individual life stories that facilitate feelings of empathy for the victims. Information resulting from individual trauma-focused narrations also facilitates the assembling of a template pattern of a region's dynamics of violence. Feeding back information about cruelties of war and torture to the public may be used to counter ongoing human rights violations. The social recognition of the suffering on both the victim's and perpetrator's side as well as the discussion of their needs may allow the community to develop their own healing process, increase stability, and make taboo torture practices and other human rights violations. For the individuals, regaining access to their biography and communicating their history to others can empower them to stand up for their rights as survivors of violence which positively extends beyond the individual into relationships and communities (Cooper et al., 2019). NET therapists are in a dual role of being a helpful listener and testimony bearer at the same time (Schauer et al., 2005).

My function in this setting is that of a companion on the eerie journey of the testimony. As an interviewer, I am present as someone who actually participates in the reliving and reexperiencing of the event. I also become part of the struggle to go beyond the event and not be submerged and lost in it.

Dori Laub (1991, p. 76)

The ethical standing and work of NET is particularly based on the UN Universal Declaration of Human Rights. One of the main therapeutic agents of NET is regaining of the survivor's dignity and satisfaction of the need for acknowledgment as well as the explicit human rights orientation of testifying.

Activating Memory Associations – NET in a Nutshell

Emotional episodes are coded in memory as networks of mutually activating information units. According to Lang, when processing the network, activity in one unit is transmitted to adjacent units, and depending on the strength of activation, the entire structure may be engaged (Lang, 1977, 1993). Reactivating consolidated memories makes them sensitive to change (Nader et al., 2000). Experience with NET has led us to believe that survivors are not always able to assess the degree to which hot memories are problematic in their life, or even the content that is encapsulated in these hot memories, especially when the memories are recalled or reenacted outside the context of the whole life story. However, individuals may be able to identify these same elements when presented with the task of confronting the memories in the context of an autobiographical exploration. Dori Laub and his group at the Archive for Holocaust Testimonies at Yale University reported the following experience with a group of Holocaust survivors (D. Laub, personal communication, 2001). In 1979, a grassroots organization, the Holocaust Survivors Film Project, began videotaping Holocaust survivors and witnesses in New Haven, CT. In 1981, the original collection of testimonies was deposited at Yale University, and the Video Archive for Holocaust Testimonies opened its doors to the public the following year. Since then, the archive has worked to record, collect, and preserve Holocaust witness testimonies, and to make its collection available to researchers, educators, and the general public (https://www.library.yale.edu/testimonies/index.html).

When the first testimony began, everything fell into place, because the power of the testimony silenced all differences. Everyone in the room was transported to another time and place, a setting that had been waiting untouched and unchanged for many years behind locked doors. No one, including the witnesses themselves, knew beforehand what the testimonies would contain; experiences and reflections came out from recesses of memory that the witnesses did not even know they had.

Dori Laub (Fortunoff Video Archive
for Holocaust Testimonies at Yale University,
http://www.holocausttestimonies.com/mainframe.htm)

People with PTSD often fail to integrate traumatic experiences into the narrative of their lives. The survivor often cannot report the related experience in a consistent, chronological order, and thus this person has no explicit links among the various events, life experiences, and the context within which the events occurred. Survivors of continuous trauma often fail to possess their biography as a whole. Not only are the threats and lifetime periods of horror and suffering not accessible, but the other memories cease to exist alongside. By using NET, we are able to carefully step forward through the complete biography of a person's life in chronological order. In telling the story, the individual is exposed to the sensory information that accompanies the memory and to the image of the events themselves. As a prerequisite for the induction of emotional processing, memory traces are reactivated, and the whole fear structure gets engaged.

The individual actually engages in their own fear network by narrating the fragments (in chronological order) throughout the course of therapy, and they are able to reweave the events back into a *cool-system framework* controlling the triggers present with the hot memories. As a result, the accompanying anxiety, which evolved from the strangeness of dissociative fragments, is defused. All somatosensory percepts (physical sensations), cognitions (thoughts), and emotions relevant to the fear network as well as the body involved in the traumatic sequences of memory are comprehensively uncovered in detail as the narrative unfolds. The course of events is established (in time and place), labeled, and transferred into speech until a meaningful and consistent narrative is reached. All traumatic events are revisited until their negative, confusing, horrifying impact dissolves.

Note that the effectiveness of the Narrative Exposure procedure can be explained by the construction of an explicit, semantic representation of the events, coupled with a defragmentation of the fear/trauma network and the overcoming of imagined fear and helplessness. As pointed out by Kaminer (2006) in her literature review, three additional factors may also contribute: (1) emotional catharsis, (2) developing an explanation of the traumatic incidence, and (3) identification of the causes of, and responsibilities for, the horror.

Individuals with histories of adverse childhood events as well as later traumatic stresses suffer psychologically and physically, and they can transmit the consequences of trauma into their social realm. NET offers a comprehensive approach to reorganize and reclaim not only the survivors' trauma memories but also their entire biography through a conscious Narrative Exposure process. The key is to deeply understand the experience and both articulate the essence in clear and concise language and distill the meaning into understandable sentences. The NET procedure is conclusive in its conscious simplicity: The most straightforward form of psychotherapy involves narrating one's entire life as a series of stories to a trained therapist, who listens and sensitively probes at significant moments, taking notes to read the experience in first person and past tense back to the narrator. This narrative path is depicted as a timeline (*Lifeline*) with both *stones* (symbolizing traumas and suffering) and *flowers* (representing cherished individuals and memorable moments). The testimony that arises from the stories documents violations of children's and human rights, suitable for community and public outreach. Moreover, it enables the victims to regain their dignity as they are heard and seen, providing them with a voice (victims' voice). In a nutshell, it works, step-by-step, as follows:

After establishing rapport and therapeutic alliance, at first, a structured identification of the person's traumatic and adverse life events is carried out in which all traumatic experiences are queried with the help of a prestructured *checklist* (example given in the THL checklist, see Appendix 1): *Have you experienced an accident? Have you experienced a robbery? A natural disaster, sexual assault etc.* This procedure provides the informed awareness and a sense of mastery on the part of the survivorso they are able to get in contact with the trauma material and then proceed to disclosure in an informed and confident manner.

In the next session, the Lifeline then traces the development in an overview, priming memory associations and shedding a first light on causes and relations. Highly arousing, meaningful, and memorable experiences are sequentially labeled and symbolized on the individual's biographical timeline.

After having prepared the ground now for the important work to come, the process evolves without further ado into the survivor relating their formative life stories one after the other from early childhood onward. The empathic NET therapist makes notes about the testimony and then reads the narration back at the next meeting, supporting mentalization, self-acceptance, and regaining of dignity and satisfaction of the survivor's need for acknowledgment.

During the following Narrative Exposure sessions, the survivor talks about the specific biographic events in detail and embeds them in their life context. This has a twofold aim: giving time to explicitly revisit the perceptions, thoughts, emotions, bodily reactions, and interpretations moment by moment of past experiences helps the hot memories to reveal their deeper denotation and the root dynamic for being such disturbing, wounding, and traumatizing agents. At the same time, survivors previously left with horrifying fragments of the past are now able to reclaim their life narrative. Furthermore, when going into the details of a story and accompanying the younger self in all the exciting and special situations of the life lived, the narrator intensely allies with the self in meaningful and existential situations of great positive and negative affect. With the guiding and directive help of the therapist, a complete narration of the survivor's life is created, focusing on the detailed context of the traumatic experiences as well as on the important elements of the emotional networks and how they go together. This process allows the majority of trauma survivors to recognize that the fear structure results from past experiences and that its involuntary activation is a memory. Survivors thus lose the emotional response to the recollection of the highly arousing previously feared events, which consequently leads to a remission of PTSD symptoms. At the same time, narrators gain access to "lost" past memories and develop a sense of coherence, control, and integration.

Indeed, these factors are an integral part of NET. Experimental evidence, however, is limited regarding whether, in the sense of posttraumatic growth, the traumatic experiences will eventually be seen as the individual's own history of resistance, survival, and thus future resilience. Expressing a high level of affect is a misconceived catharsis and will not lead to clinical improvement if it is not related to cognitive processing (Pennebaker & Seagal, 1999). However, the first deliberate activation of essential parts of the fear network will necessarily produce strong feelings that become manifest in emotionally arousing expressions which then have to be labeled and integrated. Finally, we should note that the effectiveness of NET relies not only on the trauma focus, but also on the accompanying psychoeducation about the mental suffering, on the restructuring or sometimes even building of context and cold memory, on the *putting into words*, the linguistic representation of the whole narration, and on a subsequent new appraisal of shame, guilt, and the acknowledgment of the events by the therapist.

Key psychotherapeutic goals in NET

- Active chronological reconstruction of all important, meaningful, and arousing events of the autobiographical/episodic memory: *lifespan approach*.
- In-depth exploration of the emotional memory, i.e., the hot spots connecting hot and cold memory contents: *trauma-memory focus*.
- Linking and integrating psychophysiological, somatosensory, and emotional responses and memories to time, space, and context in biography.
- Meaning making, mentalizing, and allying with the younger self through revisiting and reprocessing both negative, fearful, and traumatic events, as well as important positive moments in life.
- Compassionate and respectful care within the therapeutic relationship, allowing for reparative attachment for survivors of (complex) trauma.
- Regaining of survivor's dignity and satisfaction of the need for acknowledgment. Explicit human rights orientation of testifying.
- Challenging the culture of secrecy surrounding trauma, victimization, perpetration, suppression, and social exclusion to enable healing and reconciliation of individuals and communities and breaking the (transgenerational) cycle of violence.

3 Therapeutic Approach of NET

Basic Procedure of NET

Within a limited number of 90- to 120-minute sessions, usually about 8–12, the survivor constructs a detailed and consistent narration of their biography in alliance with the therapist. The focus of NET is on completing and integrating memories of the traumatic events into a whole, including the sensory, cognitive, emotional and physiological, emotional, and experiences of the incident. The testimony is written down and, depending on the narrator's willingness, may be used for documentation purposes (e.g., human rights work or sharing the experience with the community through NETfacts). To be as simple as possible while meeting the specific needs of different groups of survivors, the NET protocol has evolved into the following standard.

The initial step is to hold a conversation with the survivor to ascertain their intentions for trauma therapy. The therapist then conducts a diagnostic assessment with the individual to discuss their past experiences using event checklists, followed by a structured interview about trauma reactions, general mental and physical health, previous treatments and use of medication, sociobiographic information, referral history, and current somatic and psychological complaints and symptoms, such as depression and suicidality. After the evaluation conversation, the survivor is given a psychoeducational introduction, explaining their trauma reactions and affirming the universality of human rights. This is followed by a preparatory introduction, and therapy begins with the participant's consent.

In NET, survivors do not have to arrange and evaluate their life experiences in a hierarchical way, as is done in other therapies for anxiety disorders to decide in what order the events should be processed. We all carry within us numerous associations with emotional memories. In particular, experiences of any particular stressful event are intertwined in associative networks of other traumatic memories, life events, and other hardships. Therefore, it is not advisable to list events in order of severity, or to focus on an *index trauma*.

Complex traumatic experiences, including severe stressors and negative events, may have been prolonged and repeated. Such events could involve the victim having been injured or abandoned by their caregivers during childhood or deliberately could have been inflicted through organized violence and torture to humiliate the victim or their loved ones (Courtois & Ford, 2009; Schauer et al., 2017). The same applies to individuals who have survived multiple traumatic events, including witnessing traumatic events. Asking survivors to rank experiences of organized violence or human rights violations such as rape, witnessing killing, surviving trafficking and torture, and others is considered unethical and inhumane by the NET approach. Because each of these horrific traumatic experiences is part of a complex fear network that can be triggered when cues within it are activated, it is important to provide a narrative of a survivor's complete life story and to work through positive and negative events in chronological-biographical order. In addition, traumatic experiences are not just about fear. They involve the whole dimension of experiencing, including basic and social emotions. In NET, it is not recommended to weigh events against each other, because experiences build on and get connected to each other. It is only after disclosure, only after having put the various experiences in words, that the survivor will be able to separate the stressors and understand the events and the deeper meaning of what has actually happened. NET emphasizes a life span approach, and the therapist is advised to work through and guide the narration of a person's life along the developmental timeline up to the present.

To illustrate, a typical narrative of a refugee experience encompasses a range of topics:

- Personal background and individual history prior to the first traumatic event
- Experiences from the beginning of the threat to the first terrifying event
- Terrifying events
- History of escape from or ending of violent conditions
- Life thereafter
- Plans, hopes, and fears concerning the future

The initial face-to-face interview can lay the groundwork and establish a good rapport between therapist and narrator before the first traumatic life event is addressed. It is important for the survivor and the therapist to communicate with each other in a trusting manner from the outset to ensure that the participant understands the expected process of recounting life events. The therapist assumes an empathic and accepting role. Inconsistencies in the narrator's report are gently pointed out and often resolved by raising in-depth awareness about recurring bodily sensations or thoughts. The survivor is encouraged to describe the traumatic events in as much detail as possible and to reveal the emotions and perceptions experienced at the moment of the retelling, as well as at the moment of the traumatic event. The speaker maintains full control of the narrative process. In case needed, a well-trained interviewer, knowledgeable about the procedures involved, translates piece by piece.

During each session, the therapist or an assistant takes notes and creates a script of the events. The story is then organized chronologically between sessions. In the subsequent session, this report is read back to the narrator. Then the next highly arousing event that have been marked on the lifline are processed – that is, additional traumatic experiences are added to the narrative report. The process is repeated across sessions until a final version of the survivor's complete biography is created.

If the survivor's literal understanding of the document and agreement with its contents is required, or if the document is needed in a legal proceeding or human rights work, it may be reread in its entirety at the final meeting. However, in the case of complex trauma (e.g., CSA over a longer period of time, or a repeated experience of torture), rereading many similar experiences in the final session is not advisable. In any event, a final Lifeline is laid out, which is now much more complete, as all (trauma) stories have been elicited, and it reveals the pride of accomplishment. The written testimony is then signed by the survivor, the therapist, the translator, and any other witness present. A survivor who expresses interest and comfort with it will receive a copy of the signed document. Another copy may be provided to human rights organizations with the survivor's consent or request to document these events. The document may be employed for advocacy purposes or published in a way so that the testifier will not be harmed.

Basic elements of NET

A. Construction of a consistent narrative of the participant's biography. The most important, emotionally charged, and meaningful events are explored in depth (Narrative Exposure), while other periods of life are treated in a more summarized fashion.
B. The therapist supports the narration, imaginal reliving, verbalization (affect labeling and naming of emotions), and emotional processing of significant events. The therapist is a listener, a witness, and a skilled and trained ally in the work of narrative biography, assisting in the creation of a chronological structure for the life story. The therapist adopts an empathic and accepting stance.
C. The therapist writes down the survivor's account. Subsequently, the previous sessions content is read back to the narrator, who is then asked to correct it and add missing details. The process is repeated across sessions until a comprehensive version of the survivor's biography is reached, encompassing all major traumatic experiences.
D. In the last session, the Lifeline procedure is performed again, and the survivor, the therapist, and any witnesses sign the written testimony.
E. The survivor maintains a record of their life story, serving as an eyewitness account that can act as documentary evidence of human rights violations or for legal proceedings.

NET Process Step by Step

NET proceeds in three essential steps: Step 1: intake checklist and face-to-face interview, Step 2: building the Lifeline, and Step 3: Narrative Exposure (see Figure 11). NET has been tested with varying lengths of treatment. The necessary number of narration sessions depends on various factors, such as the setting, the extent of the traumas experienced, the gravity of the trauma reactions, and the age of the survivors. Ideally, the number of NET exposure sessions should be determined early – for instance, after having completed both an *intake checklist* (Step 1) and the *Lifeline* (Step 2). An open-ended treatment period can lead to increased avoidance, as both participant and therapist inevitably avoid discussing the most difficult situations, prolonging recovery and pain indefinitely.

Many survivors also suffer from comorbid, frequently also trauma-related disorders (e.g., mood disorders, personality disorders, substance abuse). If, for associated disorders, extended treatment that includes other

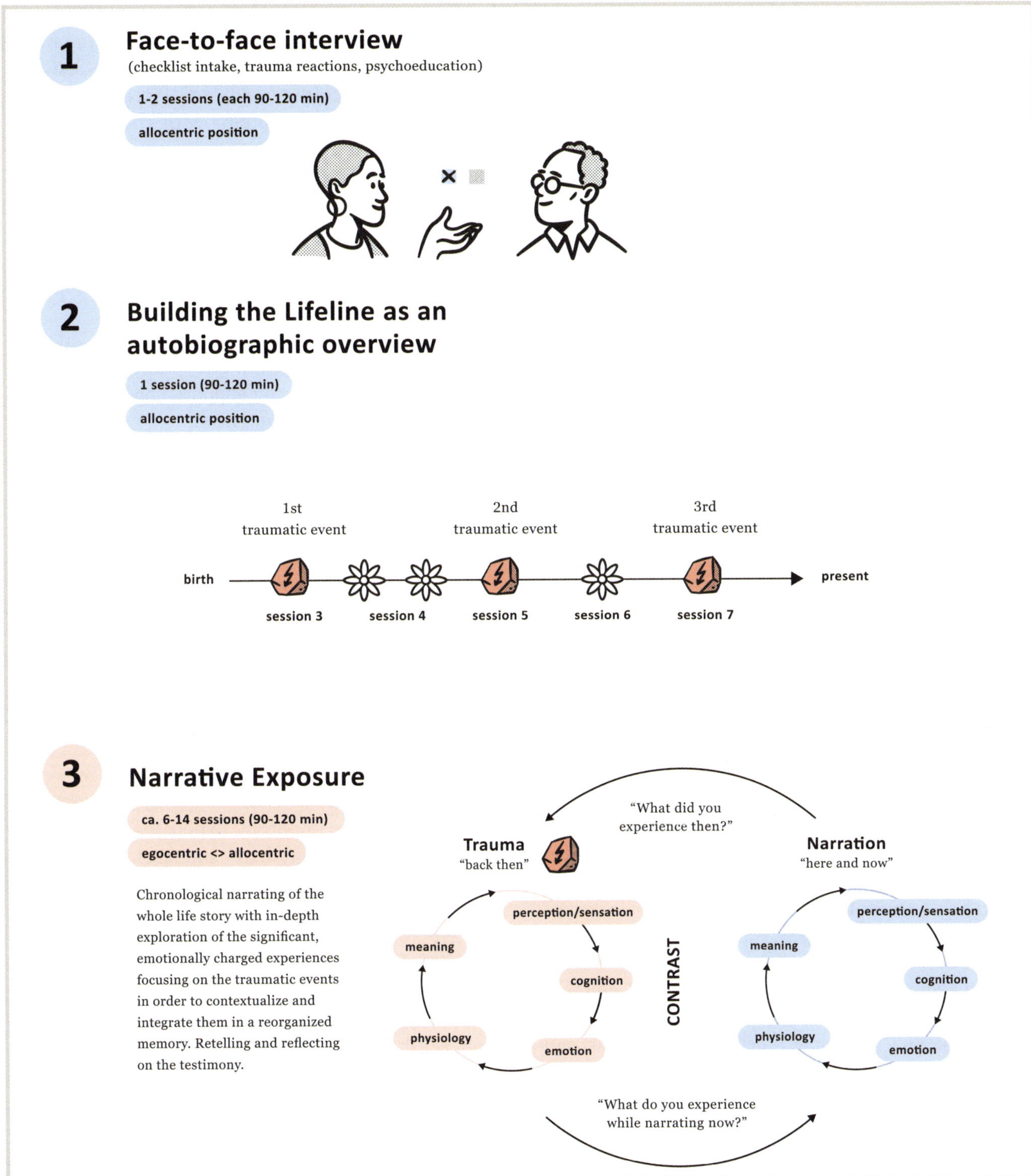

Figure 11. Illustration of the Narrative Exposure Therapy (NET) process step-by-step. NET always begins with a face-to-face personal interview between the survivor and the therapist to carefully assess life events using checklists (1), followed by an interview about trauma reactions and a thorough psychoeducation about the findings and the suggested procedure of NET. In another session, the arousing and meaningful specific events from birth to present are symbolized in their valence on the biographical timeline (2) Lifeline. The survivor is then encouraged to share their life story, focusing on the adverse and emotionally charged experiences, which are explored in depth using Narrative Exposure, (3) and those are each reviewed in the subsequent session. Also available as a handout in the online supplementary materials for this book.

specialized interventions is necessary, we recommend starting with the NET as a biographic work clarifying the developmental pathway and resolving the trauma memory problems. An exception may be detox for serious drug abuse (Hinsberger et al., 2017), which should precede the NET.

Step 1: Event Intake Checklist, Structured Assessment of Trauma Reactions, and Psychoeducation

Since trauma survivors fear a loss of control or abandonment and expect an unpredictable response, the therapeutic alliance in NET starts with a face-to-face empathic and structured conversation with the therapist who will conduct the treatment. It is advisable that the same therapist remains involved after Step 1. The initial interview (Step 1) is highly structured and predictable, including an event checklist and one checklist of adverse childhood experiences, to allow a sense of achievement. A concise psychoeducation and step-by-step explanation of the therapeutic procedure are utilized to normalize, legitimize, and articulate trauma reactions, as well as address fears, resistance, and concerns about the treatment protocol and exposure work.

When introducing the initial assessment to the participant, it is stated clearly that here is a set of questions that will cover issues common among survivors of traumatic stressors. The importance of this step is emphasized as an approach to obtaining a more comprehensive understanding of their past and current experiences. The structured interview is explained and will help establish a safe and comfortable environment for the participant while identifying whether or not the survivor meets criteria for NET. A structured interview is a critical first step in overcoming avoidance and facilitating disclosure. Thus, the intake checklist is a mandatory first step in NET treatment. Because this present manual is concerned with the treatment of trauma sequelae and related disorders rather than with the diagnosis of PTSD or CPTSD, we will not go into the details of a diagnostic interview. Note that trauma spectrum disorders seen in an integrative transdiagnostic approach include a range of mental health problems: PTSD, CPTSD, trauma-related symptoms of personality disorders, trauma-related forms of depression, trauma-related suicidality, trauma-related anxiety disorders/phobias/panic attacks, trauma-related obsessive-compulsive disorder, traumatic grief, trauma-related developmental problems, ADHD, trauma-triggered psychosis, trauma-related drug addiction, trauma-related somatic illnesses (e.g., autoimmune diseases, cancer, diabetes, cardiovascular diseases, gastrointestinal diseases, etc.), problems with social behavior, emotional problems, etc.

Practical Points

- Provide psychoeducation (acknowledgment of fear, avoidance as a hindrance that drives pathology and commitment to honesty).
- Reassure regarding confidentiality, safety, and trustworthiness of the interview environment.
- The interviewer will offer support, contain emotions, but not terminate the interview.
- Offer drinking water, juice, or tea, but avoid longer breaks during the assessment.
- Encourage the participant to ask questions and freely communicate any distress.
- The interviewer maintains objectivity and recognizes the survivor's honest reporting efforts.
- The interviewer adheres to a structured approach, asking questions as presented in the questionnaire.

Other topics must be addressed before beginning. It is possible that more memories may emerge during the process, and this is to be encouraged.

Avoidance may become apparent, and it is important to discuss all events and details, for any treatment to be successful. It is also important to note that the effects of treatment may appear gradually and that healing of long-standing injuries requires time. However, especially in the long run, NET has demonstrated significant clinical effectiveness, alleviating various symptoms and enhancing daily functioning.

It may be helpful to establish additional therapeutic bonds or agreements, particularly regarding suicidal ideation, self-harming behavior, and substance abuse. Implement safeguarding procedures and obtain informed consent to protect the individual's rights.

Note: It is acceptable for the participant to harbor ambivalent feelings, such as fear of discussing difficult experiences or doubt about the likelihood of success. However, at some point, a clear commitment to the therapeutic process is necessary, with an affirmative statement such as: "Yes, I want to work on this with your guidance." For children, this commitment must also come from their caregiver (see the section KIDNET: Narrative Exposure Therapy for Children and Adolescents).

Face-to-Face Assessment

The NET procedure is initiated in one to two sessions by the therapist in the following manner: The therapist introduces themselves by stating their name and profession.

They then provide an explanation of their interests, outlining the purpose of the ongoing project or mission. Finally, the therapist explains their ethical stance to establish a foundation for the therapeutic relationship.

The participant has a right to know who the therapist is and understand their motivation and professional background. This initial phase and the way the therapist presents themself and their work, is already a crucial trust-building step between the two of them. Before beginning the interview, make certain the individual understands the necessity of answering all questions. Ensure that the participant knows that only some of the items on the checklists may apply. Lastly, reassure the individual regarding confidentiality.

> **Example of a therapist's introduction**
>
> My name is ... I am a psychologist (nurse, psychiatrist, social worker) from the organization (clinic, organization, university, school). I am here to assist people who have experienced extremely stressful conditions such as war (rape, forced migration, torture, massacre, accidents) and to document the human rights violations that have taken place. I usually work at (in) a (treatment center, hospital) with survivors of violence (refugees) from various countries. We hope to use what we learn from you to improve the way survivors of violence are supported and respected in the future.

Traumatic Events

Trauma material must always be approached in a controlled and structured manner. It is unethical to invite trauma storytelling without providing a safe framework for containment and control. In order to understand trauma reactions and relate them to past experiences, it is important to learn about the individual's trauma history, also to comprehend the causal relationship between past experiences and present symptoms. Event checklists, such as the Life Event Checklist (LEC-5; Weathers et al., 2013) are a great help for exploring a potentially traumatizing past as types of trauma (Weathers, Blake, et al., 2013). This allows recognition of the trauma history and to foresee which events might appear in the narrations.

Adverse Childhood Experiences

The trauma event checklist is always followed by an interview about experiences of *interpersonal violence and neglect during childhood*, including physical, sexual, and emotional abuse, as well as emotional and physical neglect, using a scale like the Maltreatment and Abuse Chronology of Exposure (MACE): Scale for the Retrospective Assessment of Abuse and Neglect During Development (Teicher & Parigger, 2015; German version: Isele et al., 2014, Norwegian version: Fosse et al., 2020; brief-20-items version: Thekkumthala et al., 2023). Such a checklist asks about key areas of interpersonal trauma during childhood, such as the exposure to emotional and physical abuse by adults or parents residing in the household, emotional and physical abuse by siblings or children living in the household, emotional and physical neglect, witnessing violence among adults or parents residing in the household, witnessing violence against siblings or children living in the household, peer abuse (emotional and physical), sexual violence, and loss of parents.

> **Importance of trauma checklists**
>
> - Addressing traumatic experiences in a structured and controlled manner through contextualization
> - Using checklist as an initial step toward exploring trauma material and overcoming avoidance
> - Recording various forms of violence and neglect
> - Identifying memory traces
> - Establishing an optimal foundation for future therapeutic processing
> - Normalizing and destigmatizing the discussion of traumatic experiences

Trauma Reactions

For trauma reactions, several symptom scales are applicable, valid, and well-researched, such as the PTSD Checklist for DSM (PCL-5; Weathers et al., 2013; Blevins et al., 2015); International Trauma Questionnaire, according to the ICD-11 (ITQ; Cloitre et al., 2018); and, for children and adolescents, the Posttraumatic Stress Interview for Children (KID-PIN; Ibrahim et al., 2021) or the Child and Adolescent Trauma Screen (CATS; Sachser et al., 2017). Furthermore, available in many different languages, the Refugee Health Screener (RHS; Hollifield et al., 2013) is an excellent screening instrument (Kaltenbach et al., 2017) that can be useful for screening even larger populations and not only refugees.

Dissociative Subtype

Especially for developmental trauma we suggest the inclusion of a dissociation scale, such as the Shutdown Dissociation Scale (Shut-D; Schalinski, Schauer, & Elbert, 2015, 2016, freely available at https://doi.org/10.23668/psycharchives.4596) in the NET Checklists. It is advantageous if the dissociation scale used can discriminate between trauma reactions resembling PTSD, which are characterized by sympathetic arousal, vigilance, and sensory trauma reliving (e.g., visual intrusions and nightmares), and more complicated trauma types, which typically involve more repressed trauma material, severe derealization and detachment (i.e., flag and faint), and intense tensions and inexplicable fears.

Depending on the participants, possible additional checklists may include: questionnaires covering experiences of detention and torture, organized violence or forced migration, experiences as combatants (veterans, [child] soldiers), experiences of trafficking and slavery, etc, or active involvement in aggressive behavior (e.g., Appetitive Aggression Questionnaire (AAS; Weierstall & Elbert, 2011), or scales covering stress and adversity in pregnant women (e.g., KINDEX Prenatal Psychosocial Risk Questionnaire (Ruf-Leuschner et al., 2016), and other assessments as appropriate. Additional checklists for survivors of war, among others, are: War and Adversity Exposure Checklist (WAEC; Ibrahim et al., 2018) and, for victims of interpersonal violence, the Gendered Violence in Partnerships Scale (GVPS; Goessmann et al., 2021).

Psychoeducation After the Assessment

Following the diagnostic assessment, the respondent will be likely to be interested in receiving the results and knowing what will follow. Therefore, immediately providing explanation and psychoeducation is often recommended after the assessment. In NET, psychoeducation after the intake checklists is not a lengthy process. It is just the logical conclusion of the assessment and may take no longer than half an hour. However, elements of psychoeducation were provided before the interview (refer to the previous section Face-to-Face Assessment) and will continue to be offered as need arises throughout the entire NET.

Initial education for the participant includes explaining the condition in understandable terms, emphasizing the connection between adverse experiences or traumatic events and the subsequent symptoms. Survivors must be informed that trauma symptoms are a regular reaction to severe and damaging experiences, such as neglect and rejection during childhood, and verbal, sexual, and physical violence. These experiences affect not only the physical body but also the mind and spirit. Most individuals experiencing symptoms of the trauma spectrum find comfort in the knowledge that their condition has a well-defined conceptualization, thereby alleviating their fears of losing their sanity, and instilling hope that these emotional traumas can be overcome, albeit with possible remnant effects.

Continuing with the psychoeducational component, it is important to objectively explain to the survivor that the symptoms experienced may result from a trauma memory disturbance, and may lead to continued suffering. It is crucial to maintain a clear and concise structural progression when discussing this matter. The person should be informed that memories of the trauma may intrusively occur in the form of visual images, single sensory perceptions, or more complex internal states, affecting both the mind and body. Explain that intrusions resulting from unresolved trauma keep individuals in a vigilant state. Therapists and trauma coaches should make sure to personalize the psychoeducation and focus on the symptoms and problems the person is experiencing.

Psychoeducation points for after the structured assessment

- Normalization: After experiencing a trauma, it is common to have reactions that may be challenging to manage.
- Legitimization: Trauma responses stem from a source and arise as a result of reacting to adverse and painful occurrences.
- Description of trauma reactions: Common symptoms experienced after a traumatic event include avoidance behaviors, intrusive thoughts or memories, nightmares, hyperarousal, and emotional numbness, as well as changes in personality and mood.
- Explanation of therapeutic procedure.
- Education: Brief education presentations will be provided throughout the NET procedure.

Always adapt the language to the individual's context, to their level of formal education, culture, identity, age, etc. The therapist may want to use a simpler, an academic, or a technical style of psychoeducational language to ensure that the participant is well-informed about the origins of their symptoms as a response to the traumatic stress, and what can be done about them.

The following are examples of psychoeducational text that may be helpful to the participant:

Psychoeducational Example of Normalization

Distress is a common response following a traumatic experience; when that distress response frequently reappears later in life, it is known as posttraumatic stress disorder. Humans have evolved to ensure their survival, which causes increased perception and storage of threatening information. Currently, your body is in a state of heightened awareness, constantly on the lookout for potential danger. The best response for our vulnerable species is to be overly cautious and hypervigilant. However, using this specific method for staying alive, is costly in terms of health; it can be painful and extremely difficult, as you know. It's no longer necessary to be on guard, since the previous danger is over. It lies in the past.

Psychoeducational Example of Legitimization

The problems you are experiencing have a well-known cause. The cause can be clearly traced to the events that have happened in your life. In a life-threatening situation, people become highly aroused (not sleeping), danger-focused (not concentrating on other things), and numb (not feeling any pain in your body). During the traumatic life events, your body and mind were in a state of alert (e.g., sweating, heart pounding, rapid breathing). This is a common state – that is, remaining on the lookout after a traumatic event. [Use the survivor's specific symptoms to explain.]

Psychoeducational Example of Explaining the Symptoms – Intrusions, Hyperarousal, Avoidance, and Personality Changes

No matter how hard survivors attempt to evade them, memories persistently resurface. They infiltrate daily life, disrupting their nights and days. Abruptly, you may feel anxious, uneasy, or disconnected from reality with no apparent cause. This is because during a deeply scary experience, your organism is so aroused that your mind fails to process where and when the threat appeared. Not knowing when a danger will appear is more than one can bear. You'll become overwhelmed by repeated physical alarm and an undefinable dark fear. Experiencing the reoccurrence of emotions, images, and physical sensations suggests an attempt to process a traumatic event later and warn you. This process is crucial to understand, as it may impact one's life over the long term. Subsequently, these unresolved issues resurface repeatedly into consciousness. During therapy, it is important to explore these attempts to suppress feelings, and grant them space for examination and understanding. However, due to the inherently distressing nature of these issues, individuals tend to avoid confronting them. We will work collaboratively to investigate these fragments and offer your mind an opportunity to comprehend and incorporate them into your memories.

During the course of psychoeducation, the therapist may want to validate the individual's resources. Make this part brief but personal. Only mention positive things you truly believe in. Do not exaggerate. The survivor might be struggling with survivor guilt as well as over acts of commission or omission. And belaboring this could exacerbate the negative feelings. They are to be factual, do not minimize problems or difficult feeling. Problems are what they are at that point. It is important to bear witness and to accurately articulate the situation without exaggeration, downplaying, or apprehension, and it is crucial to maintain transparency. Trauma survivors are capable of sensing whether or not a person can empathize with their emotions and comprehend their experiences. The therapist must not judge or evaluate the particular reactions or the behaviors that led to survival. However, hindsight bias – that is, the tendency to perceive past events as having been more predictable than they actually were, given additional information available only after the trauma – can be mentioned in the psychoeducation. Hindsight bias may cause distortions of memories of what was known or believed before an event occurred; a narration may correct this problem and readjust the guilt feelings.

Participants must have a clear understanding of the process and have provided voluntary agreement to participate. They should be informed of their expected role in the NET process and should not be left with any questions about the techniques or therapeutic activities utilized.

Many people are inexperienced with psychotherapy or have never heard of it. Yet most cultures recognize the concept of a healer, elder, or counselor. Some traumatized participants in the NET process attend therapy sessions at first primarily to obtain, for instance, a written testimony that they can use for human rights work, political education, and outreach; for their asylum application; or to file a lawsuit. An autobiographical account that includes all aspects of personal experience, such as how one perceives, thinks, and feels bodily sensations, and that summarizes meaning, is highly credible and appealing to judges.

It is critical to convey that the person's involvement and awareness are essential to the process. Survivors need to know that their participation is active, not passive; therapists do not just do things to them. It is important to clarify that the process of exposure therapy can be distressing at times – a circumstance that the survivor has thus far avoided. Psychoeducation should address why the survivor is seeking treatment, how talking about the traumatic event can help them overcome their suffering, and why testifying is an important step in healing.

The following is an example of psychoeducational text that may be helpful to the participant:

Psychoeducational Example of Explaining the Interaction of Avoidance, Exposure, and Testimony

This traumatic experience you had has caused lasting emotional harm that cannot fully heal. Like an infected wound, every time you revisit this past experience, it causes pain. You have learned that distancing yourself from these memories of the past and not touching them seems, in the short-run, to be the better approach. Ultimately though, cleaning and disinfecting the wound provides an opportunity for healing. The recommended approach involves confronting the memories of the traumatic times by telling stories about past events. By sensitively framing these hot, painful memories as part of your personal story, the pain will eventually subside.

I know that you have made great efforts to eliminate these emotions. They have been tormenting and consuming you. However, we no longer wish for them to continue to control you. Together, we will understand these emotions. It is possible that up until now, you have felt imprisoned by them. This is often exactly what the perpetrators wanted. Together, we'll refuse to let this continue. We will take action. If you can recall those thoughts, emotions, and bodily sensations you experienced during the incident and put them into words, those distressing emotional reactions will eventually diminish. They will lose their hold and the effect they currently have on you. They will cease to exist. It may be difficult to conceive, but I can assist you in achieving this, just as I have helped others before you.

What has happened to you is a violation of Human Rights. No one has the authority to violate or harm you (no one has the right to harm children). By testifying about your experiences, we hope to provide an opportunity for you to seek justice through the documentation of what you witnessed and endured. Testimonies such as this have the ability to counteract forgetfulness, ignorance, and denial. This report will be provided in written form and can potentially be utilized for documentary and human rights purposes, subject to your consent and approval. However, if desired, we will maintain complete confidentiality regarding your account of suffering.

The unprocessed material necessitates conscious reworking, which is facilitated during therapy. This can be achieved when survivors narrate their life stories in chronological order. Once survivors have comprehended their experiences and integrated them into their personal history, their symptoms will decrease, and they will be able to make sense of their experiences.

Psychoeducational Example of Explaining the Narration Procedure

Our aim is to facilitate the construction of a detailed, comprehensive, and meaningful narrative of the traumatic events in your life by sharing your story. Our objective is to reintegrate your recounted experiences into your and your community's history. We strive to provide a complete testimony by assigning time and space to the threatening experiences. When you recount the events and realize where feelings of impending threat belong to, your negative emotions subside, the pain lessens, and the fear abates. We have found that a comprehensive narrative aids in symptom management. Your account will follow your life's timeline and proceed chronologically, step-by-step, as the events occurred. After each session, we will review and revise the text as needed until we arrive at a final version within 10–12 sessions. Each session will be completed within 90–120 minutes, and we will take the time at the end of each session to ensure your satisfaction with our progress.

It is honest to maintain transparency and acknowledge that when remembering a traumatic event during storytelling, it is normal to feel emotions similar to those experienced in the past – that is, fear, anger, pain, etc. The severity of the reaction to the traumatic incident can only be determined after memory retrieval, which may yield unexpected outcomes. Uncovering connections in the trauma network and identifying key elements involved in the associative network are critical aspects of the therapeutic work. Participants can rest assured that any concerns that arise during the session will be addressed until they feel comfortable once more. It should be clarified that thinking about the session's details may carry on after it ends. Individuals should keep in mind that the therapist is available if they confront challenging emotions during the session. Make certain that the survivor is aware that the therapist will stay connected during the entire healing process. There is no homework or exercises to be done alone by the participant. During future sessions, it is important for the therapist to inquire about the narrator's experiences between sessions, and address and resolve any related issues. Engaging in the healing process together is a hopeful journey that may, however, encounter setbacks and moments of crisis or stagnancy. Such instances may offer valuable insights into the individual's biography.

As previously stated, trauma treatment can impact someone's personal and professional life, as well as that of their partners, children, family, and social connections. Survivors who advocate for their rights may feel compelled to express themselves more openly. They prioritize their own requirements and refuse to tolerate mistreatment within their relationships. Some may even desire to change their way of life. During their treatment, survivors require a welcoming, empathic, and compassionate atmosphere. During some sessions, the participant may require a particularly supportive social network.

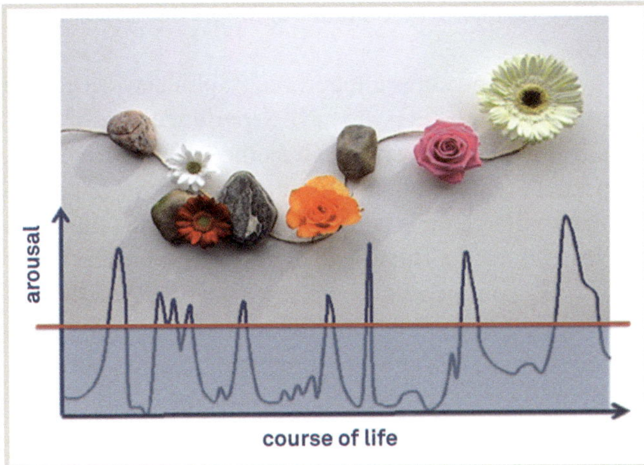

Figure 12. The Lifeline work: what, when, and where for important, arousing, and upsetting moments in a life. Just as the peaks of a mountain range are particularly prominent, emotional *peaks of meaning* are identified from the stream of life – they get named and represented when the Lifeline is laid out (Elbert et al., 2015, 2022; Schauer & Ruf-Leuschner, 2014). The horizontal axis (x-axis) displays the biographical timeline, and the vertical axis (y-axis) represents physiological arousal. This image is for illustration purposes only. It is not intended to be used with a NET client.

Step 2: Building the Lifeline as an Autobiographical Review

The past is never dead. It's not even past.
William Faulkner

In a 90-minute session after the initial interview in Step 1, a timeline called *Lifeline* will be established to represent the person's life and development from birth to the present.

Explaining the Lifeline – Flowers and Stones

The therapist will aid in categorizing particular life events within relevant lifetime periods along a time axis (spatiotemporal integration into the individual developmental context) – that is, "when, where, what", whereby the last of these just refers to a label for the event (Figure 12 and Figure 13). Understanding where events of strong emotional significance occurred can be a reparative experience for children, adolescents, and adults who have suffered trauma and have difficulty recollecting personal memories (Schauer & Ruf-Leuschner, 2014; Schauer et al., 2014, Schauer et al., 2017).

As a side note: NET typically has three parts: an initial face-to-face interview (event checklist, trauma reactions, and psychoeducation) + Lifeline + Narrative Exposure. Although most NET users include the Lifeline work as an intermediate step between interviewing and narration, it should be noted that there is some evidence showing that NET can be effective without it (Neuner, Schauer,

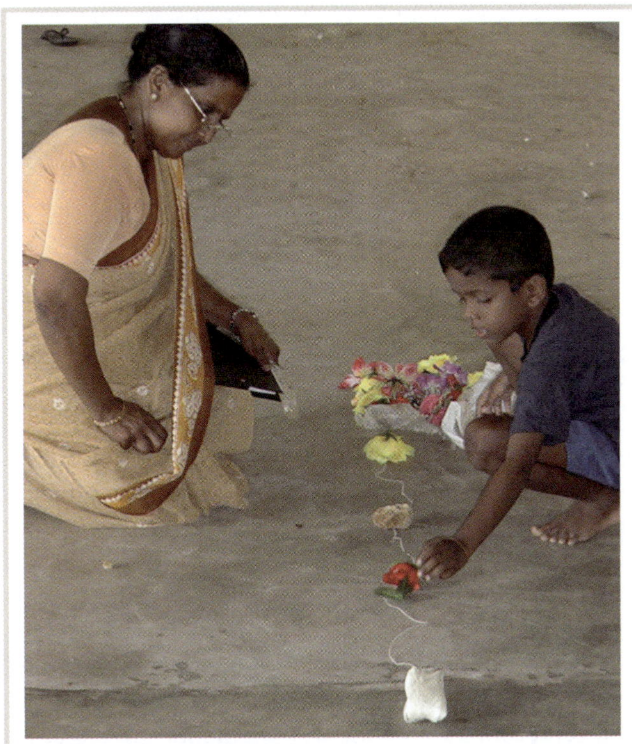

Figure 13. For both children and adult survivors, the laying out of the Lifeline can be essential to understanding the chronology of life events and how they relate – often for the first time (photo by the author Frank Neuner).

Klaschik, et al., 2004; Schauer et al., 2006; Hijazi et al., 2014).

Thorough and coherent autobiographical work can be of great benefit to kids who have experienced life-changing and disruptive events such as the loss of caregivers, adoption or foster care, life-threatening illness, or migration into exile, but it is equally helpful for adult survivors and as well for the therapists to understand more about how things connect. Lifeline work uses methods to start representing and expressing the influential events in an individual's life journey, the shaping of their personality, their core beliefs and underlying schemas, and the acknowledgment of emotionally significant events. Searching for traces of one's own history allows NET to reconstruct biographical contexts. For this purpose, the therapist, who accompanies the process sensitively and with clear verbalization, offers materials that can represent positive (e.g., flowers) and negative (e.g., stones) valence.

The Lifeline has become a widely known symbol for NET, because it symbolically represents a person's life story Survivors lay out their life's emotional journey along a cord or string that symbolizes the continuous flow of time. They place *flowers* for arousing resources in life, major happy events, and good times – for example, positive, empowering events, important people and loved ones, moments of achievement, experiences of bliss and acceptance, important pet friends, and so on. Flowers – that is, emotions of positive valence diminish perceived threat, and enhance assimilation of new information in memory. In this way, flowers facilitate and ease the response to exposure therapy.

Stones are placed to symbolize fearful and especially traumatic events such as life-threatening experiences, acts of violence, abuse, combat experiences, rape, assault, injury or harm, imprisonment, natural disasters, accidents, etc. Survivors usually also place stones for sad or difficult moments in life, such as the loss of a loved one or times of hardship (divorce, loss of a job), suffering, failure, and other stressful, unpleasant, and negative experiences that they have had to endure. Any event that caused high emotional arousal needs to find its place on the Lifeline.

Ideally, a timeline should be created by laying a cord or string on the floor or ground in order to serve as a visual representation of the developmental timeline, including all meaningful events of an individual. Symbols representing significant events are placed chronologically along the timeline. If necessary, a paper-and-pencil version can be utilized if materials are unavailable or for those with physical disabilities. The Lifeline can be drawn on a larger sheet of paper. Any flowers available can serve, either fresh ones or plastic or woven artificial ones, in various colors, shapes, and sizes. Collect stones from roadsides, mountains, or riverbeds in different textures, shapes, and sizes. Different stones and flowers are ideally offered to choose from, encompassing large and small varieties, to represent events in various ways. This allows for options such as big or small, sharp or round stones. (The therapist does not bring their holiday collection of stones and symbols with them. Rather, the material is ideally acquired from a neutral source for both the therapist and the participant.)

Creating the Lifeline is a structuring activity. The therapist helps the activity to stay as much as possible on the *cold memory* side. During Lifeline sessions, we do not engage in storytelling or in-depth immersion in events or difficult memories. We do not get caught up in detailed narration of specific events or vivid memories. The Lifeline is a rather calm activity, not at all highly emotionally charged. The focus must be on obtaining an overview of the individual's biography. The respective events are briefly named during the placement. The therapist accompanies the process empathically and briefly summarizes each event and notes it down – for example, on a sticky note: age (e.g., about 8 years), place (e.g., Milan), heading of the event (e.g., severe car accident where my mum died and my brother was seriously injured), (emotional) name of the symbol (e.g., "my world breaks"). Verbalizations help to build up contextual information: answering questions such as "At what time, or during which lifetime period was that?" "Where about, or what location?" "How would you call or label this experience? Give just a brief title for today! We will talk about it in more detail in a later session." Staying on the cold, factual side of memory does not mean that the therapist is emotionally cold. By no means will the therapist ignore the feelings of the survivor. We validate and help put into words the reactions a survivor may have in remembering their life events. The therapist helps to understand the "present" reaction in retrospect, but does not delve into the "past" emotions.

The therapist emphasizes factual information and assists with verbalizing with precise word choices. This largely helps to keep emotions and physiological arousal in check. It is important to clearly contrast the space and time when a trauma has happened from the present, the here and now. As an example, the therapist may say, "I understand that, as you reflect on your life today from London, UK, you experience sadness recollecting a painful event that took place close to Tel Aviv in 2013, when you were 20 years old."

Lifeline guidelines

1. The Lifeline intervention is done from an allocentric (an observer's) perspective. Feelings of the survivor in the room can be acknowledged, but we are not going to the past feelings or bodily reactions yet.
2. The identification of specific events for the construction of the Lifeline depends on three key characteristics: the dimensions of biographical time (when and where), valence (negative or positive), and arousal (emotional importance)!
3. Important: The Lifeline work must not exceed a single session of about 90–120 minutes.

Loss and Aggressive Acting: Additional Symbols

Stones can symbolize loss and trauma. However, *fear stones* have a different psychological dynamic and meaning than *grief stones*. For events of loss, some survivors place just a stone on their Lifeline. Others choose a small candle that can be lit, as an appropriate representation. Still others combine both, a candle with a stone or choose to place a flower in memory of a loved one who has died. These are individual and creative decisions to be made on a case-by-case basis. Some survivors appreciate the possibility of the therapist keeping the symbol (on a shelf) at the end of the Lifeline session, and later in the therapy, when the narrative reaches the time of the death of that deceased person, the candle (or flower) can be taken off the shelf and be present during the session. The candle could be lit by the survivor and kept burning throughout the session as they tell their story, and then taken home.

For survivors who have been involved in combat, fighting, or other forms of interpersonal violence, the Lifeline overview needs a *neutral symbol*. This should be neutral in terms of emotional valence, because the specific events of active involvement in acts of violence, perpetration, aggression, and delinquency can be perceived as a negative (e.g., being defeated) or as a positive (e.g., being a hero, enjoying a fight) experience and therefore should not be judged or morally examined before there is a complete narrative. Although, sticks are a symbol of active involvement of violence they can be offered as *neutral* symbols that mark the events of active participation (including fights, combat, sexual violence...), but do not require immediate attribution of positive or negative valence.Ideally, this symbol is also available as a variety of small or heavy, long or short sticks, or natural branches, to be chosen, to indicate the severity of an event.

Finding Flowers

Most of the stones in a survivor's biography were probably already identified during the intake checklist. But in contrast to the stones, the flowers cannot be uncovered with the help of a checklist. This undertaking could all too quickly become counterproductive, as the respondent might have to say no to too many positive items, and then be downhearted at the end of such a list, having found they have experienced so few positive life events. This would likely promote depressed thinking and feeling, which is already a common symptom of chronic trauma.

However, through the work of the Lifeline, we are able to discover those flowers, in addition to the stones. There are trauma survivors who cannot view their live as a positive journey. They find everything rocky, dark, and heavy. This may be fostered by depression, but it may also be a way of telling the therapist at the outset how bad things have been for them. Therapists accept this statement and summarize what they have understood, they recognize that, e.g., persistent injustice and violence have happened to the person. At the same time, the survivor is here today to tell their life story, which can show that there is some positive expectation or hope.

Flowers often hide behind stones – that is, in the time after the traumatic event(s), when it is very difficult to make it through each day and to adapt to a changed life (involving wounds, integrity violated, loved ones lost, recurring trauma symptoms, etc.). So, we can ask, how did the survivor cope with such difficult periods of life (often repeatedly)? Was it their inner strength? A neighbor who called every day? A beloved pet? Positive spirituality? ...

In this way, we can still keep an eye out for flowers during the Lifeline and later during the storytelling and ask about positive moments, people, and experiences. The following (incomplete) compilation is therefore only meant as an inspiration regarding in which areas of life flowers can be found.

Some *flower* suggestions (in random order)

- Survival moments (gratefulness)
- Loved ones
- Positive experiences with attachment figures and adults: parents, grandparents, teachers, adult family friends, and/or neighbors etc.
- Institutions (such as school, boarding school, university, convent, vocational training, etc.) that gave structure and safety

- Firsts: child-age first times such as riding a bike; teen-age first times such as first romantic kiss; first love, etc.
- Birth or adoption of siblings, own children
- Confirmation, holy communion, youth consecration, baptism, nikah, bar/bat mitzvah
- Transitions to desired independence etc. or desired belonging, initiations like leaving home for college, falling in love, marrying, children becoming independent
- Achievements in areas such as school, education, training, sports, arts; achieving a status, playing a role, outstanding performance
- Finding comfort in knowing, or having done something
- Felt blessings
- Moments of (falling in) love and connectedness
- Events that made one grow / that made one realize one's own strength
- Gain of health for self or important others
- Personal attributes that helped one overcome a stone
- Discovering interests and own gifts, talents, and abilities
- Travel experiences
- Instances of perceived support and/or people who offered that support
- Wonderful moments in nature or a nature event
- ...

Sometimes flowers seem to be mixed with stones. In cases of ambivalence, we carefully look at the chronology of things. Here are some examples:

First it was a shock when I learned that my father was not my biological father (stone), but after a few weeks I realized that I had the most loving parents who raised me (flower).

At first, receiving the job offer (flower) felt like a dream come true. However, after a year, I learned through an embarrassing incident at a public event that this profession is not my area of expertise (stone). Nevertheless, this experience allowed me to explore other opportunities and discover a genuine passion for creative artwork (flower).

I had a challenging delivery with my daughter. It was hard to connect emotionally in the aftermath (stone), but I was fortunate that the baby was healthy. After being released from the hospital, we were able to develop a beautiful bond (flower).

Biographical Overview in Action: Hands-on Doing the Lifeline

The Lifeline process is started by a short explanation of the meaning of the "line" as a timeline, as well an introduction to the symbols (Schauer & Ruf-Leuschner, 2014; Schauer et al., 2017).

The survivor is encouraged to take a string or cord in their hand and lay it on the floor (sometimes on a table). The line can be straight or curved, depending on the twists and turns of their life's course and the changing periods and stages of life. Adjustments can be made as the process evolves. But always offer a string long enough. When the line is put on the floor, the therapist encourages the participant to start placing the symbols on the Lifeline. The line is laid out proportional to the age of the person (e.g., one half meter for every 10 years of age would make a length of 2 meters for a 40-year-old client). This is just a first approximation of how this line is placed and how long it is stretched out, since it could be that there are very many important events in one lifetime period and in other years not so many noteworthy events. If determining which stage of an individual's life holds the greatest significance for biographical work, such as processing traumatic events and constructing a life narrative in therapy, childhood experiences should take precedence, since they shape our personality for the whole of the rest of our life. Therefore, ensure that significant childhood experiences (before puberty) are well-represented on the timeline, to be further explored in detail during Step 3 of the NET process.

Some survivors first want to honor their ancestors by symbolizing their legacy. This is a meaningful and respectful gesture that should be acknowledged. However, for trauma memory-focused therapy it is central to focus on the significant moments of the individual's own life and not mainly on their heritage. Furthermore, we can be sure that the effects of important events that happened in the past in the family of origin, tribe, or group, will also surface in childhood and adulthood (e.g., parents' poor mental health due to trauma in the previous generations, elders' models of how to deal with fear, recurring anniversary of enemy attacks and starvation of the village, group narratives of inequality and exclusion, missing persons, family secrets, relatives with painful fates or unfulfilled lives, etc.).

These inherited traces of the past should be placed on the Lifeline, ideally when they show up as painful, specific events in the personal experience of the participant. They should be symbolized on the Lifeline at the point in the biography when they had a more direct impact on the individual (e.g., stone for being heavily beaten with a stick as a 5-year-old child, which was triggered by the irritation of the caregiver due to a day of commemoration of the war; or a stone for house confinement at the age of 13 years by an overprotective, dependent mother who always kept the child at home, forbidding any independence, because the grandmother had suffered many losses of loved ones).

Start the Lifeline at birth. The therapist may begin, inviting a flower at the beginning of the life, symbolizing the birth of the participant. This is often well received by the survivor as a welcoming and validating gesture, and usually gets a positive response from them: "As far as you are aware, what are the circumstances around your mother's pregnancy with you and around your birth?" We write date and place where they were born, to whom they were born, and what their response was to our question. This little (sticky-)note is then placed next to the beginning of the line.

The therapist then guides the individual to name and mark important life events and transitions. It is important here to encourage the person to give each symbol (flower or stone) a label or name, and to clearly pin specific events down in time and space. The therapist verbalizes and summarizes for each item what they understand piece by piece from the survivor's life map as a symbol is placed. In this way, symbols are placed in chronological order, with a sticky note beside each of them to indicate their significance, and to note the time, place, and title (Figure 14).

Usually, a short sentence or a few words should be enough to characterize an event or a lifetime period or a distinct event without going into detail. For example, "16 years old in 2015 living in my hometown (name), I was raped by my uncle on Christmas eve" (stone); "From 35

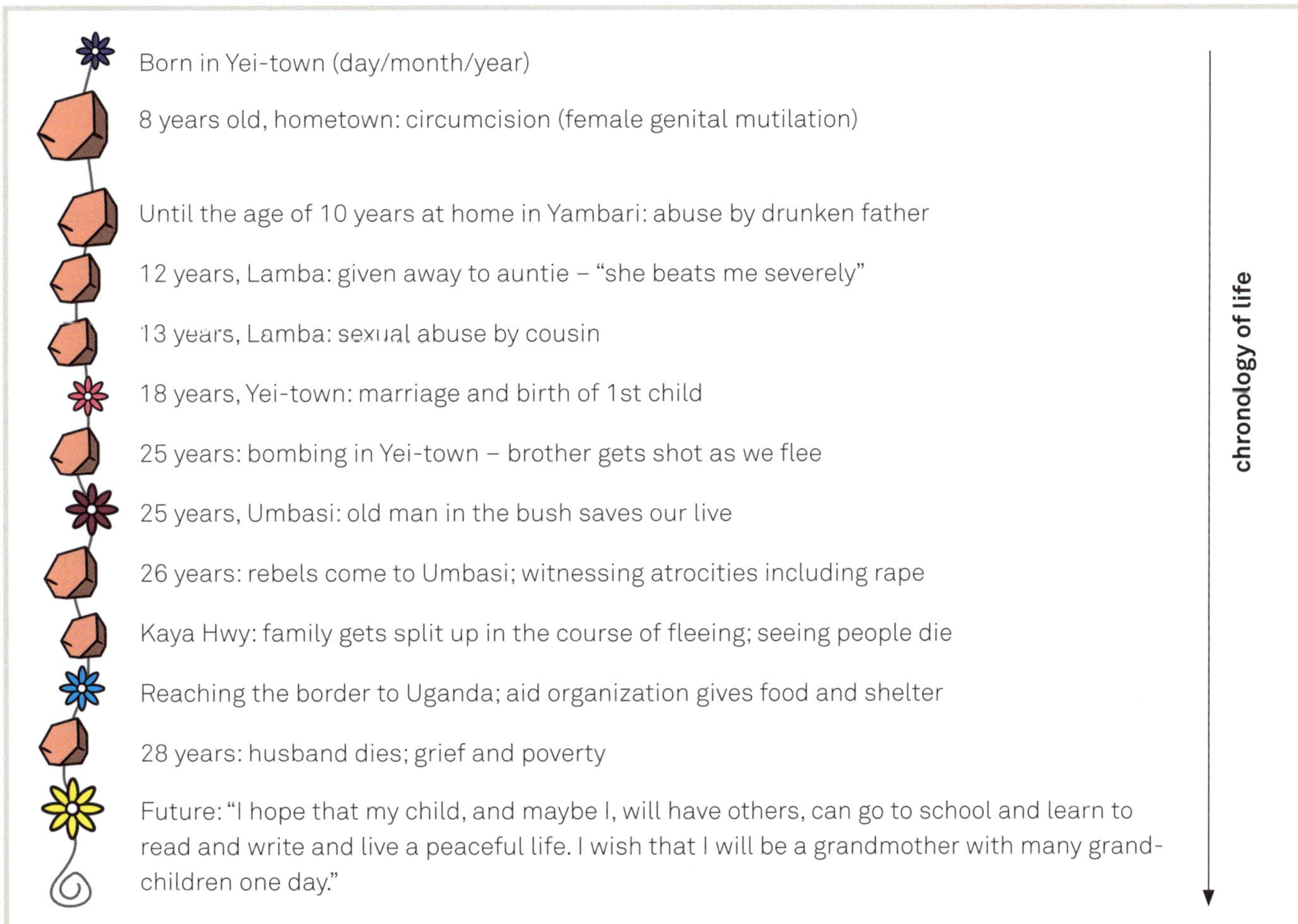

Figure 14. Lifeline of a Sudanese refugee woman. Flowers symbolize positive events, stones symbolize negative events (traumatic, stressful, or sad experiences), and sticks can indicate active involvement in violent acts if this has occured. Places and names have been changed to ensure confidentiality.

years old to present, I have been living in this city (name), enjoying a very contented chapter of my life surrounded by many close friends" (flower); "26 years old, birth of my first child, named Maria" (flower); etc.

Sometimes an initial traumatic experience is followed by a sequence of events. For example, "48 years old, terrible flooding in my village (name), we lost our house and community (stone), my wife (name) died, she drowned (candle), but our children survived (flower), after that I had a hard time carrying on as I was drinking too much alcohol and one time I aggressively beat someone so he nearly died (stick), but the neighbor woman (name) helped me to get back on track (flower)." Then a sequence of stones of varying sizes (chosen by the survivor) is placed.

Literacy is not a mandatory skill for the NET process. For some adults or children, it might be difficult to know exact dates of events in numbers. But numbers are not important. Rather, it is helpful to encourage the description of parallel events (e.g., "My first child was born in the year when the big earthquake was shaking a region next to our homeland"; "It was the winter with the terrible snowstorm when my brother broke into the ice of the lake"). Even if the survivor is unsure of the specific year or their age at the time, the primary objective is to arrange symbols in chronological order on the timeline.

Why Stay on the Cold Memory Side During LIfeline Work?

Although we should not avoid naming clearly what each stone means, the Lifeline exercise is not the time to actually process and focus on some event. It is a delicate stage in therapy where we must not encourage the survivor to disclose more information and start discussing all of their experiences at once in more detail. It is important to remember that the Lifeline session is not the same as a dedicated narrative session. As much as therapists like to overcome avoidance in traumatized people, a step-by-step process is crucial. We must not expose a participant to multiple emotionally charged experiences during a 90-minute therapy session. If we did, those experiences would become even more strongly associated, fused together in the individual's hot memories. This could impede our efforts to rehabilitate the survivor's biographical memory. So, throughout the whole Lifeline procedure, the therapist helps the survivor to stay on the cold memory side; that is, the therapist supports focusing on facts, names, dates, etc., rather than on emotions, sensory perception, or physiology, etc. As just described, this is important, to ensure that during this work, the fear/trauma network does not become strongly activated. The Lifeline is meant to be an *overview* of the whole life where important life events have their place within lifetime periods. In this regard, it is helpful to calm the mind and cool the emotions after each placement of a symbol, especially stones, before beginning to identify the next event. Helpful verbalizations to achieve this and at the same time to move the process forward are statements such as,

Yes, I see that you have chosen this large stone. I understand that the sexual abuse by your neighbor during the Covid lockdown, when you lived in Ashcroft at the house on Sutton Road, had a big impact on your life. We will take time to talk about this experience in detail later (Therapist nods for confirmation). For today, we have marked it with a representation on your Lifeline. Well done! The experience has a place there now. This was in the year 2020, you were 11 years old. Now let us see how your life has continued up to the present, Oliver.

At the end, the survivor and therapist take time to look at the Lifeline as a whole – from a bird's eye view – to appreciate the important work that has been done. Sometimes the survivor will want to reflect on the process of laying the Lifeline and perhaps highlight some of the first important insights, such as the recognition of interrelated events that have come as a surprise.

Instead of real flowers, sticks and stones, you can also draw the Lifeline on a sheet of moulded paper. The client can then draw symbols themselves or use stickers that can be stuck to the corresponding points on a drawn line (Figure 15). Zang et al., (2013) have shown that this can be equally effective.

It is important to remember, however, that the full story can only be evaluated after it has been told. It would be far too early to draw interpretations and conclusions based on this rough and often incomplete overview. Also, do not allow focusing in on distinct events at this stage. You will not have enough time or possibilities for appropriate exposure in this session. Lifeline work takes up the entirety of a NET therapy session (90–120 minutes). There is no evidence supporting its combination with other therapeutic activities during the same time. Additionally, starting imaginative exposure when both the survivor and therapist are exhausted could be detrimental, and therefore, Lifeline work is best done as a standalone activity.

It is important to end the session on a positive note. This is not the time for complaining, bitterness, or grief. If these issues come up, the therapist can suggest that they first look at each event in detail and work through it.

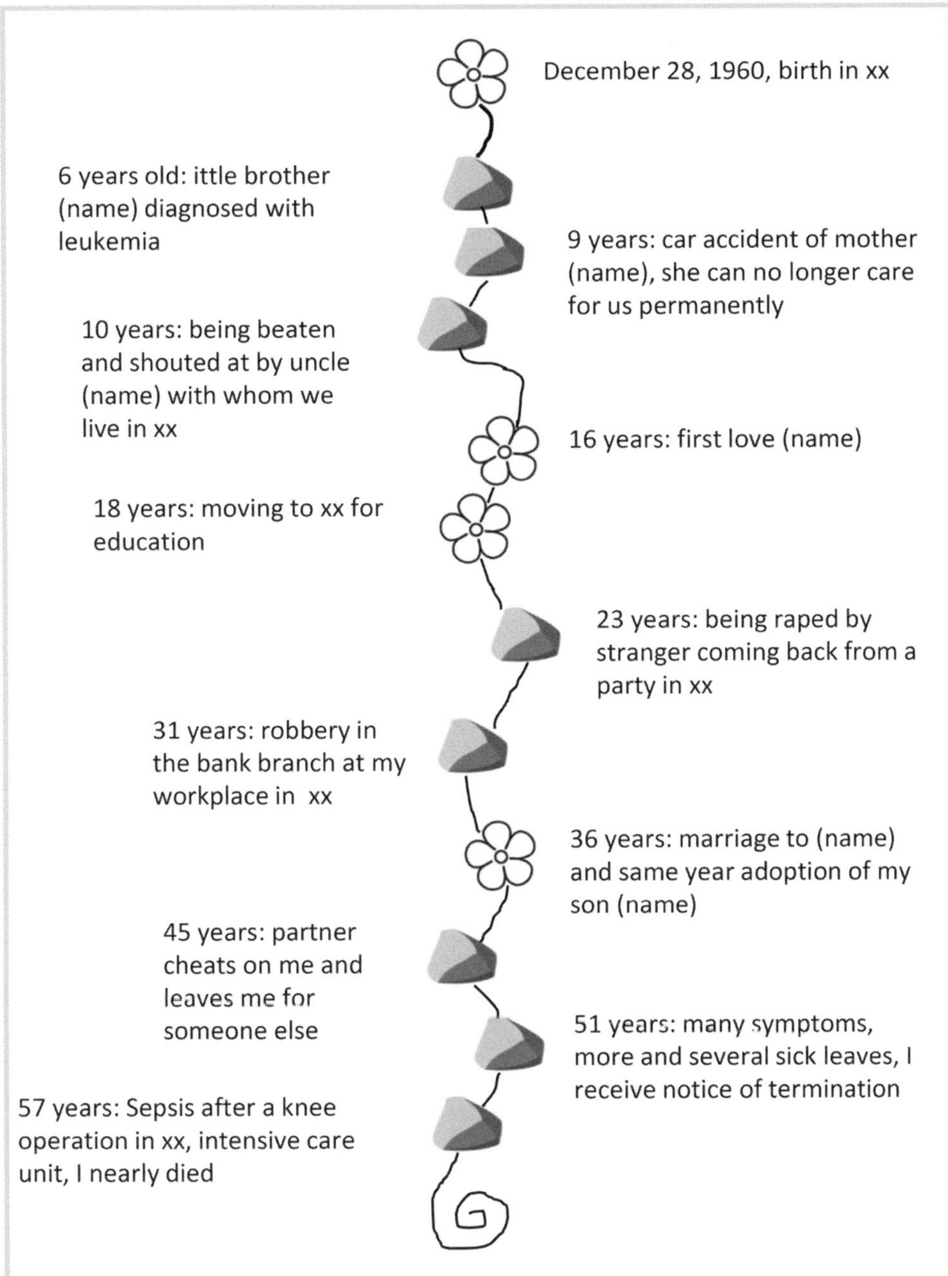

Figure 15. Trauma-intervention study participant in a primary care setting. Instead of real stones and flowers, stickers or drawings may be used. The sequence of events illustrates the building up of stressors that ultimately led to PTSD after the ICU stay. Locations and names are omitted here to protect confidentiality (study protocol in Gensichen et al., 2018).

Later, there will be time to evaluate life and particular experiences as a whole.

At the end, younger children should be offered to make a drawing of their Lifeline to include it later in their narration document (Schauer et al., 2014, 2017). The therapist will verbalize along with whatever the child is drawing, repeating the place, time, and title, and ensuring an allocentric view.

For adults and adolescents, we often offer to take a picture of the Lifeline as long as it is laid out on the floor (or on the table). This can make the cover picture of the written testimony at the end. The therapist then collects the sticky notes from the floor and stacks them in chronological order to use them to create a testimony book with different chapter titles (according to the symbols) that will be filled with stories.

Finally, the therapist and the survivor together remove the Lifeline and place the objects back in the box. The laying out of the Lifeline has to be done by the therapist and other witnesses (like a translator) with the utmost respect. It is not advisable to leave the "life" on the floor (or the desk) of the therapy space when the survivor leaves. Individuals who have gone through the Lifeline experience often report that they feel protective about their Lifeline, and they do not want it to remain lying exposed in the room. To avoid upsetting the client in the last minutes of the session, we suggest that the therapist take the stones and put them out of sight, while the client removes the flowers.

In NET with children (KIDNET), the child can quickly lay out their much shorter Lifeline each time they come back for therapy, as a kick-off for the session. Naturally, with this brief review, the child gets a welcome opportunity to see where the session continues and to realize to what point the narration has reached and where to continue. For adults, with their much longer life and more complex experiences, this is obviously not advisable. But it is generally useful to have a photo of the Lifeline or a sketch at hand at the beginning of each session, to point out to the adult survivor during which lifetime period a narration continues, how much has already been accomplished, and how much yet remains to be worked on.

Unlike survivors of multiple (different) traumatic events (such as a mugging, train accident etc.), for those with complex trauma (e.g., sexual abuse), the first Lifeline may not be very detailed or immediately conclusive. Some survivors of child abuse, sexual violence, or personality disorders may not be able to recall reliable memories of their worst past events at the beginning of therapy. This often results from severe dissociative responding when attempting to retrieve autobiographical memories. In cases where the initial Lifeline significantly deviates from the final events as they emerge during the life storytelling process, a second laying out can be beneficial at the end of the treatment as a closing ritual. This may be a gratifying closure activity for complex trauma survivors, who have endured extensive violence in a torture prison or suffered numerous similar instances of sexual abuse, to witness the restored Lifeline as a coherent whole instead of rereading all of the many single similar events. However, in cases where the testimony was given through an interpreter and the document is to be used further – for example, for human rights work or in a court case – it is essential that every sentence in the final narrative is read back to the survivor so that they know exactly what the paper says.

Lifeline basics

Creating a coherent life narrative is critical to recovery from traumatic memories, and the Lifeline can be an essential tool in facilitating this process and advancing meaningful trauma therapy.

For individuals with trauma-related conditions, a highly *structured and gradual approach* is crucial, due to their strong tendency to avoid contacting traumatic material.

To safely access and begin the process of memory rehabilitation, traumatic memories are systematically classified and recognized on a checklist before being placed on a timeline (Step 1 of NET). The Lifeline method creates then an individual profile of the emotionally and physiologically arousing life events. The *survivor's key events are arranged in chronological order* on a timeline to achieve better integration in space and time (Step 2 of NET).

"How has your life progressed? What are the most significant events within the different phases of your life?" are questions that prompt the filling in of the Lifeline with symbols, documenting significant experiences from birth to the present day.

For this purpose, for every experience, a symbol is selected according to the event's emotional *valence*, then assigned a *title* and details about the individual's *age and location* at the time of the event. The experiences are placed in chronological order, using *flowers* to represent positive events and *stones* to signify negative or traumatic ones. Symbols for violence or aggression and loss or mourning may also be added to the timeline. A brief, objective description is provided for each event.

Although the exciting, physiologically very arousing events should be identified, it is crucial not to get lost in lengthy storytelling or even become very emotional during the Lifeline work, but rather to start recognizing the physiological impact of the different interrelated experiences on the *autobiographical memory* of the participant. Therapists provides a *calming, containing presence* and gives clear instructions while holding open a space for the individual to *name* their experiences.

The Lifeline is concluded when the participant reaches the present day in their reflection.

The Lifeline can be a useful *roadmap*; it helps in structuring the coming sessions and allows the therapist to foresee the "big" stones – namely, major traumatic events or very difficult life periods.

Warning: Avoid as much as possible the mixing or confusion of memories from different events. Stay on the calm, cool memory side while conducting the Lifeline exercise. Do not mix imaginative exposure elements into the Lifeline session. Remember, the Lifeline is not the narration itself. Identifying the time and place of events, no more, is the goal of this step. *Important rule:* The Lifeline exercise *must* be concluded within one session. It is not advisable to distribute the Lifeline work over several sessions. Executing the Lifeline as a form of incomplete and superficial exposure to traumatic material would be a severe mistake. This would result in the individual's fortified avoidance and heightened anxiety. Therefore, make sure there is enough time to complete the Lifeline in one go.

Therapists' Feedback on Lifeline Work

Interested in the helper's perspective, Dix and Fornells-Ambrojo (2023) asked the question "What is the experience of therapists in delivering the Lifeline component of NET to clients who have survived multiple traumatic events?" in a qualitative study. From the therapists' perspective, the Lifeline was said to aid in building a therapeutic alliance which is fundamental for trust building in a robust human rights framework. Additionally, it serves as a containing assessment tool and roadmap, and provides a gentle introduction to the work of therapy, giving participants a sense of how the therapist responds to their history and emotions, and whether the therapist will be able to bear hearing their trauma story.

Therapists frequently referred to the power of witnessing clients' stories and, for clients, the power of being witnessed. Therapists referred to "hearing it all" as a way to allow them to bear witness to a client's testimony and noted that this was of central importance.

Dix & Fornells-Ambrojo (2023, p. 110)

Therapists also commented on the role of the Lifeline in assisting clients with the early contextualization of memories, thus helping clients begin to consolidate the traumatic events into their autobiographical narrative. The therapists further commented that pacing is as important as holding a good balance between allowing some disclosure and keeping the work on the allocentric viewpoint and cold memory side. The use of flowers seemed particularly important in facilitating a shift toward seeing traumatic experiences as terrible but discrete life events embedded in a broader context. Therapists also described how clients seemed to gain a sense of order and chronology through the process of completing the Lifeline, moving toward a coherent narrative "meeting a whole person, a whole life." The visual, physical, tangible Lifeline adds something to the verbal, taking the heat out of the task and aiding cross-cultural understanding.

Lifeline work has been found by primary care doctors to be a worthwhile tool (Sanftenberg et al., 2023), especially when the full NET procedure cannot be provided but trauma memory therapy is still necessary. Gensichen et al. (2023) laid out how the Lifeline supports and supplements the medical and personal case history which is an integral part of primary care, and helps to integrate traumatizing experiences (e.g., time in an intensive care unit) into the person's life.

Step 3: Narrative Exposure

Although there is abundant scientific evidence supporting the effectiveness of trauma-memory focused exposure in line with accepted treatment guidelines, practitioners sometimes avoid using it (Finch et al., 2020; Pearlman & Mac Ian, 1995; Deacon & Farrell, 2013; Reid et al., 2017; Wolitzky-Taylor et al., 2018; Pittig et al., 2019). Interestingly, this situation does not seem to hold true for life story telling. Both therapists and survivors equally assert that storytelling can play a crucial role in the healing process.

Clients...seeking services for a wide range of reasons. No two clients are alike. But I have noticed something that many of my clients seem to share when they first come to counseling: they all want to tell their story.... People live their lives in terms of stories. Memories are organized around stories, and hopes and dreams travel along narrative lines too.... It can be deeply affirming and validating for a client to hear their pain acknowledged, to know that what they went through mattered, and that it played a crucial role in shaping them. Storytelling is life-affirming. It coheres disparate elements of a client's life into a continuous narrative that imbues them with a sense of purpose and meaning.

Dan Bates (2022)

Since the beginning of humanity, people have shared their life stories. Humans are natural storytellers – since ancient times, they have been using stories that represent an event or series of events as ways to learn (Abbott, 2020). The Göttingen ethnologist Kurt Ranke and the Californian communications researcher Walter Fisher postulated that our species should be characterized as "Homo narrans" or "Homo narratus" (the story-telling human) rather than Homo sapiens or Homo erectus. Storytelling is a human universal that occurs spontaneously in childhood, and the universal presence and antiquity of storytelling suggests that it may be an important human adaptation, and since the times of a hunter-gatherer way of life, storytellers are preferred social partners (Smith et al., 2017). Indigenous cultural traditions and the role that cultural practices play in promoting wellness and recovery and preventing negative health outcomes include healing wisdom and have high rates of acceptability by community members and promising outcomes. As noted by Beltrán and Begun (2014), narrative storytelling is a fundamental traditional cultural practice for many Indigenous people. There are many forms of "re-storyation" in indigenous wisdom and cultural traditions (Pech-Cárdenas, 2023). It also has the potential to inform contemporary social work practice, according to Dennis and Minor (2019).

In the field of counseling, as outlined by Archibald (2008), narratives have been utilized as a tool to facilitate the healing process for those living with trauma. For numerous individuals, recounting their personal experiences through narratives can lead to a heightened understanding and greater clarity regarding painful memories (Friskie, 2020).

Individuals seeking treatment for trauma-related symptoms may benefit from treatment strategies derived from their cultural background. Recently, several innovative narrative interventions have emerged "from the ground up" based on rediscovering storytelling, a traditional cultural practice that transmits traditions, customs, and environmental, health, and community teachings and brings to life the deeply embedded sense of self (Bedard-Gilligan et al., 2022).

Evidence strongly suggests that humans in all cultures come to cast their own identity in some sort of narrative form. We are inveterate storytellers.... Narrative may also refer to psychological processes in self-identity, memory and meaning-making.

Owen Flanagan *Consciousness Reconsidered, 1992*
(cited in Steensma, 2013, p. 198)

In Step 3, which is the Narrative Exposure part and thus the core of NET, the actual life narration begins. The therapist guides the person's story one step at a time through each session – story by story and session by session along the biography with particular emphasis on thorough exploration of all of the key moments – that is, all of the highly arousing experiences in their life. Storytelling involves embarking on a journey together where the therapist can become familiar with the speaker's unique expressions and characteristics.

During the first phase, the therapist can become familiar with the speaker's unique expressions and distinctive characteristics, while also tuning in to their storytelling rhythm by actively listening, reflecting, and providing concise summaries of the information conveyed. The meaningful, important experiences are shared, while the survivor feels reassured of being deeply appreciated by the therapist.

The whole life of the individual is chronologically told from birth to the present time, highlighting the highly arousing moments of positive and negative valence including traumas, achievements, love, loss and grief, and the individual's own aggressive acts. Most of the events have already been recognized during Step 1 (intake checklist) and headlined and symbolized in their valence in Step 2 (Lifeline) of the NET procedure. Memories of other events will only become apparent when the life story is narrated chronologically now, without avoiding emotional moments on the way. By focusing on each life stage and its corresponding experiences, one may naturally evoke various arousing situations, including those previously avoided or repressed, by approaching them and activating memory associations. Emotional memory traces and their interrelated contents are explored and verbalized in the process, calming fear and revealing insight which allows for reassurance and meaning.

Lifetime periods and general events are summarized in a concise manner, whereas specific arousing events and memories of emotionally salient experiences are explored in depth. While the person's entire life is addressed, the focus is on specific traumatic events, which are described in great detail. The therapist encourages and accompanies the narrator in an open-ended and self-compassionate review of past adversities and traumatic experiences, as well as the enduring memories of joy, achievement, belonging, and love in the person's life.

Hot memories in Narrative Exposure

Note: While most memories are dealt with quickly when working along the developmental chronology of the Lifeline, the *hot memories of particular arousing experiences need to be worked through in full detail*. Significant and meaningful events of positive (flowers) or negative valence (stones) like trauma, grief, loss, or aggressive acts are to be detailed in stories. These specific events, and the moments of highest emotional and physiological arousal within them (hot spots), should receive special emphasis during Narrative Exposure, which is clearly reflected in the allotted therapy and storytelling time.

Trauma therapists should not overlook the significance of events that elicit strong positive emotions, although their training often emphasizes addressing negative experiences. For a scene in life to elicit a strong sense of positivity, including feelings of reward, self-worth, redemption, or happiness, it often requires the absence of prior hardships, such as pain, suffering, difficult circumstances, loneliness, fear, or deprivation. To the surprise of survivors, tears are often shed when delving into the heart of life's "flowers," enabling a deeper understanding during reflection on seemingly positive experiences. But before the "baby" is born, there is the pain of labor, before the exam is passed there are many months of hard work, often driven by fear, before release from prison there was isolation and detention, and there were wonderful important moments in the past with the person whose death we mourn today. Therefore, in NET we also pay good attention to the flowers on the Lifeline.

Before the narration proper is started, it is important to remember that now in Step 3 of NET, in contrast to Step 1 or Step 2, the biographic scenes are revisited and recounted from an *egocentric perspective*.

In this next portion of the manual, the Narrative Exposure procedure will be explained in detail. When working in Step 3, it can be helpful to follow a structure of moving gradually forward to well contain the situation.

Preparation of a Narrative Exposure Session

Conditions may arise in the participants' daily lives that can significantly disrupt the biographical work of dealing with the past. These need to be identified at the beginning of the session, but should not be discussed in detail. If the participant brings up what are often called *conflicts of the week* (COWs), the therapist must take into account the dynamics of *avoidance*. Avoidance as a core symptom following traumatic stress is always an obstacle lingering in the background, and it does appear in different forms. Therefore, everyday problems are documented on paper and put aside for later. They are often no longer relevant at the end of the session, especially after the traumatic event has been discussed. However, it is important to distinguish between avoidance symptoms and real-life circumstances that could pose an actual danger to the survivor; these issues must be addressed immediately and biography work must wait. Protection has priority, always.

Before entering now an exposure situation, the therapist wants to be aware of the participant's overall health and nutritional status. Adequate food and fluid intake is recommended to avoid periods of low blood sugar, dehydration which could trigger dissociation or lead to exhaustion. Water or nonalcoholic beverages should be available to encourage adequate hydration during the relatively long sessions of 90–120 minutes.

Getting Started the Right Way

At the beginning of each Narrative Exposure session, after you welcome the narrator and reconnect with the person, give a preview as a reminder of what is coming up in today's session. Beware of avoidance: Put aside until after the session any topics that might distract from the planned in-depth exposure work.

Begin by briefly explaining the piece of the timeline you are going to look at together today, giving a clear timeframe.

Examples

Today, we want to start talking about your life story, beginning at birth.... Our session today will take about 90 minutes and will end, ... let me see (looking at watch), ... at 3:30.

The next session may then begin with the following words:

Today, at the beginning of this session, I will read back to you the event we explored last time (therapist mentions title). *Then we'll continue your life story from the age of 32, when you had to go to the women's shelter with your baby....*

Birth and Infancy

During the period from gestation to infancy (approximately 0–28 months of age), developing fetuses, newborns, and infants may encounter various forms of trauma-related information that could have a significant impact on their future well-being (e.g., Caspi et al., 2016; Elbert & Schauer, 2014, 2022; Koenig et al., 2016; Merrick et al., 2017; Serpeloni et al., 2017, 2019; Ullmann et al., 2017; Provençal & Binder, 2015). It is important to understand and consider the potential consequences of such experiences for the individual. At this point, the stress axis is shaped, and experiences create physiological and bodily memories not retrievable by explicit memory retrieval later. Infants possess functional sensory systems of vision, audition, and olfaction, as well as touch. With these not yet mature predispositions from birth, they need to form strong bonds to their attachment figures. In particular, infants lack perceptual knowledge, which must be gained through experience with the world around them. All of the sensory environment leaves an imprint on the individual. Even if declarative memory develops substantially throughout the first and second years of life, the explicit memory representations we would like to have for our narrations are typically to be expected only from the age of 3 years onward.

So, in our first narration session, we rely on what the person knows about the beginning of their life, what they have been told by others, or what has been documented about them and their early months and years of life. These narratives influence the forming of our identity. Furthermore, our past experiences can unintentionally influence our emotions and behaviors through sensory cues.

Although we cannot remember our early years voluntarily, we have a second opportunity to understand their influence. Early life experiences can be linked to later representations and experiences and affiliated events in different ways.

Start the person's narration with their family background. Get a picture of how the person grew up, what the relationship to their parents or caretakers was like, and what other significant persons played a role in their life. Therapists may want to encourage the narrator to share what they know about the beginning of their life.

What were you told about your birth and first 2 years of life?

And the core question:

"Who raised you?"; "Who do you remember being around in your early years, when you grew up?"

Early childhood experiences from birth to primary school age affect the development of the personality and the brain's architecture, which provides the foundation for all future learning, behavior, and health. Since early experiences of attachment are of utmost salience, the therapeutic presence and sensitivity are highly important now (Figure 16).

In NET we begin the narration with

- date and birthplace of the survivor, as well as any relevant information regarding their parents, community, and ancestors (especially any transgenerational trauma)
- background of upbringing and whatever the individual was *told about* their birth and early life circumstances
- relationship to caregivers, attachment figures, and bonds
- brother and sisters, relevant peers, other family members living in the household
- description of context, which can include pictures and documents

This period is summarized to include important material prior to the evolvement of an individual's explicit memories and to indicate how infancy may have influenced later experiences and shaped the behavioral patterns that influence our lives.

Child survivors who go through traumatic experiences, especially physical and sexual violence and rejection by their caregivers, often struggle to understand,

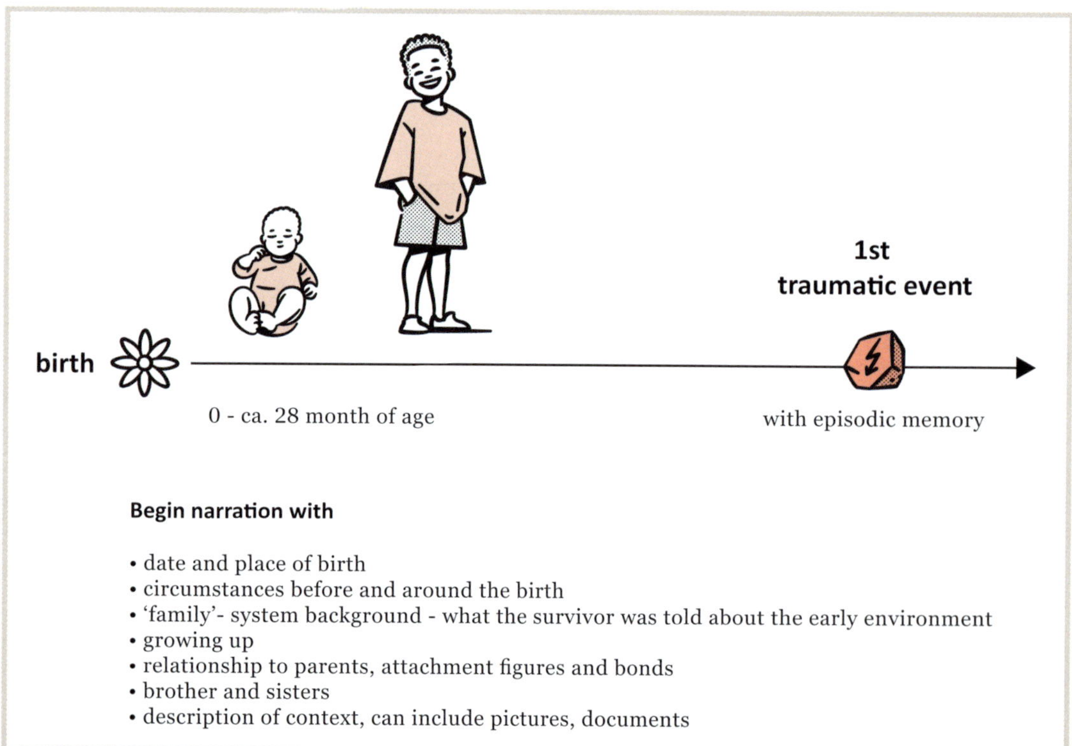

Figure 16. Narration from time of birth up to the first traumatic event.

communicate, and handle emotions. So, even when narrating a pretrauma period of life, it is advisable not only to collect the facts, but also to encourage emotional processing. When the individual is narrating some event that was particularly pleasant or some minor stressful event, they can begin to practice processing the emotional content. Children especially like to talk about happy times, and adults also like to talk about happy moments from their childhood. For many people who have been exposed to organized violence and war, the memory of good moments in their lives has disappeared along with other details from their life. This exercise in eliciting emotional content can be useful in training the participant to narrate an event chronologically. The person can learn to include emotional as well as cognitive and physiological details. Try to get a sense of how these different experiences have shaped the person's unique way of coping with stressful events, as this may help to understand the survivor's reactions, schemas, and patterns.

The amount of time spent on the pretrauma period depends on the actual number of years without potentially traumatizing stressors and the number of sessions available for treatment in total, the number of traumatic events in the individual's life, and the period of life in which the first traumatic event occurred. First order of business are the traumatic stressors, i.e., experiences with helplessness and horror, as well as interpersonal traumas in childhood for events of neglect, as well as emotional, sexual, and physical abuse. If the trauma occurred during childhood, the discussion of the pretrauma period will be brief. The narrator has mentally prepared for addressing the first traumatic event, and excessive talk about unrelated topics may cause impatience in some survivors. However, some survivors with high avoidance symptoms may attempt to extend the conversation about their pretrauma experiences as a means of avoiding the challenging subject matter that is approaching. Therapists should allocate enough time to understand and validate the time before the trauma, while also making sure to reserve enough time to discuss the first traumatic event in the first session. In the session where you address the first traumatic experiences, encourage the person to fully express and articulate their past incidents. Once complete, give sufficient time to process and reflect on the first imaginal exposure experience.

Recognizing a Traumatic Event

During the Intake Checklists, the therapist identifies most of the adverse experiences endured by the individual, in a structured manner. Prior to entering the session, the therapist takes care to remember the relevant items that were checked on the forms. Having the Lifeline in mind and being aware of the person's experiences in advance allows for listening to clues indicating difficult topics broached by the participant.

Another way to recognize when a highly charged story is approaching during the life narration is through the person's behavior. The speech patterns of a traumatized person alter as they approach a challenging period in their life. Pay attention to these signals.

1. The storytelling may become fragmented and difficult to comprehend, leading to potential gaps in the narration of the time period in question. In some cases, a traumatic event may be entirely omitted. However, narrators may provide clues to avoid or express difficulty in discussing the event. For instance, a participant may say, "In 2012, our town was affected by the war, resulting in the loss of my brother and our need to flee." In such situations where a narrator provides vague descriptions, it is important to inquire for more details. For instance, you could inquire if the survivor personally witnessed their brother's death or if they were in danger during that time.
2. The participant may exhibit symptoms of nervousness and emotional distress, which could impede their narrative if they become overwhelmed. During such episodes, survivors may exhibit absent-mindedness or engage in irrelevant discussions. Such interruptions may stem from intrusive memories that surface during sessions. It is crucial to remain aware of potential symptoms of passive or active avoidance. If such behavior is observed, including dissociative reactions, it is advisable to inquire whether the participant is experiencing any traumatic memories. In the event that a survivor discloses distressing recollections that correspond with occurrences from this lifetime period, it is of the utmost importance to proceed with caution and to engage in a comprehensive examination with the help of the Narrative Exposure cycle (Figure 17).

Once a hot memory content is revealed, there is a rapid increase in arousal as the fear network is triggered. Be aware that working with the client through the narration of a traumatic event will always take the longest part of the session (at least 40–60 minutes) and that this process should be done with great care, without interruptions. Only proceed with this part of the narrative if there is enough time left in the session to explore and discuss

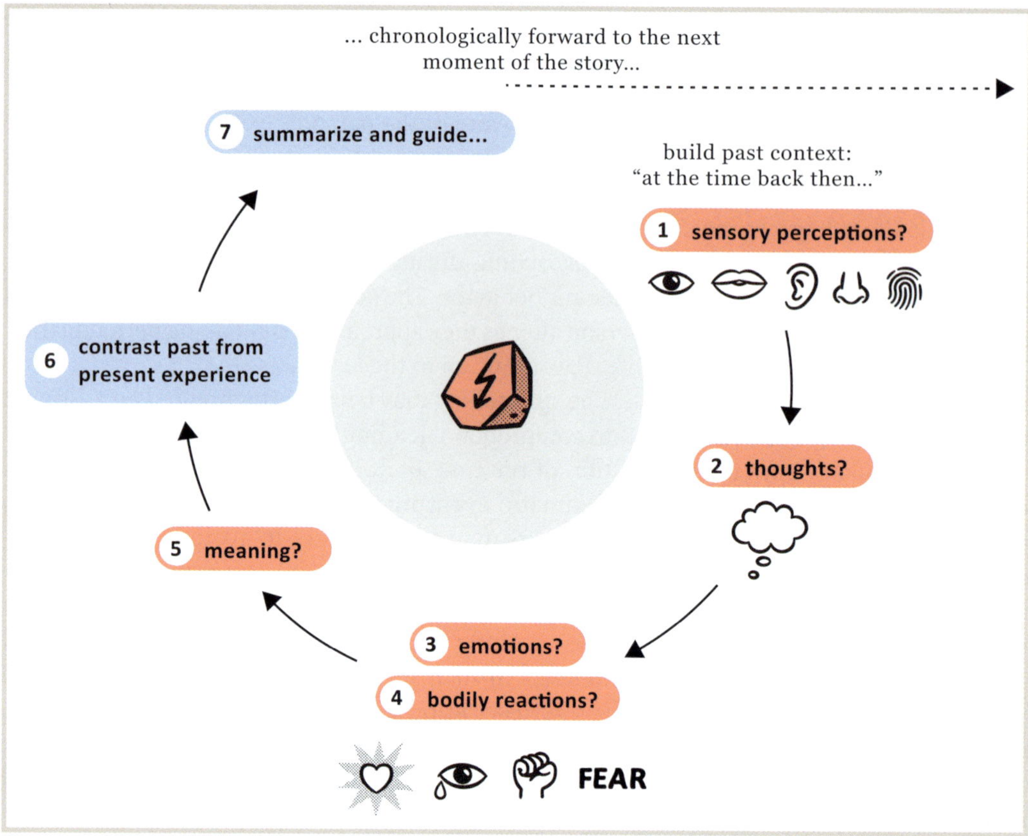

Figure 17.
The Narrative Exposure cycle is a logical exploration aid, a suggested procedure, and a reminder for the therapist to ensure that all levels of the narrator's experience are well captured. This approach allows for safe and focused exposure work that delves into the core of trauma moments as well as hidden conflicts and painful issues. Any other order of touching on different levels of experience, especially when including the narrator's reactions, can be used as needed for logical, respectful, and inclusive storytelling during the exposure process. Also available as a handout in the online supplementary materials for this book.

it, and to allow for a full reduction of aversive arousal and fear, by activating the autobiographical, cold memories.

Starting Out With a Body Scan to Ensure Grounding

When revisiting apast hot memory during a Narrative Exposure session, anchor the narrator well in the present to establish a solid grounding, before delving deeply into the past event. A brief guided body scan; that is, becoming aware of the lower and upper body, then the shoulders and head, and finally the arms and hands, can be helpful in becoming well aware in the here and now. Ideally, the therapist will help to begin scanning from the feet up, as anxiety often begins with a tensing and numbness in the legs, for example:

When you sit in the chair, feel your feet touching the floor. Pay attention to the contact they have with the floor beneath you. Can you feel your feet on the floor? Are they cold or warm? ...your legs ...any sensations in your stomach? ...your chest?...your breathing ...your shoulders, arms ...hands (temperature?) ...facial muscles, etc.?

Watch for signs of nervousness and normalize the situation by explaining that the mind and body are getting ready for the story.

The Three "S"s Approach

Whenever people become anxious, avoidant, or panicky like in an acute threat situation or when being confronted with unresolved trauma material, they cannot absorb information beyond the threatening perceptions. Their brain and body mobilize for defense. During such moments, it may be difficult for the survivor to hear and comprehend what is being said. Therefore, a therapist who is confident, calm, and fully present is required. It is helpful for helpers and therapists to remind themselves to engage in the *three "S"s approach*, as follows (Schauer & Schalinski, 2022):

S (settle in): Attend to yourself for a second, settle your mind, work toward quieting your mind in order to allow focused work. Remember: fear transmits (first energy, then strategy!).

S (speak slowly): Speak slowly, clearly, and loud enough, and in a calm manner to people in fear. Most of all: Speak little! A lot of talking will only add to their confusion.

S (say the given name): Address the person you are talking to by name (preferably given name). Do this again and again when you start your sentences and continuously mention the person's name throughout the conversation.

Under acute stress or whenever trauma survivors want to space out, addressing them by their first name is helpful.

Clarify When, Where, and What (Title on Lifeline)

Before starting the actual exposure, therapist and participant clarify which story is to be explored. Maybe the therapist invites the narrator with words similar to:

Today, Neo, we wanted to talk about the time in 2016 when you were a diamond mine worker in Botswana living in difficult conditions and you witnessed a mine explosion that killed your friend Kabelo. On your Lifeline you called this event....

When you get close to discussing a traumatic event, *clarify the period just before the incident* to enable the person to embed it into their greater life story. The therapist must never work on the incident as a fragment of the person's life. It is key at this moment to orient the events and the speaker to time and place. Ask questions such as "Where were you living at that time?" or "What time of the year/day/season was it when that happened?" and "Were you already married at that time?" After getting a general sense of the time and place, then try and pinpoint the event even more precisely by determining the day.

1. **Title of the event**
2. **Time:** "When did the event take place?" (year, month, day, or any contextual markers).
3. **Location:** "Where did the incident occur?" (name of place, context description...?). With the support of preliminary information from the Lifeline session, clarify the context and what marks the beginning of this specific event:
4. **Embed the beginning:** "What were the exact circumstances at the beginning of the incident?"
5. **Context/setting:** "Is there anything that plays into the event? Did anything important happen in the week or days before the event? How were you doing at the time? What was your mood just before the event began?" Place the incident in the context of the rest of the day. For example, if the traumatic event being described happened late in the morning, begin by asking questions about the beginning of that particular day. Ask questions such as "Do you remember what you were doing that morning?" "Who was there?" "What were your thoughts?" "How did you feel? "Was there anything special about that day?" and/or "What did you do next?" The closer you get to the traumatic moment, the slower you go – that is, the more details you get. As you get closer to the time of the incident, ask questions that relate specifically to the minutes and seconds before the incident. For example: "Were you walking your dog on the right side of the road?" Assist the storyteller in recalling specific details – for example, "I walked down the white corridor in the hospital. It smelled like disinfectant...." Remember that sensory contextual clues are crucial. Descriptions of sensory information at the beginning include simple recounting of experiences, such as "I harvested a crop in the back garden, picked beans and put them in a wooden bucket. I smelled the scent of yellow flowers and watched the sun set behind the bell tower, thinking of my baby who was with my mom...."
6. **Identify the first scare:** Find out what triggered the rising anxiety, what started the event: "What was the first thing that told you something was going to happen...something was going on.... What had changed?"

At this point an increasing number of associations within the fear network get triggered, and with it, a fast increase of arousal (Figure 18).

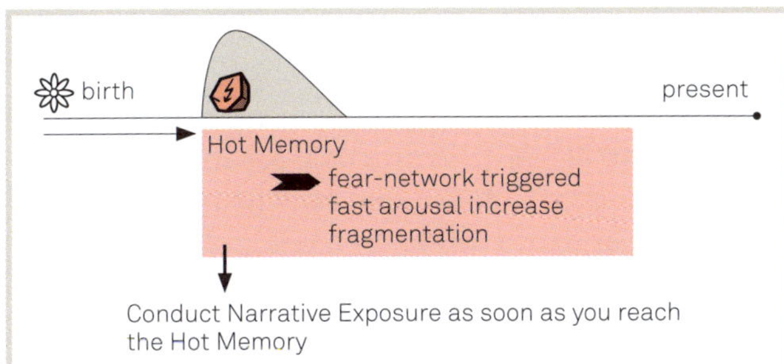

Figure 18. Upon reaching up to the traumatic event, the narrator's hot memory content is triggered.

Many survivors remember the heavy heartbeat and the surge of anxiety at the beginning of a traumatic scene, and what caused it. Ask the participant to place themselves at the beginning of the incident and to start going through the incident from that point, viewing all of it in sequence. Focus on the point that marked the beginning of the traumatic events. For example, the survivor may say, "I smelled something burning..." or "I heard a scream, and my sister was running toward the house..." or "It was suddenly very dark..." or "I could feel the car slipping on the icy road...."

Try to awake those concrete memories.

For example:

I was 8 years old and went to an international school in Qatar. We talked about this last time. It happened in the evening. I think it was in the afternoon because my boyfriend was over. We were in my bedroom in our house doing homework with my sister when I heard my father coming home from the office ... yelling with my mother ... my heart started pounding immediately as he ran up the stairs....

Or another example:

When I was 15 years old, it was during the summer break, I went with a friend, her name was Eileen, hiking the Western Ridge Trail of Rock Creek Park. It was already getting dark when suddenly a male voice spoke to us from behind. We hadn't even noticed him approaching....

Another example:

On a unusual warm day in January of 1988, I had just gotten my driver's license and borrowed my father's car to drive down a gravel road in the Patagonian Andes. I was going to the town of Bariloche to see my friend Isabella. The gravel pounded against the bottom of the car. I had to stop several times to ask for help finding the route. Around noon I had to stop again to ask the only person I had seen for many miles. My window was open because of the warmth. I was tired from driving ... as soon as the car came to a stop, this huge, dirty man reached in, grabbed my shirt, and shouted in an evil voice, "Get off the car! Now"...!

Or another example, which will be described here at some length:

It happened at the end of the rainy season in that year. My son was 2 years old then. We lived on the south side of the village of N... close to the mountains. My husband was working in town at that time. I was in the house cooking that afternoon. I prepared rice. It was hot inside, and I felt a bit tired. My cousin, who had been visiting me, had just left. We had been talking about water problems. All of a sudden, I could hear shooting outside....

The storytelling now transitions into slow motion, using the Narrative Exposure cycle (see Figure 17), asking about perceptions - thoughts - emotions - physical sensations - meaning; and, if necessary, this moment is contrasted with the present before summarizing and leading chronologically to the next moment of the story, ensuring a detailed narrative. In the example given, once the first situation had been explored, the survivor showed less excitement for the subsequent part. Here the story could be browsed a bit faster until a second hot spot was reached, which was recognizable by the visible excitement and restlessness of the narrator. The next part of this incident took place outside the village. The therapist again established the circumstances, before the narrator was asked to place herself at the beginning of the sequence:

It was already dark - after sunset. I was running together with my son in the middle of the road. I am aware that my hands were too sweaty, that I could hardly hold my little boy. Even now when I tell you about it, my hands get wet. (Narration continues....)

Methodically Working Through the Challenging Area in Slow Motion

The process of methodically working through the challenging areas is described by Watkins (1971):

> *Thus, the forgotten or pathogenic experiences which may lie at the basis of some conflict ... must be lifted from repression in all of its original vividness, its original "feelingness" ... its "beingness." Insight, to be genuinely therapeutic, must be total and must involve full visceral and muscular as well as cerebral, responses. An understanding must be "felt" as well as "known".... Thus, when repressed experiences do emerge into consciousness, they usually are accompanied by much vivid feeling and reliving.*
>
> Watkins (1971, pp. 22)

The main procedure of emotional exposure within NET consists of two processes that must be present simultaneously:

1. Activate the hot memory (associations of the fear network).
2. Verbalize the relevant elements of the experience, recognize thoughts, label emotions and bodily sensations, phrase the meaning, and include everything in the narrative of the traumatic experience.

To put this into practice, opting for a slower pace may appear counterintuitive; however, it is, in fact, more tolerable for the narrator. This allows them to work through the experience in small portions, and the event can no longer unfold with the same vehemence as before. Processing the experience gradually in chronological order, reduces the emotional intensity and keeps the arousal within a window of tolerance, allowing for a reliable interweaving of hot and cold memory contents.

Working through hot and cold memories

- Ask the survivor to imagine the beginning of the incident and work through viewing it in sequence.
- Go in slow motion!
- Support the processing of the material by following the emotional reactivity.
- Generate the physiology of that emotion and pursue memorial associations.
- Reinforce reality to prevent avoidance, dissociation, or flashbacks. Ensure the person stays focused on the present while discussing the past. Keep the survivor grounded in the present.

How to Do Narrative Exposure – Narrative Exposure Cycle

A safe way to interweave cold and hot memory content is to put all memory elements into words and thus into episodic memory. But it can be quite a task to establish a coherent chronological account of a emotional arousing and traumatic event, because associative elements in the emotional network emerge in unpredictable and nonlinear ways. For example, in the following, a young man from a South African township recalls an instance where he was challenged by someone carrying a knife. He describes his experience during the encounter at the following levels:

- Cognitions: "It is too late!...I'm going to die."
- Emotions: fear, anger.
- Behavioral responses: duck and cover.
- Verbal responses: "No, no...please don't!"
- Visceral responses: heart racing, muscles tensing.
- Sensory perceptions: hearing screams, seeing the crowd around the man with the knife, smelling alcohol and smoke....
- Body position: squatting, bending sideways.

In this situation of seemingly randomly linked associations lacking a temporal structure, employing a process rooted in the Narrative Exposure cycle can offer a safe approach: narrating – re-experiencing in greater depth – labeling in more detail – integrating into the narrative again – further narrating – continuing this sequence.

The Narrative Exposure cycle (see Figure 17) offers a structured wheel of exploration that enables the narration to proceed in a safe way through highly arousing events that are very hot and where recall is fragmented. This step-by-step exploration in great detail is empathically supported by the therapist walking through the imagined scene shoulder to shoulder with the narrator. The stones and sticks in particular, but sometimes the flowers as well, are revisited in the present and contrasted with the past (see the section Activating Memory Associations – NET in a Nutshell). The therapist asks primarily closed questions in an exposure-conversation style, being clearly active and directive, mirroring the experience, reflecting back, and giving direct feedback of what is observed, as well as paraphrasing and clarifying verbalization of sensory perceptions, cognitions, emotions, bodily experiences, and meaning content that the narrator experienced at the time and in the present moment. Therapist repeatedly offers a summary of the narrated content – ideally after you have explored perceptions, thoughts, emotions, and bodily sensations first – since this allows mentalizing and reflecting on the meaning making. It helps to modulate intensity supporting grounding by *contrasting the levels of experience in the past with those in the present*. By providing an occasional summary when needed (e.g., as a means of demonstrating warmth and connection, or as a means of countering detachment), the therapist can enable the storyteller to sit back, catch their breath, and listen for a moment from an allocentric (observer) perspective. The Narrative Exposure cycle can best be defined as a spiral that progresses toward the aim of a thorough and meaningful narrative of the traumatic incident (Figure 19 and Figure 20).

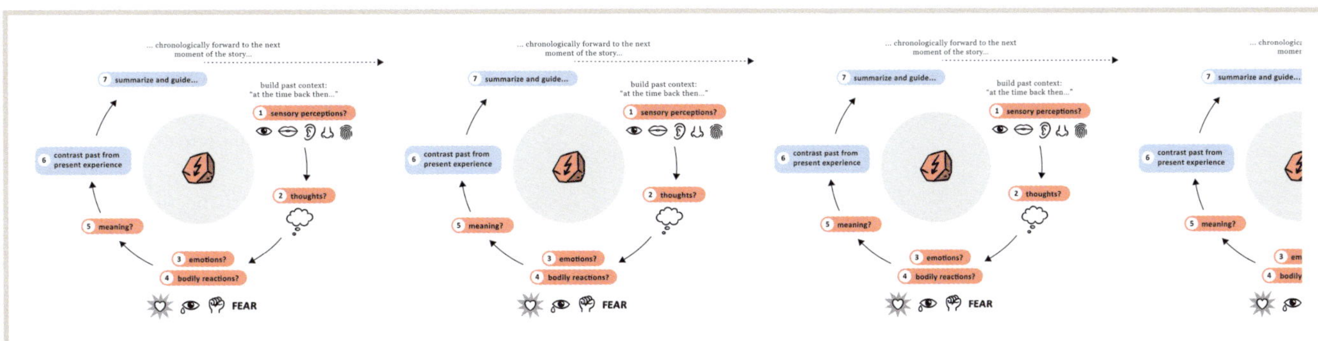

Figure 19. The schematic flow of the *exposure conversation* demonstrates the continuous forward "rotation" of the Narrative Exposure cycle, through which the various levels of experience are worked through, contrasted, and summarized while exploring a stone, stick, or flower, as well as other significant life moments such as the loss of a loved one. Employing a safe and structured work is particularly important during challenging and emotionally charged moments in the narrative.

NARRATIVE EXPOSURE

Exposure – Conversation Style

Imagination of the past trauma scene

experienced
<then and there>

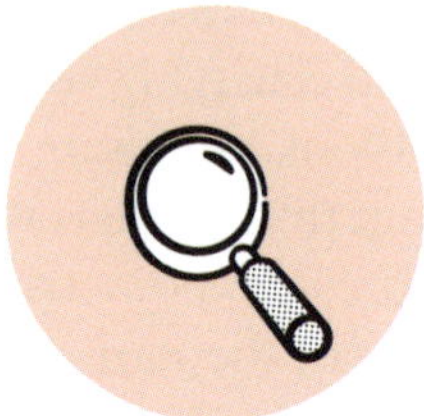

What/how...

- ... did you perceive?
- ... did you see, hear, sense, taste, smell?
- ... was your body position?
- ... did you think?
- ... did you feel (emotion/body)?
- ... what did this mean?
- ... did you react?
- ... did you want to do?

And what ...

- ... happened next?

The therapist helps to move back and forth in time between the past and the present situation

PAST **PRESENT**

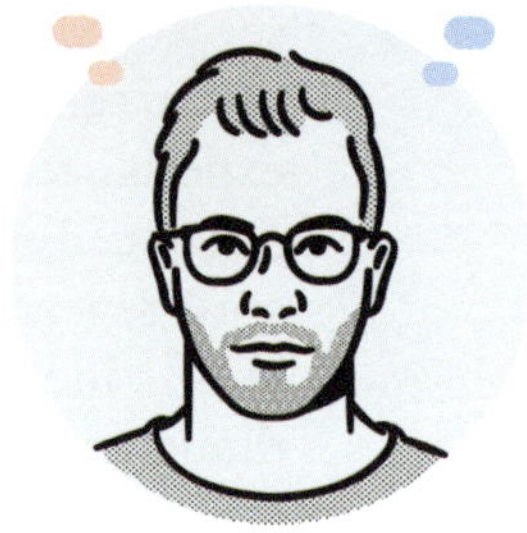

Imaginary contrasting past with present

Grounding in the therapy room

experience
<here and now>

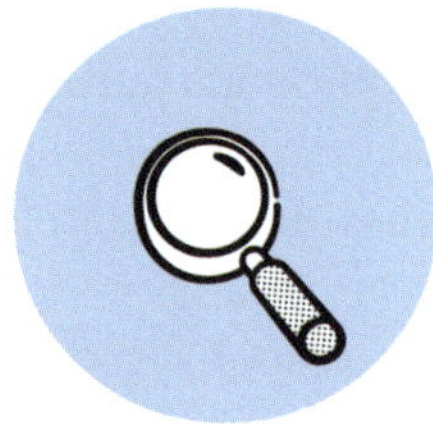

What/how...

- ... do you perceive?
- ... do you see, hear, sense, taste, smell etc.?
- ... is your body position here and now?
- ... do you think?
- ... do you feel emotionally and in your body?
- ... what does this mean for you?
- ... do you interprete this?

Especially in case of dissociation: emphasis on the past tense of the narrative, sensory stimulation in the present, good contrast to the trauma event (dual awareness), anti-dissociative counter-maneuvers.

Encourage introspection, mentalization, self-acceptance and self-care.

Meaning making.

Figure 20. Exposure conversation style – contrasting past with present, moving back and forth in time. Also available as a handout in the online supplementary materials for this book.

Listening Basics for the NET Procedure

Mindset Principles for Listening and Being There for the Storyteller

NET therapists are active participants in the narrative endeavor. They show lively, interested reactions to the story and refrain from merely listening to someone's account without providing a response. If there is too little reaction from the therapist, the narrator may stop sharing, out of shame and embarrassment, or avoid the topic altogether. In addition, if participants are not helped to maintain their connection to the present moment, trauma survivors may dissociate (refer to the section Etiology and Treatment of Trauma-Induced Dissociation in Chapter 5). Narrating and witnessing the account is a constructive dialogue – a joint, cooperative activity.

Ask clarifying questions when *actively listening* and make affirming statements to support and build the other person's self-esteem and confidence. The other part of active listening is the listener explaining throughout the conversation what they have understood in their own words. This allows the client to know what you are thinking and to check whether you are an interested partner in this coconstructive activity. Do not shy away from suggestions that help with verbalizing the contents of the hot memory, but leave the telling of the cold memory to the survivor. Show that you are thinking along as a listener, imagining how the scene unfolds and how the other person must have felt. Suggest wording and phrasing if the storyteller is having difficulty putting feelings, thoughts, or emotions into words. But do so in a clarifying, challenging, offering way. Watch closely how the other person makes use of your offers. As an active listener and witness of the life story, speak your truth, but be very careful not to hijack the event. It is not your story, not your life. The therapist's interpretation may be correct, but sometimes the survivor is not ready to accept a difficult truth. Do not force or lecture the other person. First, the narrator is the expert; they have been there. Second, the emergence of trauma material takes time. Some realizations may have been avoided for a long time in order not to have them come into consciousness. All you can do is be present and offer the opportunity to dare to look at the past and face the seemingly unbearable.

Create a *relaxed interpersonal environment* in which the narrator feels at ease and comfortable talking about difficult things and being vulnerable. Get in sync with each other. Create a safe space for the survivor to open up and talk about what happened.

Never judge, criticize, argue, or compete when you listen. If you need to question content react in a spirit of cooperation and help. One possibility is to repeat slowly and thoughtfully verbatim what the person has just said. You may then invite reflection by saying: "How does this make you feel?" "What do you think, when you hear your own words?" Allow time to reflect. You will review the testimony again when reading it at the beginning of the next session. Revisiting a past episode enables reflection and consideration of features that were previously neglected. Moreover, it is possible to highlight specific details from the survivor's account that were disregarded or evaded. The therapist may invite the participant to perceive their own emotions without judgment, which could be initially challenging if they still feel guilt or shame (see Chapter 5). Listening with intention and curiosity can foster resilience and mindfulness. The therapist should model attentive self-respect by refraining from making judgments while actively listening to the survivor's experiences.

Work Thoroughly Through the Avoided and Painful Content

For trauma spectrum disorders, passive and active avoidance is a core symptom. Activation of one element or level of experience can trigger the activation of other elements or levels of perception, thoughts, emotions, bodily reactions, and meaning content in a person, together with behavioral patterns, schemas, coping styles, etc. The therapist's task is to carefully address the emotional structures at all levels of experiencing then and now, when exploring specific events in-depth such as threats to human life and integrity, adversities, and situations of social pain, among others.

It is helpful for therapists to imagine the highly charged situations themselves to determine if a description is complete. For example, if an individual was emotionally rejected as a child by a caregiver who looked at them with hate and contempt, or if a victim had to witness grotesque scenes such as mutilated bodies, the visual details of these scenes are likely to become a significant, painful and feared sensory element in the fear structure. It is important to note that the traumatized individual experiences this involuntary and painful reliving, and engages in unintentional automatic behavior and reenacting, until these experiences are put into explicit memory. The compassionate therapist asks for a thorough depiction of these feared memories, even if the narrator (and possibly the therapist) prefer to avoid it. Thus, it is vital to aid the survivor in verbalizing these images and hurtful moments.

Here are some suggestions for what you can do to *help in activating elements of the emotional memory structure, while being attentive and empathic.* It is important to employ these interventions only with an authentic and sincere desire to listen to and care for survivors, to show concern and empathy:

- **Active listening while regulating your emotional response as a listener**
  A skilled NET therapist practices looping back by reflectingthe narrator's words and emotions. It is important to closely follow the sequence of the other person's story and echoing what they are saying, including the emotional state they are experiencing, to confirm understanding. This process of reflective listening enables effective communication and builds rapport between the therapist and the narrator. This demonstrates that you are present and attentive, allowing the speaker to express their emotions, particularly in emotionally charged situations. Confirm to the survivor that you comprehend what they are conveying. Providing even small reflective confirmations like this can help the other person feel heard and understood. Another way of looping back is to summarize every now and then, especially after having completed one round of the Narrative Exposure cycle: "Let me give a 'playback' of what I've heard you say, so you can tell me if I've understood you exactly." Be more curious and follow up with questions guiding chronologically forward to the next moment of the story.
- **Feedback of observation:** Some elements of the hot memory – especially its expression in physiological and also behavioral responses – can be observed by the therapist. Direct feedback and statements are helpful, such as: "I can see your hands are trembling" or "Your eyes are tearing up now" or "I imagine, you must have felt so desperate in this situation...." Feedback like this can help the survivor to better sense their feelings and inner state, leading to a clearer understanding of the experience.
  Interestingly, the appropriate naming and labeling of emotions and facts can reduce (!) the intensity experienced and help to moderate arousal during tense states when in a hot spot. Note that putting feeling into words regulates negative emotional responses. Linguistic processing such as *affect labeling* and naming of emotions control amygdala activity (Hariri et al., 2000; Lieberman et al., 2005). Affect labeling, not just the recognition of the emotion as such, disrupts the affective responses and diminishes activity in the limbic system that would otherwise occur in the presence of negative experiences, a process that may ultimately contribute to better mental and physical health (Lieberman et al., 2007). In NET, there is no skill training phase or qualification for the participant before treatment begins. This comes as a natural integral agent that helps the process (see section Does NET Require a Stabilization Phase?). With the help of an active listener, there is a *stabilizing* and containing quality to engaged storytelling itself. Research investigating affect labeling has found it produces a pattern of effects like those seen during explicit emotion regulation, suggesting affect labeling is a form of implicit emotion regulation. To put our feelings into words, we must first identify what those feelings are, requiring a degree of *self-reflection*: being aware of and observing our own experiences. Investigating narrative affect labeling has demonstrated a modulation of emotional output effects in the same experiential, autonomic, neural, and behavioral domains as found in other forms of emotion regulation (Torre & Lieberman, 2018). Throughout the Narrative Exposure process, the therapist helps the verbalizing, labeling, and clarifying and integrating of emotional and physiological responding. Survivors are invited to alert the therapist if there has been a mislabeling. In reality, receiving feedback or suggestions can be beneficial as it allows for a brief moment to pause and clarify.
- **Make an effort to use apt wording:** Describing what has happened in detail and using language courageously can destigmatize and break the haunting secrecy. In an effort to be with the narrator in the past, when they are physically aroused and the story seems horrific, the therapist should not hesitate to use accurate and precise language, even to describe horrific situations, and to help verbalize all of the details experienced. This will in fact effectively help to contain the situation! The attempt to avoid addressing or naming things only conveys to the narrator that one should be afraid of them.
  Victims feel extremely lonely during overwhelming, humiliating, or horrific traumatic events. The effort to understand and describe in appropriate language what has happened to them helps the survivor to regain dignity and self-worth. Through empathy and testimony, the social pain, and confusing taboo, together with a sense of shame and stigma are lifted.
- **Direct questions:** During Narrative Exposure work, the therapist can use direct questions to address the

elements of the emotional network at different levels, such as asking, "What and how exactly did you feel when ...?" The questions serve as an exploratory tool to gain a full understanding of the happening (Table 2). Avoid making this sound like an interrogation, and instead use each chance to continually verify that you are truly understanding the situation. Tentative guesses that clarify understanding demonstrate that the listener is attentively following and attempting to fully comprehend the narrative. Direct questions aid to verbalize and express feelings. The therapist praises efforts to reveal and gives assistance in the struggle to be articulate.

- **Modulating the narrator's arousal:** The tense of the questions can help modulate arousal (Table 3). Anchoring the focus in the past, with deliberate use of the past tense, will increase the contrast to immediacy and help calm overactivation. And the opposite, anchoring the focus in the present, with the use of an intentional present tense, will be effective in engag-

Table 2. Sample questions used to target elements of the fear structure across different levels of processing

Element of fear structure	Past	Present
Sensory (perception)	"What did the mutilated body look like?"	"Do you have the images of the mutilated bodies in your mind now, as it was then? What do you see?"
	"Could you see the soldier? His face? How did he look at you?"	"Can you remember the soldier now as you talk about it? How does this look?"
	"Could you smell the bodies?"	"Is there a smell in your nose right now? Similar to then?"
	"Could you feel the gun in your back?"	"Can you feel a sensation in your back right now, reminding you what you felt then?"
	"Could you hear the others screaming?"	"Any acoustic sensations right now? You remember the screams?"
	"Did you feel the pain in your legs?"	"Can you feel some reminder in your legs now, just like it hurt then? How does that feel?"
Cognitive (What was it? Thinking about? Considering what has been perceived)	"You thought it was too late.... There was nothing you could do?" "What did you think when you experienced this?"	"At that time, you were afraid that it was too late to change the situation. You felt helpless. What do you think now?"
Emotional (How did it feel?)	"Did you feel intense fear at that moment?" "How was that moment for you?" "What was going on for you at that point?"	"How do you feel about your perceptions and thoughts (of the past)?" "Can you remember the terror now, in this moment, as you felt it then?"
Physiological (How was your body reacting? What did you [want to] do?)	"You felt your heart racing fast at that moment?" "Did you have trouble breathing?"	"Can you feel your heart beating fast now, as it did then?" "Can you catch enough air right now as your body remembers the shortness of breath?" "Where in your body can you feel this?"
Meaning	"At that moment, did you fear that you will have to die?" "How did you understand this?"	"What changed in that moment of life-threat?" "What was that about?" "What did it mean to you?"

Table 3. Modulating the arousal during treatment

Anchoring questions in past trauma *increases* intensity	Anchoring questions in the present *decreases* intensity
• Ask affect questions • Ask for trauma content • Ask for sensory (visual, kinesthetic, auditory, olfactory) memories of the event • Ask what happened to their body and focus on the fear • Focus on same body position as in the traumatic moment	• Ask content questions about the context (e.g. "How old were you?" "Can you describe the room?") • Ask for thoughts in the present (metalevel of awareness) • Repeat and rephrase what the client has just said • Get client to open eyes and describe the current setting • Use breathing out (!) techniques in the session • Ask to focus on anger, feelings of opposition • Focus on different body position as in trauma • Ask the client about activities before and after present session or other events not related to the trauma

ing the narrator more emotionally (see also the section Etiology and Treatment of Trauma-Induced Dissociation in Chapter 5).

Linear Storytelling – Résumé for Narrative Exposure

One method for monitoring the therapist's focus on storytelling is to assess whether the survivor's descriptions could be turned into a compelling movie or a fairytale. The survivor's recollections and explanations must be thorough enough to provide a vivid depiction of events throughout the narrative. However, narrative structure is about two things: the content of a story and the form in which the story is told. The two parts of the narrative structure are the *script* and the *plot*. The plot is the action of the movie, and the script is *how* the story is told. The narrative structure can be either linear or nonlinear. A movie with a nonlinear structure starts in the middle, also called *in medias res* (Latin for "in the middle of things"). Such a story is told in flashbacks, turns and twists, leading up to the end of the movie. Depending on how the script and plot are used in a movie, this can be exciting for a cinematic film, but we do not do this in NET. With Narrative Exposure, we move along the timeline in a linear, chronological order.

Moreover, analogously to the structure of a classic cinematic film (Reich, 2017), the *context* in Narrative Exposure is established at the beginning of the "movie," where the main characters are introduced, and the audience learns about the setting. This is followed by a marked increase in the complications, threats, and pain that the protagonist must face in the story. The action that follows is a series of important developments when approaching *key moment(s)* as the protagonist moves toward the heart of the crisis. Finally, the *climax* is the culmination of our narrative in which the protagonist contacts and verbalizes the most traumatic moments of the past event, works through the hot spot(s), and resolves the trauma by holding the imaginative memory long enough (with, e.g., the help of the Narrative Exposure cycle, Figure 17) to allow for a detailed narrative interweaving of hot and cold memory content. Eventually, the *falling action* ties up or resolves any minor loose story ends by the end of the session. Resolution and reflection conclude the story.

It is helpful for the therapists to see these videos in their minds. Most likely, there will be gaps and inconsistencies in the narrative, which will then become more apparent when it gets difficult for the "audience" to imagine what happened. At these times, it is the therapist's job to kindly but actively engage and intervene. The therapist may want to say something like, "Maybe we can stop here for a moment. I am having trouble understanding what is going on in this sequence. Can you help me visualize....". If there is still confusion about the critical point, further insight can be gained by asking specific questions such as "What was the most challenging moment?" or "Which perception, thought, bodily sensation, or meaning ...had the most significant impact?" for further insights.

In addition, the therapist may try to retell as much of this stuck or gaping story moment as possible, clarifying the situation and making sure to be closely present in the story. If the therapist cannot comprehend the scene, it indicates the survivor feels lost, distressed, and requires support. Consistent efforts are made to keep up with the narrator and provide substantial support during periods of uncertainty, avoidance, distressing emotions, or intense tension.

Although a person's entire personality, including their complex and conscious intelligence, life history, transgenerational elements, and deep psychological responses to extreme and life-threatening events, contributes to the complexity of a particular narrative, the therapist ensures a linear storyline during the Narrative Exposure work: Narrator and therapist stay on a chronological path, working in depth, distilling and then going deeper until all elements of the highly charged moment(s) are experienced and made explicit on all levels. Then move sequentially to the next moment.

If elements of a different experience unexpectedly flash up during the narration of a particular event, the therapist briefly helps to identify the *time*, *place*, and *title* of these vivid hot memory contents in order to frame them and postpone further detailed narration of them until the next session.

How to Behave in NET

The therapist:

- *Does not interpret for the narrator.*
- *Does not judge for the narrator.*
- *Should make sure that they comprehend what the survivor is saying.*
- *Does nothing in a session that counteracts the process of narration.*
- *Acts in predictable ways and with integrity.*
- *Will always respect the survivor's boundaries.*
- *Takes complete responsibility for the session, without dominating or overwhelming the survivor.*
- *Must not transfer care to another therapist without preparation.*
- *Assures fidelity and confidentiality.*
- *Assures the survivor that their working relationship will be cooperative.*
- *Is explicit and transparent in all actions.*

Does NET Require a Stabilization Phase?

One of the essential responsibilities of a trauma therapist is to provide psychological support, or "guardrails" as clients commonly refer to them. This involves helping participants maintain client resources for engagement and a sense of safety during exposure therapy sessions. Several authors write about the debate and scientific evidence on the topic of *stabilization* prior to exposure (De Jongh et al., 2016; Foa et al., 2002; Neuner, 2012; Ruzek et al., 2014).

In NET, we do not exercise skills, special emotion regulation, or stabilization techniques. There is no training period for survivors to be eligible for the NET treatment process, i.e., to qualify for narrating their own life story. However, NET as it is composed naturally, provides what has been referred to as *stabilization and emotional containment elements:*

- **"Inner helper"**: Rather than establishing imaginary figures as a source of help or setting up some "other" within (animals, supernatural beings, heroes, etc.), the therapist is present with the narrator throughout NET. Participants are not advised to do any tasks alone (e.g., with eyes closed and being still, not sharing), or after the session as homework. Instead, whatever is worked on, is done together during the sessions. In addition, the special exposure conversation style in NET reassures the storyteller that they will be shoulder to shoulder as the events unfold. The narrator has a companion that is there with them throughout, seeing through their eyes, being aware of their thoughts, emotions, bodily sensation, and interpretations one moment after the other. This close support serves as a helping hand in moments of need and provides relief in difficult circumstances; support that was not available during the traumatic events, but is now available during Narrative Exposure. Due to the lack of emotional support in the past (especially in attachment trauma), many survivors are not accustomed to relying on another person for compassion, comfort, and sincere assistance. Therefore, at the start of therapy, the therapist can be used as a role model for self-compassion through empathic and nonjudgmental behavior. As therapy progresses in NET, survivors increasingly develop self-acceptance, particularly when viewing their younger selves within the context of their past experiences and expressing compassion toward their difficult, fearful, joyful, or sad experiences. The hurt, abused, rejected child or adult; that is, the narrator themself as a younger person, is perceived with understanding, forgiveness, and self-care for the first time when the life stories are told to an empathic counterpart and read as testimonies by the therapist while listened to by the survivor. In particular, during the retelling of the reported story by the therapist, when the narrator then turns into the listener of their own life story, mentalization and succoring to the younger ego is naturally encouraged. This creates a secure connection and a kind relationship with oneself. The victims did not have control during the event, whereas the survivor has agency during the reading.
- **Dosing the load – preventing being flooded and overwhelmed:** The stress for both participant and therapist typically associated with the use of exposure ther-

apies is mitigated in NET by an absolutely stepwise approach to the trauma material, a containing allocentric perspective in Step 1 (event checklists) and Step 2 (Lifeline), and an unobtrusive but constant accompaniment with every breath in Step 3 (Narrative Exposure). In addition, the therapist helps to safely modulate arousal through sentence-by-sentence verbalization, by being an extremely close, path-guiding listener, and by supporting a constantly shifting focus of attention that alternates between the past and the present time throughout the Narrative Exposure. The use of this narrative technique, which involves imagining and talking about the experience during the "then and there" moments, and then returning to the experience in the "here and now" from time to time while remembering, has been shown to be very helpful in being safe and stable as a narrator (see Figure 20).

- **Counteracting flashbacks and dissociation**: A survivor can become trapped in the prison of the past through a flashback, triggered when the consolidated memory (associative network) is activated. This can transport the person back to the perceptions, thoughts, emotions, actions, and bodily sensations of the traumatic event as if by a time machine, leaving them disconnected from the present. A dissociative reaction is a detachment from reality because a shutdown process (shutdown dissociation, detailed in Chapter 5) is initiated. Derealization and depersonalization are barriers to treating trauma, but tend to be the rule rather than the exception. In NET, these phenomena are expected and counteracted by the close exposure conversation style with constantly very controlled moving back and forth in time, which ensures the contrast between the trauma setting and the therapy context (Figure 20). If special "skills" need to be used (antidissociative strategies, detailed in Chapter 5), they are employed and most effective *while* the narrator is in contact with the trauma material during the session, not after or between sessions and not as homework.
- **The buildup of resources:** In NET, the flowers – our favorite past moments – aid in identifying positive experiences and accessing resources, such as situations where the survivor felt strong, confident, loved, and safe (see section Finding Flowers, above). During Step 3, it is recommended to narrate some of the flower events in detail, using the Narrative Exposure cycle, similar to how a stone or stick is explored in depth. Reorientation and reflection are useful at the end of the session. What does the narrator take away from the flower? With a physical anchoring (e.g., "Where in the body can you find the sensation of happiness, love. ...?") and a detailed description of the beautiful, happy feeling, the narrator can come away from a flower session with intense positive emotions and take that "gift" home with them, owning their experience and drawing on these resources later in life.

The Human Condition and How We Relate to Our Experiencing

Humans seem to have a deeply ingrained urge and ability to share stories. To do so, people can fully immerse themselves in a past event and – being the narrator – step back to view it from an external (allocentric) perspective, like watching a movie about this event. This enables individuals to become aware and reflective of the past and its recollection. When we engage in storytelling, we connect with our past selves, recalling and reflecting on our experiences, considerations, emotions, and actions, both then and now. Moreover, we can relate to ourselves as narrators – think and feel about "seeing" ourselves (Figure 21).

Very young children experience the world without conscious evaluating. As we grow older (5–6 years of age), we shift away from an *egocentric* being (Plessner, 1975, 2003) and start becoming aware and relating to ourselves and our experiences (usually during primary school). At that stage, we need close contact with other humans to become fully human. To learn to speak, to relate adequately to ourselves, and to understand and integrate our experiences and the world, we need to be with our caregivers and our social group. If our social others do not explain the world, and validate and normalize our emotions and reactions, but instead punish, betray, and confuse our experiencing, thinking, and self-referencing (e.g., when a child is frozen in fear and disgust, but the abuser praises the child for giving him sexual pleasure; or when a caregiver ignores and humiliates the child for expressing emotion), we begin to devalue ourselves – that is, our very own experiences. Only a felt sense of acceptance, coherence, and belonging calms and stabilizes the stress axis and allows us to accept all emotions and thoughts without censorship. Not so, if we cannot form beliefs about the mental states of those with whom we interact and constantly have to watch out for danger or rejection.

This is why children depend on their attachment figures to learn how to be empathic and to verbalize their experiences authentically and truthfully, and furthermore, to be reliably sensitive and approachable. The acceptance and validation of the child's emotional experiences by the attachment figure is key to the child's self-accepting

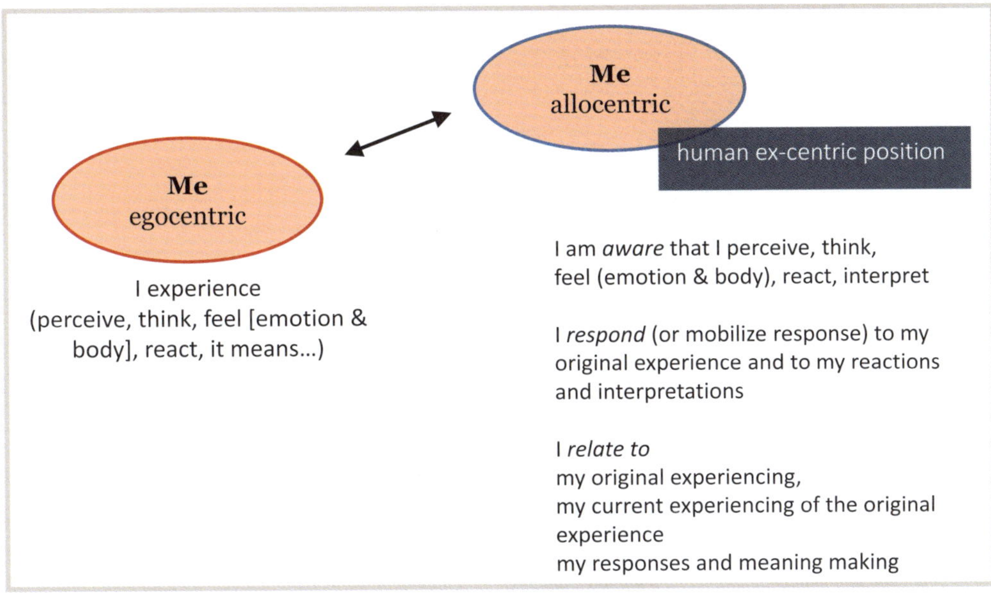

Figure 21.
This essential aspect of humanity, the ability of adaptive self-relating, is a defining characteristic for humans and their mental health. We effortlessly navigate this highly complex situation during the narrative process, when experiencing ourselves, while experiencing and talking about these levels of experiencing. When we narrate our stories, we can report from these different dimensions. Under traumatic circumstances, however, this ability can be compromised (Brewin et al., 2010; Schauer et al., 2005).

social and interactive learning in order to develop proper mentalization (Bateman & Fonagy, 2013; Gergely et al., 2002) about emotional and physical states of self and of others, as well as self-acceptance. Only with a healthy imaginative mental and emotional activity can we master self-relation and relation to others.

This allows us to feel safe in a world we can understand, to connect with others, and reflect on our personal experiences in a meaningful way. However, this development is susceptible to disturbance, as it is shaped by interpersonal learning. Traumatic stress, violence, and insensitivity from attachment figures disrupt this complex and potentially vulnerable self-balance, resulting in bewildered and dysregulated emotional states, as well as an increasingly maladaptive memory representation.

As a consequence of traumatic stress, individuals may develop a distorted view of themselves and their past (Figure 22). Exposure to aggressive, neglectful, and

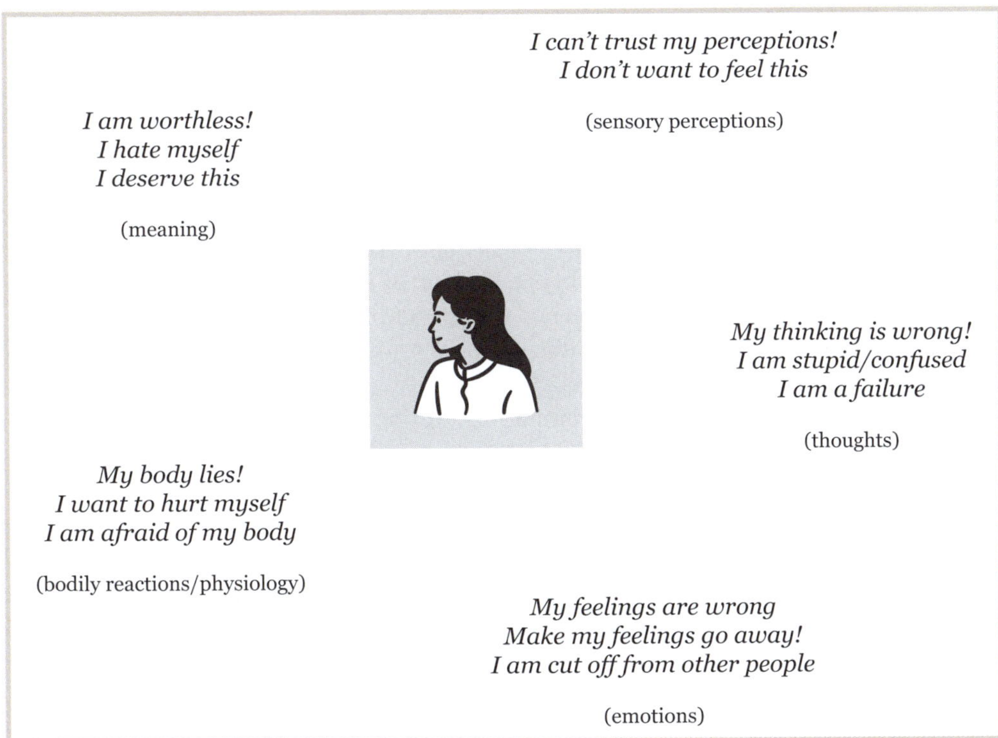

Figure 22.
Some or even all aspects of an individual's original experience may be negated and confused (e.g., in developmental trauma), including thoughts about sensations, emotions, bodily reactions, and the meaning behind them all.

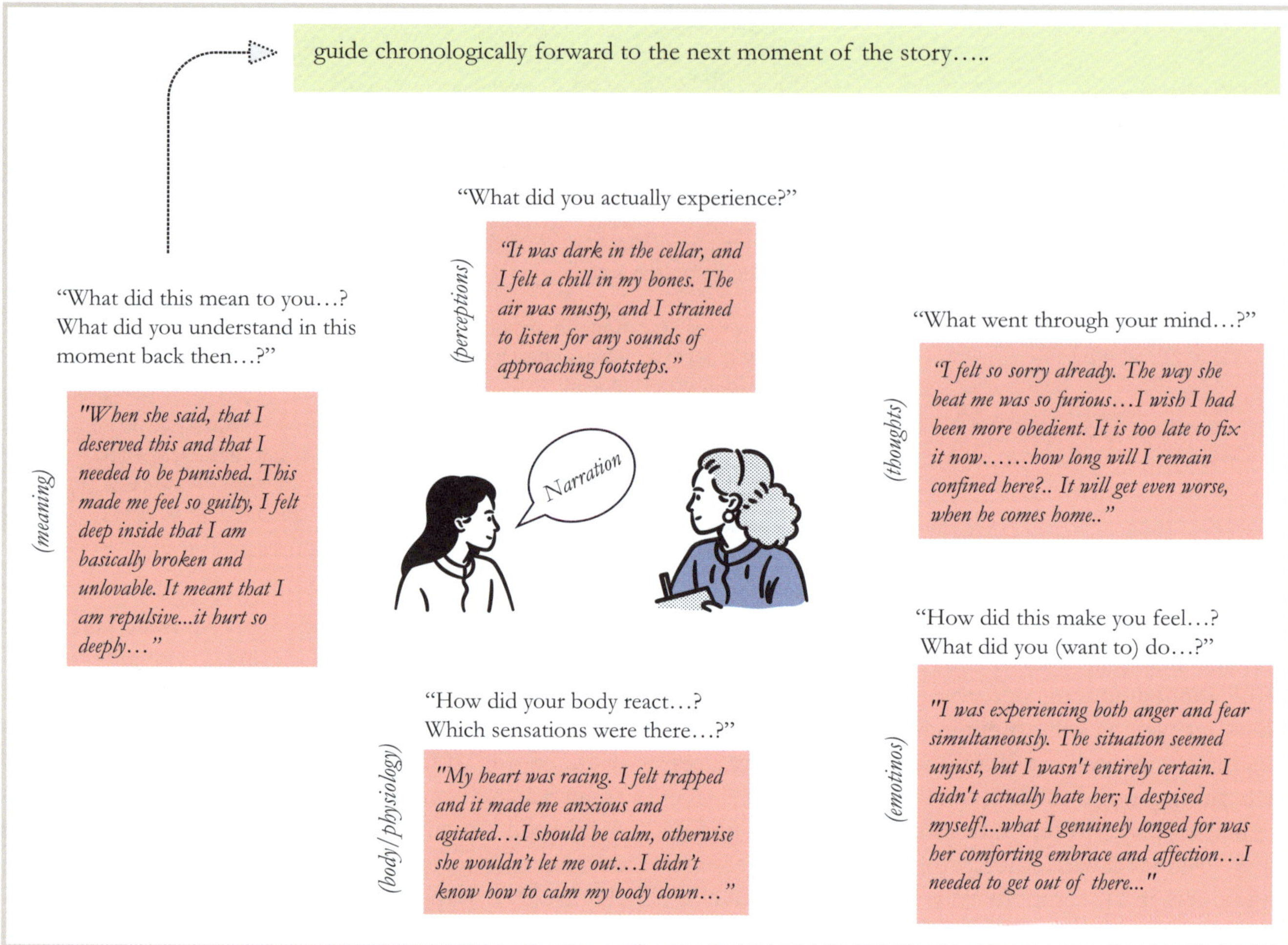
guide chronologically forward to the next moment of the story…..
"What did you actually experience?"
(perceptions)
"It was dark in the cellar, and I felt a chill in my bones. The air was musty, and I strained to listen for any sounds of approaching footsteps."
"What did this mean to you…? What did you understand in this moment back then…?"
(meaning)
"When she said, that I deserved this and that I needed to be punished. This made me feel so guilty, I felt deep inside that I am basically broken and unlovable. It meant that I am repulsive...it hurt so deeply…"
Narration
"What went through your mind…?"
(thoughts)
"I felt so sorry already. The way she beat me was so furious…I wish I had been more obedient. It is too late to fix it now……how long will I remain confined here?.. It will get even worse, when he comes home.."
"How did this make you feel…? What did you (want to) do…?"
(emotinos)
"I was experiencing both anger and fear simultaneously. The situation seemed unjust, but I wasn't entirely certain. I didn't actually hate her; I despised myself!...what I genuinely longed for was her comforting embrace and affection…I needed to get out of there..."
"How did your body react…? Which sensations were there…?"
(body/physiology)
"My heart was racing. I felt trapped and it made me anxious and agitated…I should be calm, otherwise she wouldn't let me out…I didn't know how to calm my body down…"

Figure 23. To facilitate the recovery and recuperation of the survivor's original experience, the therapist provides a warm, empathic, non-judgmental, and encouraging presence to support and guide self-exploration and narration. Through this mindful and in-depth storytelling that deliberately includes all levels of experiencing, the narrator is enabled to ally with the younger self.

reality-distorting communication can contribute to the development of various forms of psychopathology throughout the lifespan.

Trauma survivors often cannot consciously know what happened to them, since a coherent narrative structure gets lost in the process of generalizing the increasing number of stressful experiences. As a result, individuals may find it challenging to regain control over their responses to stimuli, situations, and their innermost experiences. In stressful situations, in the face of danger, or when seeking the approval of significant others (e.g., attachment figures), we may disregard our own feelings and thoughts, and instead adopt the dominant narratives; we adopt the narrative of the abuser, of the person who holds sway over us as a victim, guiding perceived reality. This incongruity can lead to long-term emotional suffering, struggle, and self-hatred.

Narrative Exposure, with the help of an empathic therapist, carefully allows the recovering of the original experiences of the survivor, so that the important process of truthful exploring of past events can confirm the perception and interpretation of the individual and counteract confusion and a sense of inferiority caused by trauma (Figure 23).

An empathic, chronologically structuring listener allows for a corrective relational experience that rehabilitates healthy self-referencing. The distorted and incomplete process of attainment can be clarified, recovering the underlying, original truth.

Survivors of adverse childhood experiences often lacked supportive empathy and warmth from those closest to them when experiencing intense emotions. Their desire to be liked, approved of, and soothed went unmet, and in some cases, they were even punished for expressing negative feelings. As a result, social interactions can be particularly challenging for them. Ensure that emotional support is provided to the narrator throughout the conversation. The therapist should moderate the survivor's arousal level and continually bring them back to the present moment, ensuring good grounding and orientation. Ensure that the social interaction is safe for the survivor, and always show the utmost regard for their feelings.

In Narrative Exposure, the therapist should adjust the pace and detail of the narrative to match the narrator's physiological arousal. If the narrator is experiencing higher levels of tension, emotionality, or confusion, the narrative should be slowed down, with careful gradual progression and sensitive, but unflustered, direct support for clarifying and verbalizing. Pacing the stone effectively is critical. One should be cautious not to slow down too much before the event truly commences. In instances where not much changes or happens during extensive events, it may be necessary to accelerate between hotspots. This approach is necessary for session time and energy management.

Throughout the narrative, the therapist should closely monitor the survivor's arousal, and seek to contrast the present with the past, adjusting the tense used. This is significant for the narrator's sense of control, protection from overload, and consequent participant engagement.

The process behind the dynamics of human self-awareness is amazingly complex, but the intervention to recuperate and fortify the self is straight forward. The storytelling encompasses all dimensions of the person's own experiences: the original past situations, the experience and the reactions during event(s) and during the current narration (mental time travel), as well as allowing control in the storytelling process and the reading experience.

Moments of silence, but never left lonely: Storytelling in NET is done in a relational manner of patience and pace. Deep listening means giving a person space to think and say things that people only add in a moment of brief silence. There is almost always more in a moment of self-exploration than is said out loud. If the therapist can maintain therapeutic presence, this more will come forward. At the end of a segment, the therapist wants to hold their breath for a moment and wait. From time to time, the therapist needs to have the skill of not speaking. Only then does the survivor have an opening, a space they normally do not have. This is very valuable. When people come to a point where they feel comfortable with what they have said, the next step will probably be more revealing, something that will come from a deeper place. Give the signal to listen as a therapist and then remain silent, but not for too long. As a testimony bearer you want to allow enough space and moments of silence to let the narrator come forward even with difficult contents, but being highly engaged and alert to recognize dissociation and act fast enough to prevent it (see the section Etiology and Treatment of Trauma-Induced Dissociation in Chapter 5).

Sample Transcript of a Narrative Exposure Conversation

The following conversation was with Demi, a 35-year-old woman, who had a stone on her Lifeline: an almost fatal mountain accident with her son Lino in the Swiss Alps. This is a sample scene from a NET in-depth work, demonstrating the levels of narrative detail and the underlying complexity of human experience that need to be expressed by the survivor and received by a carefully listening and emotionally present therapist.

Demi recalls a mountain accident she had when her son Lino was 7 years old. They slipped off a trail and plunged down a rocky, dangerous slope onto a narrow ledge. The mother was trying to save her son from the ledge and climbed down to him.

This piece of therapeutic dialogue is only the climax of a specific event narration ("mountain accident"). Demi, the survivor in treatment, had already worked through highly arousing experiences of her first 35 years of life when reaching to this stone. The spatial and temporal context of the experience was set, and the story had been ongoing when it reached the peak of emotional arousal (the levels of exploration during the Narrative Exposure session are indicated by the headings):

Context and First Perception

Narrator: "... There he was. ... I saw him on a narrow ledge."

Therapist: "What could you see?"

Narrator (holding breath): "... I saw him barely able to sit, on the wet, narrow mountain ledge. There was a deep gorge below. Lino was crouching and clinging to the gray narrow ledge. I knew, I had to climb down from higher up to get to him. The clouds were forming a dark mass now. It started to pour with rain...."

Senses and Perception

Therapist: "Demi, you saw him crouching and clinging to a narrow gray ledge. Could you tell in what state he was in?"

Narrator: "I shouted to Lino: 'Stay where you are!'... I heard his frightened voice... and I was so scared that he could not hold on for any longer."

Therapist: "What exactly did you hear from Lino?"

Narrator: "He was screaming!"

Thought

Therapist: "What were you thinking when you heard his scream?"

Narrator: "I thought, he is losing it, he needs to calm down or he will do something stupid ... a move... unthinkable!" (Narrator covers face.)

Emotion

Therapist: "I see you covering your face, Demi. The thought was so intense that you could not look at him barely able to hang on to the rock for any longer?"

Narrator: "Oh, yes, I felt so incredibly helpless. He was too far away... I am his Mum ... I must help him ... I was feeling desperate!"

Body

Therapist: "So there was this great helplessness and desperation in you. Where in your body did you feel it?"

Narrator: "Oh, oh, my heart was beating so fast! Just like now!"

Meaning

Therapist: "Yes, your heart is beating now as well. Your body reacts to your memory. When you had all these thoughts and feelings and bodily sensations at that moment, what was going on in your mind? What did it mean?"

Narrator: "I knew his life hang by a thread! He needed to calm down to be safe and it would give me time to get to him ... or else he could do something unpredictable ... like trying to move closer to the edge of the rock ... and then ... then ... he would fall ... and he would ... die ..."

(Arms of Narrator fall into her lap; she becomes motionless and seems weak.)

Here and Now

Therapist: "This moment was so terrifying for you Demi. And as you sit with me now, I can see that your body has gone weak. You are sitting so still, and your arms have fallen into your lap. Thinking that he might die, at that moment back then, seems to have taken away all your energy. Is this what you also feel right now?"

Narrator: "Yes...no energy, as if nothing makes sense anymore.... I have never thought about it before, but now I realize I felt so alone at that moment."

Comparing and Contrasting the Past With the Present

Therapist: "At that moment back then, at the cliff you were alone, Demi, there was no help available. Right now, I am here to sit with you and to listen to you."

(Narrator nods and starts crying.)

Narrator: "Uhhh, yes... ah there is so much sadness now....at this moment back then I could have lost my son. I never realized that the feeling of loss is still in me...."

Therapist: "Where in your body do you feel this loss and sadness now?"

Narrator: "It is here in my heart." (Narrator puts hand over the heart area.)

Therapist: "Yes, there it is.... At the time back then you could not allow yourself to think you could lose your son, or allow yourself to feel your emotions. But now, I want to invite you to feel your sadness deeply."

(Narrator cries, keeps holding hand over her heart area.)

Therapist: "It is good to take time now to stay with the pain in your heart. ... This is the pain that comes from that time back then when you thought you might lose your child.... Losing a child – could there be worse? What did it mean for you, to possibly lose Lino, Demi?"

Narrator: "I love him so much.... Mmhhh, this is the pain I still feel even nowadays.... It is...actually the truth is, that I need him more than he needs me...he doesn't know that, but without this child...."

Therapist (repeating the last words): "...without this child...?"

Narrator (looking to the therapist): "...He gives meaning to my life... and if he wasn't there, I wouldn't have any. I would be nothing...Just now, it dawns on me that before he was born, I had often felt lost...."

Summary

Therapist: "What an intense moment this must have been for you, Demi. It sounds like your whole existence hung in the balance, in this moment: you could lose your son and you could lose your life's purpose."

Narrator (nodding): "Mhmm, that is right.... I wasn't aware of this."

The therapist prompts the narrator to reflect on this new realization for a moment and asks to explain their insight.

Therapist: "Can you put this into words, Demi?"

Narrator: "Well, I am just beginning to understand, that my child had helped me to find a life worth living!"

Therapist: "A life worth living!"

Narrator smiles and takes a deep breath.

Therapist: "That got through..."

Narrator places feet firmly on the ground ready to continue the story.

Therapist: "Let me summarize what I understand, Demi, and where we are in the story. Your child, Lino, had helped you to a purposeful life, and now you both found yourselves in this life-threatening situation. So, when you climbed down, the sky had gone dark, it was pouring rain, and you saw your son sitting on that narrow ledge, barely able to hold on. At that moment, you had to fear that he would slip and die. Tell me, what happened next?"

Context

Narrator (getting more frantic again): "Yes, it is true, the sky was getting dark, and the rain was pounding down on us. I looked at the climb down to him and saw that there was no path. The rock face was slippery and so wet. But I just had to take action. At least try to do something! I tried to step further down with my right foot. But immediately I lost my footing...."

Senses and Perceptions

Therapist: "So the rock was so wet that your foot just slipped off?"

Narrator: "I lost my footing! I lost my grip. I felt that even my hands could barely hold onto the rocks. Uhhh, that icy coldness. My body was stiffening."

Thought

Therapist: "Your fingers couldn't hold you, and your feet were not supporting you? What were you thinking at this moment?"

Narrator: "I am paralyzed!"

Therapist: "So you thought you could not move anymore? How did that make you feel?"

Emotion

Narrator: "Ahh, no time for feelings ... I had to stay calm, or else I would start to panic!"

Therapist: "I understand. When it is about life and death, feelings get in the way.... They are disturbing?"

Narrator: "Concentration now! I need to get to my son.... Uh, the thought of not making it gave me so much fear."

Body

Therapist: "I get it. So inside, you were close to panicking at this moment?"

Narrator (exhales): "Yes, yes ... my feet slipped. I accidentally kicked off stones with my feet. I had no support. Only my hands were holding me.... I was basically hanging.... This surge went through me like an electric shock!"

Therapist: "That must have been terrible"

Narrator (grimacing and looking toward therapist): "It still gives me the creeps!"

Meaning

Therapist: "So it felt like a shock went through your body, as you were dangling from the rock face?"

Narrator (stops breathing): "...I did not dare to look...."

Therapist: "What happened then, Demi?"

Narrator: "I don't know.... I don't remember.... There was so much confusion."

(Narrator breathes heavily and clutches the arm rests of the chair with her hands.)

Therapist: "I can see that you hold on very tight to the armrest. Is this how you were trying to hang on to the rock? ... This must have been exhausting?"

Narrator: (silent, almost contemplative): "There was a deep regret.... I should have never come here ... but, at the same time I knew that staying like this would not help.... I would just lose muscle power...every second you lose power...and I was not sure if I could move my limbs.... I will have to let go.... I did not want this to be the end, yet....!"

Comparing and Contrasting Here and Now

Therapist: "At that moment back then, on the cliff, you realized that you were in a situation so dangerous that your life might end, and you regretted going there? I see your hands clasping the armrest. How do they feel right now?"

Narrator (exhaling): "Ahh, yes, this is better now.... My hands were behaving as if they had to hold on to something."

Therapist: "As if you where there holding on...."

Narrator: "Oh, yes, the blood is pumping back into my hands now...they are warming up."

(Narrator massages her hands.)

Summary

Therapist: "Ok, so let me see if I have understood correctly, as you tried to make your next move and climb down, you placed your right foot, and it slipped off the rock immediately. You were now only able to hold on with your hands. You were dangling, and you thought this might be your last moment of life. A serious moment of threat. Let me understand how you kept coping with this moment."

Context and Perception

Narrator: "Oh, my hands were all sweaty! And cold ... I could not see well, I only saw the rock face in front of me. I could see the colors of the stone, dark, wet ... and under me was a shadow to my left ... my son sitting on the ledge ... he must have seen my predicament."

Senses

Therapist: "How did you know that he watched you dangling?"

Narrator: "Ahh, there was an urgency in his voice as he was screaming, 'Mommy... Mommy... I am scared!'"

Thought

Therapist: "I understand. What were you thinking as you heard Lino scream 'Mommy'?"

Narrator: "Oh, I knew that my wet hands wouldn't be able to hold my weight much longer ... and I thought: God, please let my son not see me slip off. The thought of him watching me die was unbearable."

Emotion

Therapist: "That must have been a very helpless situation, not being able to control your body and wanting to protect your son from seeing you fall at the same time. Do you remember how that felt?"

Narrator: "Oh, I couldn't feel my fingers anymore. Only the icy coldness that hurt so much. I could not stop the panic, so much fear...."

Body

Therapist: "... and in your body?"

Narrator: "... my body was out of control ...."

(Narrator starts to tremble.)

Therapist: "I see you starting to tremble, Demi, and you just held your breath for a moment. What was going on for you?"

Meaning

Narrator (breathing heavily): "I felt like I will have to let go.... I realized I was going to fall... I'm going to fall off this cliff... I can't do anything!" (She takes time to verbalize the feeling.) "I... I felt lightheaded... defeated..."

Therapist: "Defeated... What did that tell you?"

Narrator (nods sadly, sighs heavily): "You know... like I have to let go of my life. Oh, now I realize that all my battles in life seemed lost at that moment.... I was strong for so many years ... but now...."

Therapist: "...so at this moment back then you realized that you have already worked through many challenges in your life ... that you had to be strong for such a long time already. ..."

Narrator: "Exactly! But now I couldn't keep going,..." (showing signs of shutdown dissociation).

Comparing and Contrasting Here and Now

Therapist: "Demi, let's come back to now for a moment. Can you compare the situation in the mountains 8 years ago to how you feel right now in this room telling the story?"

Narrator: "Phew, that was pretty intense...I nearly forgot where I am. ..."

Therapist: "Can you feel your body? Any numbness? What do you notice about yourself?"

Narrator (focusing on her perceptions): "Oh my arms ... I can feel them again ... Look, they are trembling and my legs too. ..."

Summary

Therapist: "So, let me summarize where we are at this point of the experience. As you were dangling from the rock face, you realized Lino could see you and you were panicking since you did not want him to see you fall. And you were getting too tired to struggle.... Take it further, Demi: and then ... what...?"

Context/Perception

Narrator: "I knew it was only a matter of time. My muscles grew tired ... my feet felt for support. Then stones came loose.... I can hear them now, falling into the depths ... how terrible...."

Therapist: "... to hear the sound of the stones fall down?"

Narrator: "Now that you ask.... I realized how deep the abyss was when I heard the sound of the stones falling into the void..... And my right hand had no strength left.... (Narrator gasps from the effort) ... I thought it was too soon to die ... but by then, I was already slipping.... I saw the rock wall pass close to my face.... I felt my skin being torn.... I heard it scraping, it was sharp rocks ... but I didn't feel the pain ... I remember wondering for a split second...." (Narrator ponders.)

Thought

Therapist: "What was that thought?"

Narrator: ".... in a flash a thought came to me that I had heard from my parents as a child: 'Always protect your head!' I imagined my skull hitting the rock down in the gorge and cracking." (Narrator makes a disgusted face.)

Emotion

Therapist: "Oh, of course, the head ... can you describe the image you had there.... I can see you are shaking now."

Narrator: "Uhhh, it was a horrible feeling of fear and nausea.... I had forgotten that I had this picture."

Body and Grounding

(The Therapist can see that the Narrator turns very pale.)

Therapist: "There was this feeling of fear and nausea. I can see that even now you feel unwell thinking about it. You are very pale."

Narrator: "Yes, I felt so sick ... lightheaded ... and like fainting."

Therapist: "That image of your head cracking caused you to feel like fainting?"

Narrator: (speaking with a weak voice): "Yes ... ah.... yes ... I keep fainting ever since ... oh!"

Therapist (invites counter maneuvers as narrator becomes dissociative): "Demi, can you hear me well? Can you put some tension on your muscles like moving your legs up and down ... good! Then press your palms together please ... very good! Then stamp your feet ... very good! Can you tell me whether you see me well?"

Narrator: "Yes, I can see you well."

Therapist: "Good. We really want to give your body a chance to stay well-grounded and for you to be in control!"

Narrator: "Yes, phew, my head felt very light."

Meaning

Therapist: "There was a frightening image in your mind, and this caused your body to shut down. A normal reaction of the body when we are disgusted. Can you describe to me what you were envisioning exactly at that time?"

Narrator (speaking slow and looking at therapist's reaction): "I have never told anybody.... For a moment I saw my skull cracking and the brain spilling out ... my body lying down there at the bottom of the gorge all disfigured."

Therapist (looking at narrator steadily): "In your mind's eye you saw your brain spilling out of your skull and your body disfigured. Oh, that must have been a shocking image! What did that mean to you at that moment, Demi?"

Narrator (gulps): "It would be a nasty heap of flesh and blood ... and oh ... my child would remember me like this...."

Narrator (getting more lively): "I had no time to think further you know, all of a sudden, I fell. And I hit the ground with my legs! I fell on my feet and heard a crack in my left leg."

Comparing and Contrasting Here and Now

Therapist: "How does it feel right now to relive that moment of landing hard on the ground?"

Narrator: "Au, uh, I must have been seriously injured, I felt blood running down my leg, but could not feel the pain at first."

Summary

Therapist: "I see, even now you feel the horror of that moment when you realized that you must have been seriously injured. So, do I understand correctly, just after you had this image of the broken head and body in your mind, you hit the ground. You must have hit with great force, since your leg cracked. Were you able to orient yourself?"

Context and Perceptions

Narrator: "Yeah, oh, I was afraid I would faint, but I realized that I had landed. ... I was screaming and gasping for breath.... It took time, but I managed to drag myself to a safer place.... Flashes of pain began to run through my leg. It took me forever to get myself together."

Thoughts

Therapist: "Oh, ... so you gathered all your strength. What do you remember, when you allow yourself to connect to that moment in the past?"

Narrator: "Oh, it is difficult.... I felt bad because Lino had been watching. He wailed. He stared at me. It is saddening that he had to observe my fall and see me getting injured ... yet at the same time, I realized that I could now reach out to him!"

Emotion

Therapist: "You realized you could get to him now? What do you notice? I can see your face brightens up. How did this make you feel?"

Narrator (now overcoming her paralysis): "Oh, so relieved. I felt so deeply relieved...!

Body

Therapist: "I understand. You could now reach out to your child, to Lino. Where in your body could you locate the feelings of that time?"

Narrator: "In my stomach ... in my shoulders ... and my head was intact!! I was incredibly grateful!"

Meaning

Therapist: "Let's go deeper, Demi. What did this moment mean to you? What changed there?"

Narrator: "We would not die. We will be rescued ... this is not the end of our life!..." (starts tearing up).

Therapist: "I can see tears in your eyes."

Narrator (waiting to respond): "... My father isn't right. He always said to us as children, that we deserve to be punished...."

Therapist: "You connect now to your traumatic childhood events, the physical violence by your father?"

Narrator: "... Mhmm, ... but deep down ... someone meant well with us, back there on the mountain...."

Therapist: "You felt protected...."

Narrator (nodding): "It feels good that you can understand."

Comparing and Contrasting Here and Now

Therapist: "And how does it make you feel right now, when you think of that moment back then, when you were reunited with Lino again?"

Narrator: "Oh, I can almost see Lino's presence now. When he was a smaller child, he was so skinny and young. I can feel the love we had."

Therapist: "Where exactly do you feel the love right now, Demi?"

Narrator: "Ah, it is here in my heart (places hand over heart area); it is warm. There is space now."

Demi has now overcome her paralysis and faintness. Therapist gives her a moment to anchor the relief and emotion of love she feels right now.

Step by step the end of the whole story is further recovered. The therapist helps the client narrate the experience to the end. He assists in expressing and identifying what Demi experienced. How the pain became excruciating, how the helicopter came, how they were rescued, and how they both received medical care. The event ends at a safe place in their hospital beds, where they were lying side by side in the evening.

Therapist: "How are you doing now, after having explored the whole story?"

Narrator (spontaneously): "Well now, I can feel that it is over. My leg is healed. We both survived! Which is truly miraculous."

Therapist: "You both survived and healed. You say 'truly miraculous,' so you still feel gratitude. How do you feel about having told the story, Demi?"

Narrator (leans back a bit and gasps for air): "Phew, it's better now.... I wasn't prepared to remember everything so clearly ... even that moment with the shocking image ... only now I realize that's why I've been feeling so nauseous at times and my circulation has been weak ever since."

Therapist: "Yes, this is how we can get stuck in unresolved past moments. You reclaimed and narrated an important event in your life today, Demi. You were even able to connect this experience with other events in your life. We did good work today, I can see you are proud of yourself (smiles). It is remarkable how you were able to recall in such detail. Very well done!

"So how will your day end today? ... How will you spend the afternoon and the evening...?"

The therapist briefly asks the narrator about planned activities after today's session (no drugs after a session) and arranges a new appointment in a couple of days, reassuring connectedness from now until the next session. They say goodbye to each other.

After the narrator has left, or in the following days after the session, the therapist uses the notes he drafted during the narration, to write out the account in the form of an essay

Immediately After the Event Narration – Ending a Session

The storytelling process typically commences with the period before the traumatic incident, develops into the experiences during the actual event, which constitutes the core section, and concludes shortly after the occurrence in a time of comparative safety in the past. This methodology enables the trauma to be embedded within the context of space and time, and helps the narrator to appreciate and comprehend the circumstance of the incident. The "speechless terror" will subside once these hot memory contents are put into words. After the arousal has been reduced noticeably, the narrative is brought to a close for this session.

Speaking of relief, the point of successful trauma therapy is that the tension and anxiety subside because of a detailed exploration of the dreaded, worst moments, and not because that point was quickly skipped or avoided. That would be real malpractice! Therefore, it is essential for a responsible therapist to mentally review the sequence at the end and check with the narrator whether the "worst moment(s)" have been captured in sufficient detail.

Even if time is limited during a session, it is essential to provide closure to a traumatic event that is being addressed. One critical principle is to avoid concluding a session while narrating *toward* a hot spot or when already in the midst of a vivid imaginary exposure.

After successful in-depth work, closure is achieved by moving forward to the period immediately after the event. To do this, the therapist has the narrator verbalize in at least a few sentences what happened in the period following the incident. This can be accomplished by summarizing the minutes, hours, and days following the traumatic event to allow the survivor to integrate the incident into the larger life story. The therapist may use questions such as the following: "What happened next?", "Where were you?", "What did you do after the event?", "Whom did you meet next?", and "What were your expectations at the time?"

Before ending a session, the therapist will assess whether the individual's level of arousal has decreased and ensure that they feel more peaceful, positive, and relaxed (see Figure 24). Objective assessments are made to ensure the person's calm state. It is normal to feel tired after completing an exposure session.

"Looking back on today's storytelling, are you still left with anything now?"

"What is showing up for you talking about it now?"

Note: During exposure, both the level of arousal and the intensity of the feared emotions increase. But at this point in the session, during "closure," the arousal is decreasing, and the therapist supports calming down. Consistency in the direction of the session, without mixing exposure and closure, is imperative!

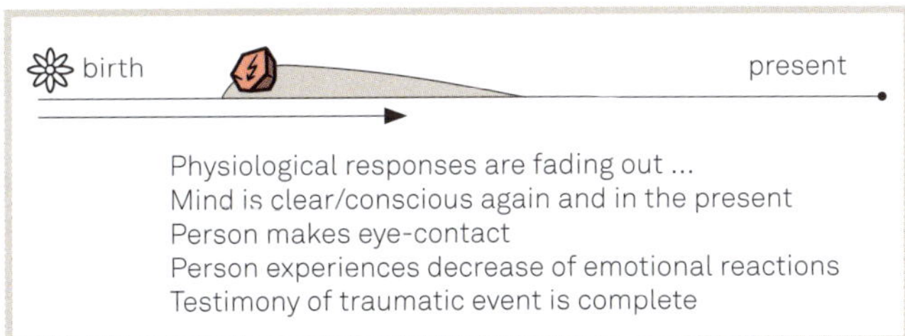

Figure 24. Hot memories have now been integrated into the autobiographical memory.

We can verify this by looking for the following signs (see also Bisbey & Bisbey, 1998):

The emotional state of the narrator has improved: The narrator's emotional state has improved. They demonstrate improvements through good facial color, stating they feel better (relieved and peaceful with a smiling expression), disappearance of muscle tension, a more relaxed posture, and relief from negative physical sensations, such as pain and headaches.

The survivor's attention transitions from its internal environment to an external awareness: The individual establishes eye contact with the therapist, observes their surroundings, acknowledges the passage of time, notices external sounds, and fully experiences the here and now. The participant may discuss future activities or comment on observations regarding the therapist.

There are indications of a shift in the survivor's cognition (see Figure 25): Their perspective on the significance of the traumatic experience appears to have altered.

The narrator has gained insight and is making connections with other experiences in their life, resulting in a greater understanding of the event. The survivor discusses the meaning behind their experience. Finally, the participant states that the traumatic experience now appears to be more resolved and holds less significance than it did previously.

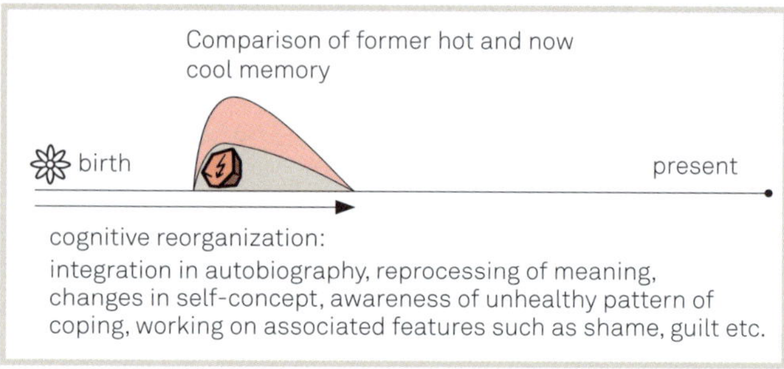

Figure 25. The relived and completed comprehensive story as a tool for insight at the end of session: enhancing meaning making at a deeper level.

This final safeguarding should conclude the treatment session. The ideal time to end a session is when the narrator experiences emotional relief from the most recent stimulating or arousing memory, because resolution has been achieved. The session's duration varies between 90 and 120 minutes, contingent upon the individual and their trauma, and whether there are any other fixed time frames. While the therapist may aspire to cover extensive ground, it is crucial to consider the individual's capacity within a given appointment. It is important not to start working on a new focal point if there is insufficient time to complete the exposure process. A narration session ends at a contextually appropriate moment, such as after completing a chapter of the biography, a certain lifetime period, and/or after strenuous work on a significant event.

The therapist (or another witness who was present during the session taking notes), writes the narrative promptly after its conclusion, arranging the account in chronological order. The narrative is reviewed for completeness, and any gaps are examined and discussed at the start of the next session.

Reading Back the Narrative

The story is read back to the narrator at the beginning of the next session. The therapist retells the previous story slowly and respectfully in first person and past tense with the help of the written testimony. This time, the hot memories are linked to the episodic memory and the arousal peak will be much lower (Figure 26). If this is not the case, an essential part of the story may have been missed, e.g., due to avoidance or shame. The therapist makes sure that the survivor has a chance to listen carefully, to emotionally take on the situation again, while mentalizing, correcting, and adding details. Reviewing the narration during the retelling can be supported by questions like:

How do you feel now when hearing this bit of the story?

Is there a shift of anything inside, when you hear your words?

What do you get when you experience yourself in the past?

What do you feel for your (younger) self? Or: ... for the younger person you have been?

Can you find that in your body?... Does it sit with you somewhere?

When you hear what you reported last time, how does it resonate with you?

How do you view the event now?... with the meaning that you would attach?

Testimony Reading Example: "Mountain Accident"

Background information about what happened before the event called "mountain accident": During the school holidays, Lino got bored being at home, so we often went hiking. Lino was a very active 7-year-old boy who loved being outside, in the mountains, running around, and exploring new places. It was the summer school holidays, July 2015, and we had already spent 3 days hiking in the scenic mountains of (name.) On this particular warm sunny day, we looked out our cabin window at the stunning peaks of Mount (name) and got ready to go on a hike.

The story unfolds up to the traumatic moment, how they walk up the mountain, get lost, the boy tumbles down, and his mum is searching for him. Verbatim from Demi's testimony:

... And then, suddenly, I saw Lino who was barely able to sit on the wet mountain ledge. There was a deep gorge below him. Lino was clinging to the ledge. I knew, I had to climb down from higher up to get to him. The clouds were forming a dark mass now. It was the afternoon, and we were both already so tired. To make matters worse, it also started raining. I heard Lino's frightened scream. And I shouted back: "Stay where you are!"

When I heard him scream, I thought he is really panicking and needs to calm down or else he would do something stupid, maybe try to move. That was an unthinkable thought.

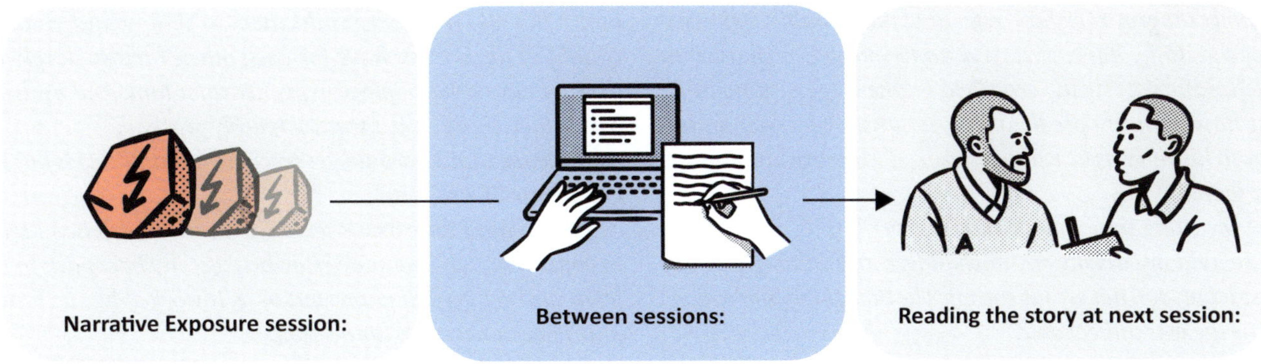

Processing of traumatic events: The arousal decreases during imaginal reliving and the therapist makes a transcript of key points.

The therapist structures the narrative, transcribes the oral account and brings the draft document to the next session.

After the survivor is back and the session is initiated, the therapist provides a retelling of the last Narrative Exposure.

They read the written down narration from the previous session sentence by sentence. The narrator is now the listener and can review their past in this way from the presence and from the present state of mind. The survivor let's the reading-aloud sink in and may want to comment and add more recovered parts of what happened then.

This is a very active, co-constructive process. The therapist encourages the survivor's support, self-care and compassion for her/his younger self in the stories. If indicated, some passages are reworked in more depth with Narrative Exposure.

Then the entire event is read again.

Figure 26. Read back is a mandatory step in NET. Be sure to use the survivor's own words and idioms as much as possible. Allow mentalization when reading and further reflection on the testimony. Also available as a handout in the online supplementary materials for this book.

I felt so incredibly helpless. He was too far away. I am his mum, I must help him. I was feeling desperate. Helplessness took over. He was too far away at that point. My heart was beating so fast.

I knew that he needed to calm down to be safe, and I needed to get to him, or he could do something unpredictable and move closer to the edge of the rock ledge. I thought he could fall and die. In my body the energy faded. I felt so alone at that moment without help.

It started to pour with rain, it was pounding down on us, and the sky had gone dark. I saw my son sitting crouched on this narrow, small ledge, barely able to hold on.

I looked at the climb and saw that there was no path between us. The rock face was now wet and slippery. But I just had to take action. At least try to do something! I tried to step further down with my right foot. But immediately I lost my footing. I felt that my hands could also not hold on. I kept losing my grip. There was this icy coldness. My body was stiffening. I had to concentrate. I needed to get to my son. But I was terrified by the thought of not making it.

Then my feet slipped. I accidentally kicked off stones with my feet. I had no support. I was only gripping on with my hands. I was basically hanging. Fear surged through me like an electric shock!

Then I realized that I felt deep regret. I should have never come here. At the same time I knew that staying like this for longer would not help. I knew that every second I would lose muscle power. I was not sure if I could still move my limbs. I knew I would have to let go. I did not want this to be the end of my life.

My hands were sweaty. It was very cold. I could not see well now, only the grey rock face in front of me. I could see the colors of the stone, dark, wet. And under me was a shadow to my left. Lino was sitting crouched on the ledge. I thought he must have seen my predicament, because there was an urgency in his voice as he was screaming, "Mommy...Mommy... I am scared!"

At the same time I knew that my wet hands wouldn't be able to hold my weight for much longer and I thought: God, please let my son not see me slip off. The thought of him watching me die was unbearable.

I couldn't feel my fingers anymore. Only the icy coldness. I could not stop the panic. My body was out of control. I was trembling.

I knew I would have to let go. I realized that I was going to fall. I was going to fall off this cliff, and I couldn't do anything. I felt lightheaded at this moment and defeated, because all my battles in life seemed lost at that moment. I had been strong for so many years, and now I couldn't keep it up.

My arms and my legs kept trembling. I knew it was only a matter of time. My muscles grew tired. My feet felt for support. Then stones came loose. I could hear them falling into the depths. That was terrible. They fell a long time before reaching the ground.

My right hand had no more muscle strength left. In the last moment, I thought it was too soon to die, but by then, I was already slipping. I saw the rock wall pass close to my face. I felt my skin being torn. I heard it scraping, it was sharp rocks, but I didn't feel the pain.

Then I dropped.

I remember wondering for a split second. In a flash a thought came to me that I had heard from my parents as a child: "Always protect your head!" That's when I imagined my skull hitting the rocks down in the gorge and cracking. I was overcome by a terrible feeling of horror and nausea. I felt so sick, lightheaded, and like fainting. For a moment I had seen my skull cracking and the brain spilling out with my body lying down there at the bottom of the gorge all disfigured.

Immediately I thought of Lino. It would be a horrific death and my child would remember me like this.

I hit the ground with my legs. I fell on my feet first and heard the sound of a cracking bone. And when I felt the blood on my left leg, it almost made me faint, but I realized that I had landed. It took me forever to get myself together. I was gasping for breath. I dragged myself to a safer place.

The first thing I thought after the fall was that Lino had been watching. He wailed as he stared at me. He had to observe my fall and see me getting injured.

However, I realized that finally I could now reach out to him. Lino was a smaller child then, so skinny and young. I could feel the love we have for each other. I felt so deeply relieved. I have a warm place in my heart for him. And my head was intact. Suddenly, I was incredibly grateful.

It meant that we would get rescued and that this is not the end of our life!

I told Lino I only broke one leg. Not too bad. Then I tried to control myself and move slowly to get my backpack to the front and get my cell phone out of it. It worked like a charm, and I had a network connection!

I was able to call mountain rescue. They told me to send a location. The man was very calm and reassuring. I was sure it would not take long. I told Lino to lean on the mountain and not to look down. The helicopter will be here soon.

The helicopter came, we were rescued, and both of us received medical care. We were in a safe place in our hospital beds, where Lino and I were lying side by side in the evening.

It took several weeks of recovery and also physical rehabilitation for me.

Once reread, the final narrative of this experience will be integrated into the testimony of Demi's whole life.

How to Deal With Loss and Grief – Stones

Having to let go is the painful reality of loss. Grieving requires rituals to adjust to a world in which the deceased is missing, and physical representations to find a lasting connection. This dynamic is quite different from that for an anxiety that interferes with memory, such as an alarm response. It is possible to mark the experience of death with a stone, as the Lifeline can be established on the time axis through the dimensions of arousal and valence. However, a cold and hard stone may not adequately represent the love felt for the deceased as a symbol. Some survivors decide to of use small candles or flowers to symbolize their mourning; however, this is not mandatory in the NET procedure.

Individuals may experience the loss of a loved one due to a traumatic event, such as in a war, an accident, natural disaster, or organized violence, among others. First, an imaginal exposure is carried out, and the entire narrative is created. This detailed work often brings to light many new levels of experience and insight in memory of the person who was lost. In the aftermath, individuals often create cherished memories and engage in rituals and rites to facilitate the grieving process. For instance, one might dedicate a home shrine featuring a photo and symbol, or launch a self-made paper boat downstream while making a wish. The effectiveness of these interventions can vary based on factors including age, religion, and cultural background.

It is very common that survivors feel guilty about the death of a loved one. This is often in hindsight and based on rumination, with the wish that they could have changed what happened (control!). Often the realization of shared responsibility and the understanding from the narrative of the (illusionary) desire for control bring relief. Guilt wants to give back. Perhaps you can work out a plan for how the person can support other similar groups, even though their own loved one has died.

Bear in mind: A person we mourn was part of our life. We had a deep relationship, spent quality time with them, cherished every moment, and shared many events. In the context of NET, it is essential to offer the survivor the opportunity to revisit the past by narrating a flower situation with the departed loved one. This allows individuals to fully immerse themselves in the memories of their loved one and engage with their senses, including scent, voice, touch, thoughts, and bodily sensations, as well as participating in shared activities. Again, work through the specific events on the Lifeline as they chronologically happened. Experiencing such an event may provide comfort to those grieving, and foster a positive memory. For instance, "On a summer day, my family and I swam in Crummock Water where we laughed and splashed in the water while throwing a ball. Afterwards, we rested on the grass where my son gave me a warm embrace...." This is very beautiful situation on that particular day, in a particular year, at that particular lake, etc. To go deep in those specific moments leaves an intense warmth and loving feeling in the body. It makes clear why we cherish them so much. This precious gift (sensations, thoughts, emotion, bodily feelings, meaning), can be carried with the survivor forever.

Be sure to carefully read the experience(s) back to the narrator. And perhaps the client may have personal sentences to add.

A New Understanding and the Days After the Narration – Beginning to Change

Narrators typically utilize the cooling-off period at the end of a session to comprehend the trauma and assign significance to their experiences. After a session, trauma survivors often take time to reflect and gain new insights about the meaning of the event for their lives. They may realize that their negative emotions and behaviors (such as anxiety, helplessness, mistrust, or anger outbursts, among others) stem from the adverse childhood experiences and the traumatic event(s). The narrative's explanation and understanding offer a deeper comprehension of experiences, which is emotionally satisfying and subjectively true (Figure 27). It provides meaningful insight into existential relevance. Additionally, an elaborate account of the event can provide better insights into the individual's behavior and self-assessment of their actions. This may result in a reduction of feelings of guilt and shame, as the individual gains a novel understanding of the underlying motives, patterns, and forces at play during the traumatic experience (see Chapter 5 and the section Shame and Guilt).

The next step is to compare the memory when it was difficult to manage, with how it is now when it is easier, and talk about its meaning. However, if the narrator needs more time to understand the impact of an exposure session, they can delay this step until the next session. After an exposure session, many survivors need time to process it mentally and emotionally. Much of the helpful advancement in awareness and integration of past events, known as memory reorganization, continues to happen further on its own after the session, throughout the following days, and while sleeping. When the therapist and the survivor meet again, the therapist should listen attentively to any thoughts or concerns the individual has had since their last meeting. The therapist can explain that it is typical to have new insights when understanding information, indicating progress toward healthy growth. If the person wants to talk about these things, the therapist can assist by suggesting more realistic beliefs and supporting the consideration of changes to their daily life, home, and social life.

If the survivor brings it up, we can talk about topics related to ethics and human rights. They may also want to work on getting back their self-respect or taking action, like getting involved in politics. The NET protocol is relatively brief. We recommend completing the biographical work before delving into political activism or facing trauma-related topics in public relations or legal proceedings. Take a few months to recover from symptoms and make overall adjustments and strengthen your mind and body. The participant may mention topics related to healing, such as joining a support group or seeing an alternative therapist who specializes in bodywork or massage. These ideas may or may not be helpful during the NET procedure. Currently, there is no systematic scientific evidence for the effectiveness of such combined approaches. We would expect meditation practices or body-related therapies to work better once the person has faced

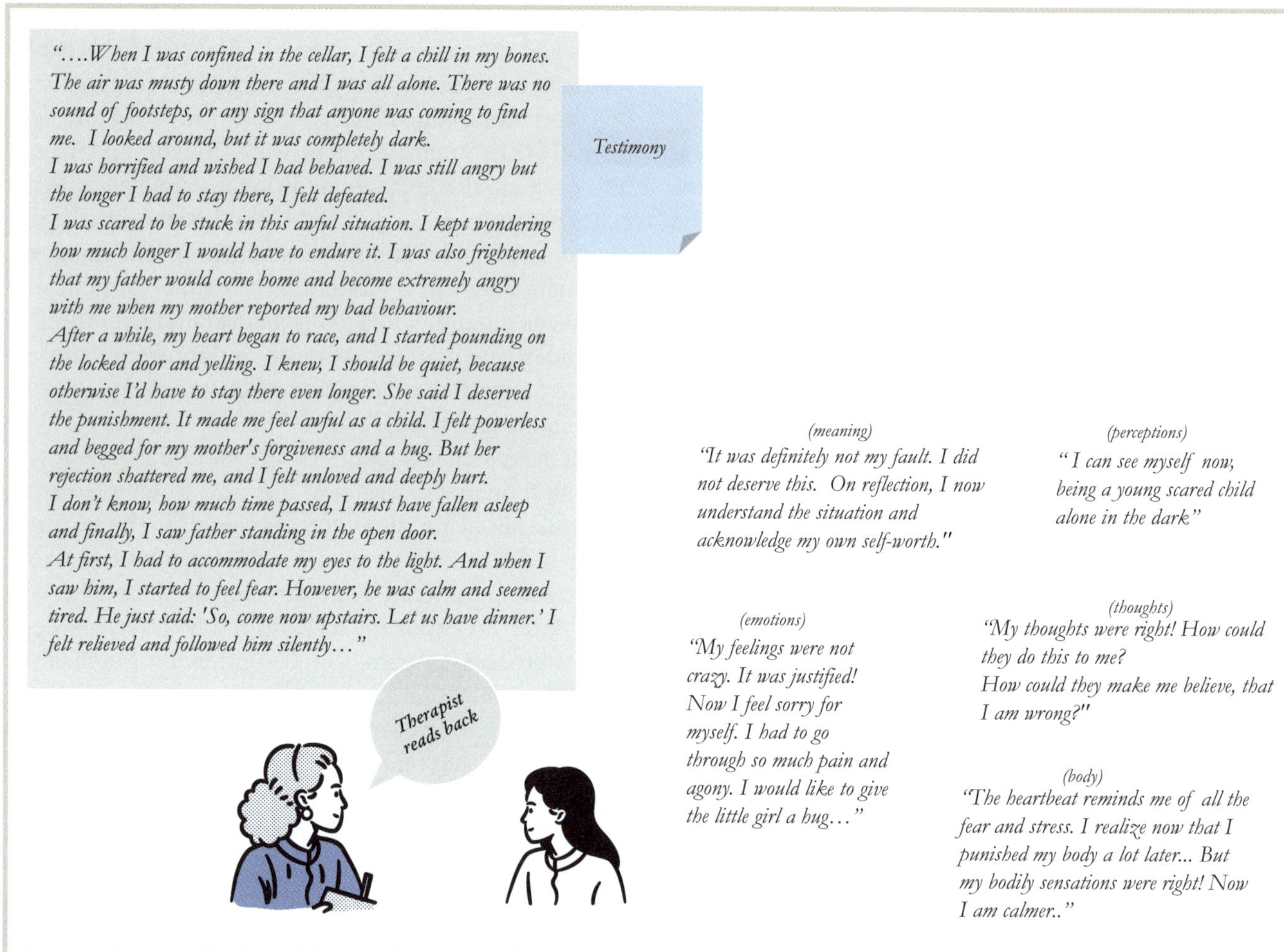

Figure 27. Reading back the stories, is a key element of the NET procedure: rereading and retelling can be seen as a powerful and effective way of feeling seen, heard, and validated, transforming the narrator into a listener and historian of the event(s).

their trauma story, overcome avoidance, and is no longer afraid of internal reminders.

After the Narrative Exposure sessions, participants will undergo various processing steps. They might face thoughts or feelings they had been avoiding, which could lead either to increased sensitivity or to more courageous behavior. As a result, participants may feel heightened levels of emotion and make new experiences for themselves. It is important to inform the survivor that these experiences are normal and part of their healing process. Encourage narrators to carefully note anything they observe. This will bring about transformation changes in their inner world and in how they interact with others.

Frequency of Session Scheduling

Due to the demanding character of the work and necessary processing, sessions should not be spaced too far apart. There is ample empirical evidence to support the effectiveness of one to two NET sessions per week. While less frequent sessions are possible, some survivors may have difficulty coping with longer intervals between sessions.

For clients who have reported experiencing severe traumatic incidents and interpersonal violence at various points in their lives, it is crucial to establish a consistent and dependable schedule of appointments. This approach will help prevent avoidance behaviors that can lead to prolonged suffering. There are even some recent developments in NET scheduling of sessions much closer together (Schalinski & Ardino, 2020; Strijk et al., 2020).

However, much of the memory reconsolidation requires sleep or at least a relaxed period with a nap in between sessions. But to our knowledge, it remains to be investigated how closely sessions can be scheduled.

A definitive exception to scheduling sessions close together is for the last session. It may be beneficial to schedule the final session a few days later than usual in order to give the narrator time to reflect on and reconsider the entire testimony process.

Important rule: Never schedule a vacation or extended break *before* major events are showing up (on the Lifeline) to be talked about next session!

Tenses of the Narrative – Emotional Impact

In a Narrative Exposure session, the survivor should become fully engaged in the controlled reliving of the event. However, it is important to note that reliving the event must always be approached in an *as if* only manner. We aim for the individual to emotionally process their past experiences while staying grounded in the present moment. It is crucial that they maintain a strong connection to reality and do not feel abruptly thrown back into the *there and then* without awareness of the present here and now.

In NET, we use verb tenses in speech as needed to modulate the process: present tense is helpful when a narrator is underengaged or cannot connect to the past, because they cannot retrieve memory content well. Present tense intensifies the experience, brings it to the forefront, and helps stimulate memory connections to fully recapture the scenes.

Past tense pushes our experience further away from immediacy and therefore cools it down or reduces the excitement, which is helpful for better structuring when a narrator is flooded with memories or overly activated by arousal.

When *underengaged*: use the present tense and an egocentric viewpoint to make the scene more vivid and to get the full activation of the fear/trauma network (e.g., "You are lying on the grass.... Can you feel the hand on your body now? Where do you feel it touching you? ...").

When *overly aroused* (or panicky): use the past tense and an allocentric viewpoint to achieve a lower level of autonomous activation, to reinforce reality, and to point out that the threat is (long) over (e.g., "Take a moment and experience [sensations in the here and now] how you are sitting on your chair now in the room with me here, while we are *thinking* about that moment in the past 10 years ago, when he had his hand on your ..."). Explicitly *compare and contrast* then and now responses, sensations, emotions, and cognitions during the session (e.g., "Your heart was beating in that moment then, how is it now? ...).

Finally, in the written testimony, everything is phrased and read back in the past tense (because it happened in the past).

Levels of Parallel Processing During NET – Therapist's Tasks

There are different processes going on in parallel that need the therapist's continuous monitoring during and between NET sessions:

1. **The incidents** (past) – perceptions, thoughts, feelings, bodily sensations, and meaning content at times of incidents
2. **he here and now** – perceptions, thoughts, feelings, bodily sensations, and meaning content while recalling the event during sessions
3. **Gaining cognitive and emotional control** – as cues that trigger memories can be identified – *during and between sessions*
4. **The narration** – keeping a chronological and comprehensive testimony
5. **Therapeutic contact** – as in any psychotherapy, the nature of the therapeutic relationship is crucial, and establishing a rational and effective connection between the therapist and client is essential for the success. Checking in with clients about their experience in therapy and seeking feedback helps to address any concerns or issues that may arise – *during and between sessions*
6. **Therapist and other witnesses to the narration** – as well as the interpreter's reaction and psychohygiene – *during and between sessions*
7. **Admin** (red tape, set time limits) – *during and between sessions*

Following Session(s)

Figures 28, 29, 30, and 31 depict how the following Narrative Exposure sessions should be structured.

Reading the Story to the Survivor

As mentioned above, an important aspect of creating the testimony is writing down the story behind each stone. So, in the session following each Narrative Exposure, the written narrative from the previous (!) session

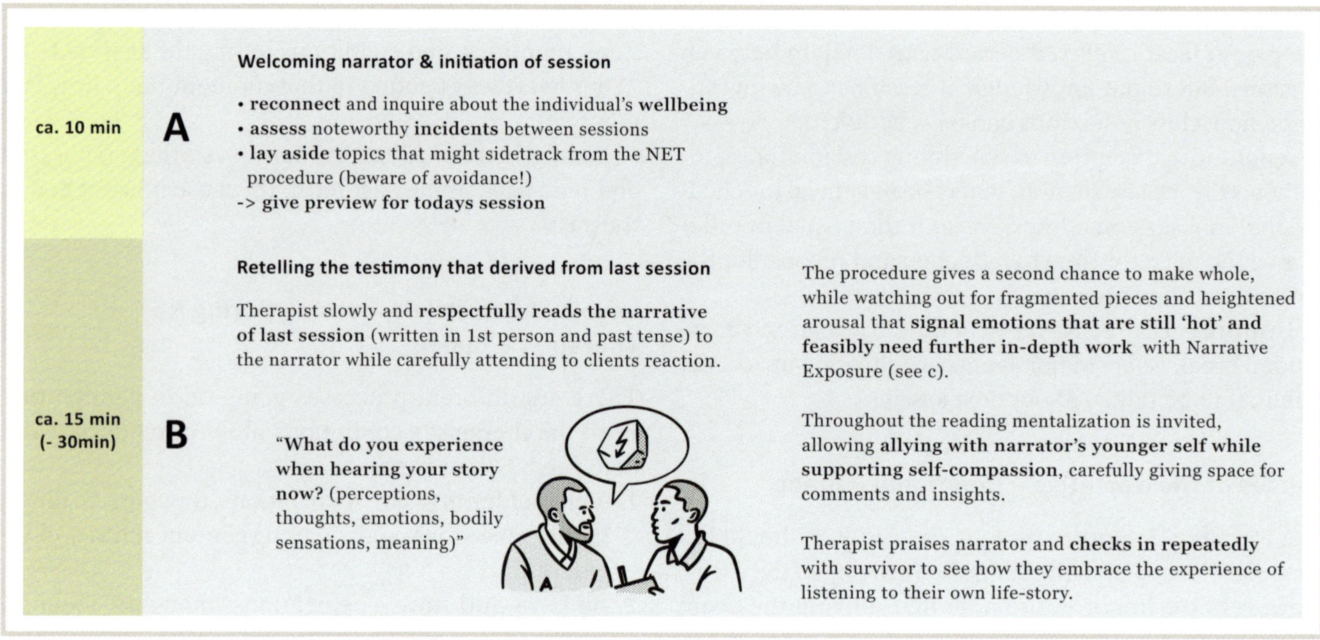

Figure 28. How to structure the beginning of the following Narrative Exposure session(s). Also available as a handout in the online supplementary materials for this book.

will be read by the therapist – sometimes in abbreviated form – to the participant. Session by session, the life story becomes more complete. The reading back of the stories facilitates further emotional processing and expositioning (stepping out of the position of the victim) during the review. "When you compare with what you faced then, is everything shown correctly, what happened? Is anything missing? ... Do you want to add anything?"

The therapist is careful to ask about changes in the survivor's perceptions. "What do you experience now, when you hear your story...?" If the material is still highly charged at the time of reading, the survivor is asked to reimagine and retell the incident in slow motion, using the text from the last time to understand and digest what happened and what it actually meant for cognitions, emotions, body, and change of meaning. Sometimes there is an underlying theme that needs to be uncovered; other times there has been an avoidance of accepting some aspect of the story, or great fear has made it impossible to allow an important missing link to be filled, etc. Often the tension and anxiety will subside only when the situation is fully understood, and these things can be put into words.

During the read back, the narrator is invited to mentally and emotionally move back and forth between the experience of the younger self and the current experiencing with its more mature views. "...So, how do you feel now when you see your younger self in the past?"

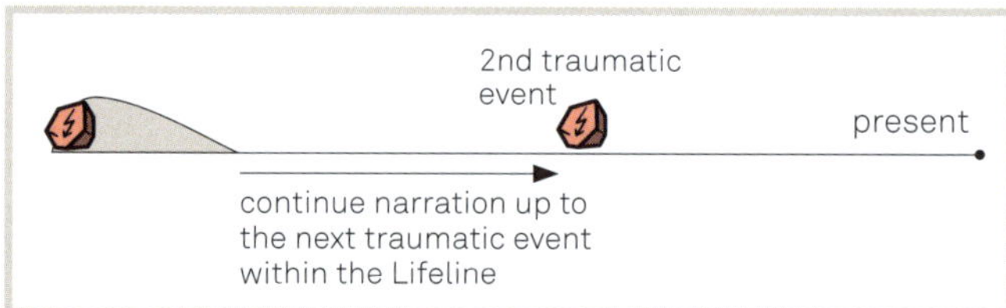

Figure 29. After reading at the beginning of the next Narrative Exposure session(s), the first-person chronological narration is resumed until reaching the next hot spot on the Lifeline.

The observation of our younger self's experience of past situations with compassion naturally supports mentalization and self-acceptance. In addition, stepping back as a listener to our life story allows us to make a connection between the dynamics of past situations and the patterns and schemes of current life situations in which the same forces may be controlling or influencing our emotions and actions in previously unrecognized ways. This can help in comprehending our past, have a preventative effect, and be a safeguard against unconscious repetition and reenactment.

ca. 45 min **C**

Narrative Exposure with significant events

Chronological narration along the biography in first-person is **resumed until reaching a 'hot spot'. Therapist helps** narrator to recognize the specific event ("title on the lifeline? time and place?") and invites **grounding (brief body scan)** to ensure a good sense of control. **Exposure is initiated** through a good situational **past context description.** Both engage in a **detailed 'exposure-conversation narration'** (see figure) with the non-judgemental emotional presence of the testimony bearer throughout.

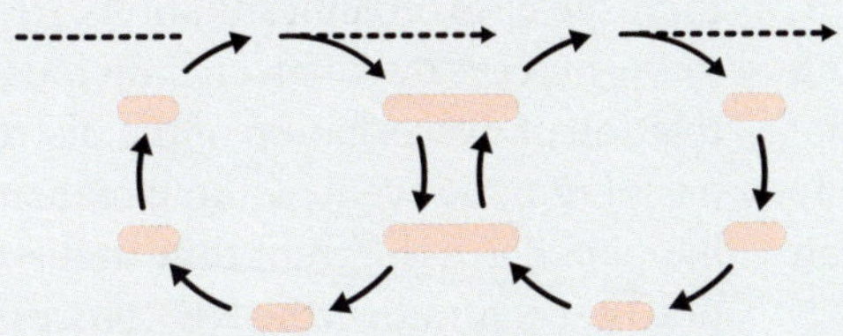

The *Narrative Exposure Circle* offers a structured wheel of exploration that enables the narration to proceed in a safe way through highly arousing events where recall is fragmented. The step-by-step exploration in great detail is empathically supported by the therapist walking through the imagined scene shoulder by shoulder with the narrator.

The "stone" is relived in the present and contrasted with the past.

To set Narrative Exposure in motion means supporting the **verbalization of sensations, cognitions, emotions, bodily experiences and meanings** that the narrator is experiencing both then and now. In difficult moments, the therapist asks primarily closed questions, is clearly active and directive, mirrors the experience, paraphrases, immediately reflects back and gives direct feedback on observations. All of this means that the therapist remains emotionally close at all times and thus enables grounding. The therapist repeatedly offers a summary of the narrative content, helps to modulate intensity, and supports grounding by **contrasting the levels of experience in the past and present.**

Figure 30. Once more, Narrative Exposure is employed through the verbalization of the different levels of experiencing. This offers a structured *wheel* of exploration that drives the story forward and enables a comprehensive, safe, and revealing in-depth narration. Also available as a handout in the online supplementary materials for this book.

ca. 10 min **D**

End of narration & end of session

Storytelling is completed at the temporal end of the past incident. The hours, days, and weeks that followed the event are wraped up. Provide your appreciation and invite ventilating of todays work.

Allow **meaning making** about the significance of the recovered memories.

If need be, topics that where laid aside at the beginning of session are discussed now.

Therapist **guides out:** "what will the rest of today look like for you...?"

Goodbye: set appointment for next session, therapist communicates connectedness between sessions.

Figure 31. Ending a Narrative Exposure session. Also available as a handout in the online supplementary materials for this book.

By going through this step-by-step process of reading back the narrative to the narrator and having the details filled in, an entire narration or eyewitness testimony will be completed, including all traumatic events of that person's life in chronological order (see Figure 32; examples of testimonies are available in Appendix 2).

When the timeline concludes in the present, the narrative delves into the individual's current and prospective life paths, including their aspirations and desires for the future.

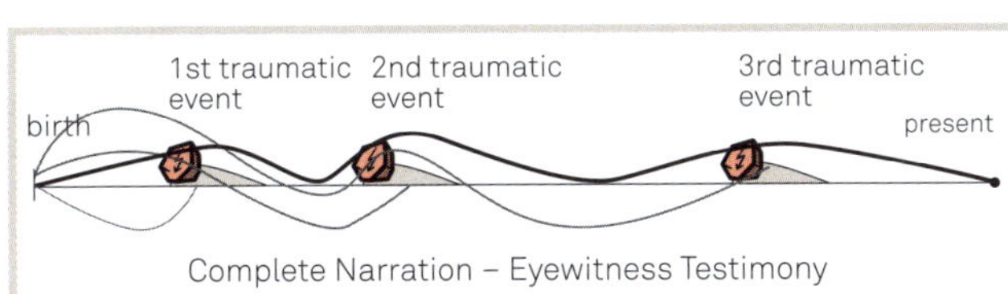

Figure 32. When all the significant specific events have been covered (typically in about 6 to 14 double sessions), the entire narrative is completed. In the last session, a final Lifeline can be laid out.

Last Session

At the last appointment, the final printout of the testimony is brought to the session.

First, a final Lifeline is laid out, now much more informed and complete, including the recovered parts. Only if needed (for human rights or forensic purposes) the whole testimony might be reread to the narrator, and all final corrections are made. Sometimes the content of nightmares can also be helpful in understanding the individual's current stresses and strains. In this way, the therapist ensures that the criteria for closure are reached. By the final NET session, the recall of life events during the Lifeline or rereading should have lost its highly arousing effect. Some survivors, upon review of the work, may comment that they have reclaimed their lives and had an important personal growth experience.

Finally, the participant, the therapist, and other witnesses such as the interpreter sign the written report. The signed document is given to the narrator if the narrator feels comfortable with it, combined with the advice to think very carefully about who and when others may and should receive this narration. At the individual's request, the testimony may be anonymized and used for human rights or political and public awareness work.

The final Lifeline reveals the *gestalt* of the life (Schauer et al., 2011; Merriam-Webster Dictionary: Medical Definition: "gestalt: a structure, arrangement, or pattern of physical, biological, or psychological phenomena so integrated as to constitute a functional *unit with properties not derivable by summation of its parts*" [emphasis added]). Working through the whole life in NET provides a framework that emphasizes acknowledging the survivor's whole life story. It is a respectful and significant moment to reflect with the survivor on their journey at the conclusion of treatment.

Trusting Narrative Exposure in the Face of Typical Trauma Memory Dynamics

We need stories in order to understand ourselves.
Salman Rushdie

It is beyond question that it is beneficial to explicitly recover traumatic situations that one has suffered and to know what has happened. But, what should we do when there is no story, only an involuntary intruding piece of memory of immense negative power that is overwhelming? Or the other way round, when many doors open at once, and one memory network ignites the next and the one after that, and various fragments and pieces of memory hijack the survivor's mind?

During NET it is rare for earlier events to emerge unexpectedly, because we work chronologically, touching on each important situation at a time during the Lifeline exercise. Then, during Narrative Exposure, the story is told from earliest episodic memory onward.

Avoidance and momentarily insufficient access to memory content can interfere with desired construction of a narration, and survivors and therapists can find themselves in difficult situations. *Retraumatization* refers to the process by which an individual experiences a reactivation or exacerbation of the distress associated with a past traumatic event, without realizing that this event has happened at a different time and space – that is, a situation that contradicts the NET process. There are two such situations that are typically feared by therapists: (1) having to work from memory fragments to complete recall, and (2) handling the sudden emergence of unexpected, older memories.

Working From Memory Fragment to Complete Recall

The situation of working your way from a memory fragment to complete recall and narration of the whole episode involves overcoming seeming memory blankness following trauma. The being confronted with extremely isolated fragments of intrusive perceptions, such as a single image, can cause great distress, but does not provide any indication of context, of who was there, and what was happening. With this problem, the individual remains tremendously stressed and trapped in the past. Creating a chronological narrative seems impossible, since the memory fragment is not presented as part of a story.

Survivors suffering from trauma spectrum disorders have impaired access to episodic memory. This state is characterized by the inability to connect intruding hot traumatic memories to an episode. Often referred to as *psychogenic amnesia,* it typically occurs due to a traumatic situation that individuals wish to consciously or unconsciously avoid through repression.

To overcome the destructive dynamics of unrecovered trauma material and make it accessible for reprocessing, it is helpful to know how to activate the dissociated episodic memory content to allow full retrieval of past events. Therefore, in the case of missing cold, autobiographical memory, we need to follow the trail that leads to the time and place where a traumatic event has happened. Because of the way memories are encoded and stored, memory retrieval requires the brain to revisit the neural pathways formed during encoding, and the strength of these pathways determines how quickly the memory can be retrieved. In particular, survivors of traumatic experiences during childhood (e.g., repeated CSA) often do not know the sequence of trauma scenes that allows for a straightforward chronological narration.

The three steps of the NET procedure each gain access to the memory pathways differently, and more and more of the meaningful life events become chronologically retrievable to the individual participating in the procedure. At the beginning of Step 3, Narrative Exposure, when the life story is told from birth, the survivor has already gained a fairly good overview of stressful experiences through the intake checklist and the laying out of the Lifeline. They have become aware of people, situations, and contexts that were important, and which patterns and schemes of coping and consequences have emerged.

As we proceed chronologically along the biographical timeline in NET, we automatically encounter seemingly amnestic gaps in memory as well as moments of fragmented recollection and unbearable tension that may indicate a hidden place of trauma on the timeline.

Identifying and Uncovering Traumatic Life Moments and Filling Memory Gaps

First: Build Context

When memory gaps occur, it is advisable to first walk through the spatial environments of this life period (typical places, scenes, everyday contexts). Explicitly describing the spatial contexts is an imaginary revisiting.

Here is an example:

Paul is in psychotherapy and talks about being plagued by an intrusive image that is causing him great distress. On his Lifeline, the therapist had already seen that there was a gap at the age of 10–12 years that he could not fill. Then they moved on and recounted the first 10 years of his life until they reached the period in question.

To move on from here, helpful questions can help evoke memory associations, such as "What was a typical day like back then?" "What sort of person were you at 10 years old?" "How did you look?" "What did you like to wear" "Who was your friend at school?" "What was your school environment, the classroom like at that age?" "Can you describe your leisure activities?" "What did your house look like? Let us walk through the different rooms of your family's home together...."

Second: Watch Out for Physiological Arousal

During the explicit description of the different areas of life, the therapist pays careful attention to the places where the narrator's arousal increases. As soon as unpleasant sensations or tensions arise in the recollection of certain places, people, activities, etc., a more detailed exploration is needed. This creates space for visual memories to emerge (using antidissociative strategies if necessary). If the memories are traumatic, the emergence is often accompanied by obvious emotional upset and physiological arousal (e.g., increased heartbeat, sweaty palms). To explore the environment of the past situations, the therapist may prompt with questions such as "What did it smell like?" "What did you see there?" "What did you hear at that moment?" "Who was there?" "What were you thinking?" "What did it feel like to be in that place in the past?" "How did your body react?" and "What did it mean to you?"

In Paul's case, he described in the session how his heart started beating more and more strongly, as he explored the first floor of his parent's house from that time.

Third: Apply the Narrative Exposure Cycle to the Memory Fragment to Recover the Whole Story as a Motion Picture

Contextual cues and focus on perceptions trigger memory connections that involve primary sensory areas becoming active. In our experience, survivors with blank memories of highly arousing situations may have an isolated physical sensation or a single visual fragment, such as a static image, a sound, or a voice only, at first. Whatever it is, the therapist starts the storytelling with the narrator from this moment. Since it is impossible to know the beginning of the event, both explore this snippet. Staying with these pieces of information that the narrator's body is showing can be used to get a good description with the help of a focused Narrative Exposure. The whole sequence of that specific event will become accessible.

The therapist must be very careful not to specify anything here, so as not to suggest false associations, but instead to allow space for the narrator to connect with all of the details they can recall. The therapist is simply providing a safe framework for the memory to come to the fore.

Case of Paul: From a Visual Intrusion to Accessing the Whole Story

In the example of Paul and the therapist working through his frightening image (he calls it "dark energy") coming at him without knowing what it is and whether there is a real story from the past behind it, the therapist uses the Narrative Exposure cycle (perception, thoughts, emotions, physical reactions, meaning) to defuse and pause for a moment and help Paul to respond to the activation and allow time for activating neural assemblies connected to this network.

Paul (as narrator) starts the Narrative Exposure with a visual perception that haunts him. After some initial psychoeducation he starts to describe:

Narrator: "As I told you, I believe I am upstairs in my parent's home in this scene. Again and again, I see a face in front of me ... and ..." (Paul makes a sad grimace, sniffing). "I don't want to look at it ... it's painful...."

Therapist: "Yes, Paul, this is the picture you keep seeing. I can see this is very frightening for you and just how much you don't want to see it again.... Can you describe for me which rooms are there on the first floor. Take me along and we will walk through shoulder by shoulder. OK? What do you see, when you come upstairs?"

Narrator: "Well... (Paul is fidgeting on his chair), I don't remember which city we lived then, or what the place looked like from outside the house. My mother kept changing locations, and we moved a lot. But I know the blue carpet, and I can tell you the rooms. To the right there was a bathroom with brown tiles, next a guestroom with a strong smell of room freshener, at the end of the corridor, there was a little window, and opposite, on the other side there was my parent's bedroom and our children's nursery" (Paul takes a sharp breath and closes his eyes.)

Therapist: "What just happened Paul? I can see you closing your eyes, you really don't want to see it, I understand, but we can do it together."

Narrator: "Yes. There is the picture again! Her face is distorted with pain. She is crying. Her face is all red...." (Paul covering his own face with the hands.)

Therapist: "That must be a horrible sight. You covered your face. Perhaps there's something embarrassing? Can you take the handle and go into the kids' bedroom?"

Narrator: "Yes! She is trembling! I can hear her hear crying now, indeed. And now I see a hand.... The hand is grabbing her waist...."

Therapist: "You see a hand touching 'her'? Do you recognize the hand?"

Narrator (waiting): "...No... It's a dirty hand."

Therapist: "Can you see rings on the fingers of this hand?... hair on the hand or arm?... anything particular?"

Narrator: "I can see a tattoo now! ... I know this hand. Ugh, my stomach hurts!"

Therapist: "What did you think? What was going on for you?"

Narrator: "She is in pain and fear. I can't help her.... It is my sister."

Therapist: "Your sister. Can you see why she is in pain? What is happening?"

Narrator: "I don't know ... my heart is beating." (Paul presses his fist to stomach.)

Therapist: "I can see you pressing your stomach? Do you feel disgusted right now? Is that how you felt back then? Something very disturbing was happening.... What is your sister's name, Paul?"

Narrator (whispers): "It's Louise."

Therapist: "Can you look to your right and left where you are with Louise there?... Was it in a room?"

Narrator (breathing heavily): "It's in our nursery.... I can see a pair of jeans pants behind my sister.... I mean legs, with the pants down.... Oh, no!!" (tormented)

Therapist: "This is a difficult moment to remember, Paul. I can see you are terribly worried. Who is it? Who wears the pants?"

Narrator (grimacing in disgust): "... Now I ... now I see what he's doing ... Oh, my God!"

Therapist: "What do you see? What is so disgusting?"

Narrator: "I see my stepfather now moving back and forth ... behind my sister. He is having sex with my sister. He is forcing his penis into my sister!" (Paul begins to cry in distress.)

Therapist: "At the time you had to watch this and you were crying. Where were you, Paul? What was going on for you in this moment?"

Narrator (bursts out): "I had to sit on the sofa in front of her, and I had to watch. He always did that to me. I hate him! What he did was so sick! I wanted to kill this bastard! I can see it all now.... I hate it to be true." (Narrator's face flushes with anger.)

Therapist: "There were a lot of emotions, and you had to hold them back. You felt for your sister, and you hated that your stepfather raped her right in front of you.

Narrator: "Yes, I felt so helpless, and he grinned and moaned and enjoyed the situation."

Therapist: "What a malicious intent to have you watch your sister being horribly abused...."

Narrator lowers his head and nods in despair. "Now I know what this face that appears in my nightmares means.... It is my sister suffering. I will always hate him. I hate all men!"

Therapist: "That's a terrible crime, Paul, that he committed. Nobody may inflict sexual violence on children."

Paul looks up.

Therapist: "Now, that we have found a place for this isolated picture of your sister's face, can you remember, how this traumatic event began?"

Narrator: "...Yes, very well. I remember that my mother was away on a business trip that day. I didn't want her to go. I had begged her to stay...."

Therapist: "Your mother was on a business trip, and you were how old?"

Narrator: "I think I was about 10 years old. It was springtime, because I remember my T-shirt. It had short sleeves. The sun was shining in the window."

Therapist: "Good. Where did this happen, Paul? At what time in your life?"

Narrator: "We were living in Portugal at the time. I remember the street (name). My stepfather (name) came home earlier that day. I heard the door slam into the lock and knew immediately that I had to pay attention. It was in the afternoon. We were alone with him. No one would come until the evening...."

The whole story is now being told, from the beginning to the end, just as it is in a typical Narrative Exposure session.

At the end, Paul is shaking his head again and begins to rock back and forth in his chair in the therapy room: "I can't believe it was my stepfather. I didn't know that anymore. I didn't want to know, hoping this was not ..."

Fourth: Be Supportive and Allow Time to Accept and Evaluate the New Insight

When repressed trauma material appears explicitly for the first time during an exposure session, it may be perceived as alien to one's own biography. Previously, these memories have always been fended off through avoidance and dissociation. To avoid the insertion of *false memories*, the survivor's uncertainty about the credibility and authenticity of such memories must be respected. Typically, gaining these insights is difficult and has serious consequences. In NET, the therapist empathically summarizes what has been understood, validates the important work accomplished at the end of the narrative, and supports the survivor in taking time to understand the new memory content. Even if the content of the newly remembered experiences does not initially seem to be a part of one's own life and feels foreign to one's sense of self, it is all right to leave the story as is until the next session. The therapist tells Paul,

You did an incredible job today, and I feel honored that you trusted me to accompany you. Take time for yourself and be patient if any emotions or thoughts continue to resonate with you after our session. I'll see you next week for our appointment. Until then, there's no need to do or think anything specific.... You do not need to evaluate or verify the story for accuracy. Your brain and body will process the information during rest and waking hours, and we will reassess your progress next week, all right?

The NET session is now ended as usual. After some hours and days, the reclaimed past feels much more owned.

Case of Tarik: From a Bodily Perception to Recovering the Trauma Memory

Tarik who had witnessed a war massacre stopped his narration during the Narrative Exposure session at one point. He had lost the thread of the story. He did not know what to say next. Without realizing it, he had been bending forward in his chair for quite some time. The therapist noticed the posture and asked him: "What do you feel in your body, Tarik, when you lean forward like that?" Because he had been sitting like this for a while, he noticed that his back was hurting. As he became aware of this sensation, he also noticed that he was experiencing a feeling of suffocation. In response to the therapist's question, "Where do you feel it?" the narrator suddenly commented, "It's in my neck. And my heart is beating up to my throat." The therapist encouraged him to continue to be aware of the perceptions, emotions, and sensations of his body. Describing it in more detail, he mentioned that there was very bright light around him, and this meant that he would have to die. Staying with this, Tarik became very agitated, and his body stiffened. He was barely breathing. A few minutes later, as he continued to observe and name the sensations of his body, he realized that the various elements of sensory and bodily information he was experiencing were coming together to form a whole. They were part of a traumatic scene he had experienced. Tarik had panicked during that traumatic event in which he had expected to be killed in a mass execution. The victims had to huddle in a courtyard for many hours without being allowed to move. Many had already been shot, but the others had to remain in a squatting position. After some time, he was in great pain and completely focused on whether footsteps were approaching. Now all these bodily reactions made sense: a strong heartbeat, not being able to breathe properly, a feeling of paralysis, heat from the sun, and a thirst for water. Other trauma reactions, such as nightmares of screaming people and blood, were also linked to the previously inaccessible experience, which was eventually recovered.

In NET, the therapist does not judge to what extent the memories are based on objectively recordable events. It is the personal experiences that count. The subjective truthfulness (!) is what matters for the healing process. However, the therapist needs to take care to not support the creation of false memories. As soon as an individual presents with a memory gap and the wish to fill this gap in therapy, it is wise to inform the survivor that a narrative process as described below can be effective in recreating memory traces that seem to be lost. However, the success of this attempt can not be guaranteed. Even though the connection of hot and cold memories is essential for healing, it is preferable to leave memory gaps rather than invent false recollections.

The truth must not be blurred by associations created by the individual's imagination or external suggestions. While such false memories can be very vivid, making it difficult to distinguish between what is real and what is not, the client ultimately will be left in a state of uncertainty when false memories become interweaved with the real memory fragments. Therefore, in particular, the therapist should be aware of the following sources of false memories:

- **Misinformation or suggestion:** Do not suggest any details about the event, as these might be incorporated in the story.
- **Imagination inflation:** When people repeatedly imagine an event that never occurred, it can lead to the creation of false memories, as the imagined details become incorporated into their recollections.
- **Confirmation bias:** People tend to remember information that confirms their existing beliefs or expectations, and may unknowingly create false memories to support these beliefs. It is not the task of the therapist to confirm expectations or beliefs or confirm that events had actually happened in this way.
- **Forgetting source of memory:** Finally, individuals may remember a fact but forget where or how they learned it. For instance, a reader may know that the capital of Spain is Madrid, but not recall where he has learned this fact. It is not the task of the therapist to attribute this information to a source (e.g., do not say something like, "You must have learned this in primary school"), as this can create false associations.

The creation of false memories may have important implications in various fields, including the private life of a person or the legal system.If Paul (see the section Case of Paul: From a Visual Intrusion to Accessing the Whole Story, above) had attributed the wrong room or house to his horrible experience, later information or memories might then be incompatible with their story, which may invalidate the experience and make the survivor doubtful, putting them back to the situation of unpredictable horror. In addition, false memories can create real life suffering – for example, in the cutting off contact with alleged perpetrators or witnesses, in legal complaints, lost court cases, relocation, or loss of community, etc. Then again, psychotherapy is never without side effects. Some people may want to free themselves from the confining circumstances of their lives once the anxiety disorder is overcome, and they have more self-confidence, and the biography work also leads to new insights and thus new behaviors and new life plans. All we can do is provide survivors like Paul and Tarik with a safe framework and therapeutic support so that they can venture into their own memories. With a recovered past, the person has the freedom to reclaim their life.

The therapist should therefore help with imagining the individual's situation at the time of the trauma and attempt to understand how the incident is being remembered. The therapist wants to be particularly aware of the following factors, all of which are known to shape the representation of an event memory (Baddely, 1990; Reviere, 1996; Schacter, 1996, Schauer et al., 2011):

1. **What were the characteristics of the individual at the time of the event?** How old was the individual at the time of the incident? What is their gender? What are the current emotional state, physical condition, and circumstances of the speaker, as well as those at the time of the incident?
2. **What knowledge base did the narrator have at the time of the event?** How would the individual comprehend and make sense of the events that occurred to them, their family, and others? How could they effectively incorporate this understanding into their existing knowledge and past experiences?
3. **What is their current interpretation of the events?** How does the narrator attempt to make sense of the things that happened? Which aspects of the event do they connect with other information? How are symptoms that arise from the trauma interpreted?
4. **What retrieval strategies does the narrator use, and what is the context of recall?** How does the participant attempt to remember objective facts, individual emotions and physical sensations, or thoughts at the time? The therapist aims to utilize the Narrative Exposure cycle to comprehensively cover all levels of experience, including the narrator's current emotions. Sometimes the memory content returns

only after accepting gaps and not trying too hard to force memory.

Handling Sudden Emergence of Unexpected, Older Memories

Being involuntarily "beamed" from one memory to an earlier one along unexpected pathways of association is the other challenging situation.

What to do when memory traces – that is, neural connections to situations in earlier times and places, are evoked during Narrative Exposure work? Watkins (1971) called these emerging associations *affect bridges* to repressed experiences that can take a narrator from the present to a past event connected by a shared affect. The earlier experience, typically a childhood memory, becomes vivid and comes to the fore.

When this happens, the narrative of that day's session that has already begun may be interrupted because the person is experiencing sensory intrusions or intense bodily sensations and physiological arousal and somatic reenactments that they do not (yet) recognize, understand, or associate with any event. In these moments, instead of talking about these impressions on a metacognitive level, it is important to stay with the sensory elements to be able to cross these bridges. The therapist shall help the narrator to fully experience and be in touch with the affect and bodily experience, and give the narrator the opportunity to find out what the feeling means and what the source of the feeling is.

What to Do When Traumatic Fragments of Other Events Flash in Unexpectedly During a NET Session?

When working with a hot memory, the therapeutic goal is to help the person become aware of what is happening and to help the narrator sort through these perceptions. The therapist will support the narrator in trusting their reactions and experiences, which may be confusing and seem to make no sense.

The first step is to identify the sensation. The therapist would help with questions such as for example:

What does this sensation feel like?

Where in the body do you feel that? Where else? Is that the same feeling or different? What else is there?...

What quality does the sensation have (cold, warm, fast, slow, heavy...)?

From there, the therapist will help, but never force the person to assign these perceptions and integrate them into the narrative. To build the survivor's trust in their own inner feelings, the therapist will gently, but unwaveringly, guide, reinforce, and encourage the narrator to explore more about what they are experiencing, in order to fully connect with these emerging memories. Whatever comes forth is perfectly fine, and there is no need to cognitively critically analyze, judge, or fear it, or even be worried to go too far into memories and uncover things that might upset the current relationship with a person or the constructed self-identity. The priority is to perceive, feel, and explicitly describe the sensations.

Stimulated by similar feelings or bodily sensations or other resemblances, such unpredictable *bridge crossings* to places in the past can open up. This can happen when the survivor is triggered by similarities between two stories, by similar bodily sensations or emotions, or especially during the increasing physiological arousal as a *hot spot* approaches, because then decontextualized fragments from other trauma situations can be activated.

Ibrahim's Case: Dangerous Mediterranean Crossing After Childhood Physical Abuse in African Village

A 16-year-old unaccompanied minor was registered for treatment at a refugee outpatient clinic because he was so distressed by a past incident in which he had crossed the Mediterranean by boat while fleeing. After the crossing, Ibrahim developed nightmares about water, about panicking, and people on boats. He often woke in the middle of the night drenched in sweat, and began drinking alcohol in an attempt to calm himself. He had described his boat experience several times to different people who asked him about it, pointing out that he had not experienced any fear of death during the crossing. For no apparent reason, he felt guilty, became more socially withdrawn, and stopped attending language classes. Ibrahim became increasingly paranoid about people, and those around him soon viewed him as "strange." Refugees who lived with him talked about him behind his back and avoided him. His social withdrawal led to subsequent stigma and isolation.

First Memory: Sea Crossing on a Boat in the Mediterranean

After an assessment that included a structured intake checklist and diagnosis, he was provided with psychoeducation and completed the Lifeline. Ibrahim was then invited to recall the experience as part of his overall life narrative in Step 3 of the NET procedure. Narrating the stone he had put down on his lifeline labeled "sea crossing on the boat in the Mediterranean" revealed the connection of the boat event to an older traumatic event in the past that had occurred much earlier in childhood. The discovery of this previously hidden antecedent event using Narrative Exposure went as follows:

Ibrahim described sitting in the front of the overloaded wooden boat. The crossing was from the North African coast to the island of Malta. It took 2 days. There were 200 people on the boat. Ibrahim was guided by the therapist to imagine himself back in the old boat, remembering the waves and the sounds on board that day. As he told the story, he was closely guided to feel the burning sun and salt water on his lips and to catch the intense smell of the sea, the sweat of the other people, and the pressure of the human bodies against his own. He soon remembered the tension of realizing that the hull of the boat was constantly leaking salt water. The anxious thoughts from that past were accessible again, as was the nausea in his body from the rocking of the boat. He had become increasingly frightened and remembered his heart beating in his throat.

Second Memory: Physical Abuse as a Child

At that moment in the narration, Ibrahim was bent over, remembering clutching the wood with both hands. The therapist observed that he became visibly agitated by this memory, breathing rapidly, grimacing in pain, and becoming increasingly silent, until he stopped speaking altogether. Invited to stay with this experience and verbalize what was happening, a completely different scene suddenly emerged with full intensity. Ibrahim moaned in pain and said: "My father, he's beating me! It hurts so much! I'm so scared...."

After this utterance, the therapist realized that another scene from the past had intruded. "It is as if you have been taken from one place and deposited in another moment of your life," the therapist to then said to help explain what had happened. Then, she immediately caught up with the client's experience and gently helped him to verbalize the newly recalled event, to contrast it with the present, and to understand that it belonged to a different time and space – namely, to his time in his childhood village.

It turned out to be a scene from when he was 8 years old. Ibrahim had been abused by his father as a child. At that time, he had to bend forward in fear, clinging with trembling hands to a chair instead of the edge of the boat, having heart palpitations, feelings of guilt, and sweating while his father beat him several times on his buttocks, on his back and legs.

The posture and physiology, the bodily feelings, the helplessness of the life-threatening situation on the boat had so many similarities to the earlier scene that this old trauma (physical violence) was activated in his memory and tormented him, but he had not been able to distinguish it from the threat on board during his flight.

By understanding the experience on all levels and integrating the contextual elements (time of day, escape, living room, etc.) as well as the contextual differences (chair vs. boat, blows vs. fear of water, etc.) and similarities (both times fear, body position bending over, heart palpitations, clinging with hands, helplessness, etc.) with the earlier scene, the ongoing intrusions and his personality change in the present suddenly made sense to him. In both situations there was a strong physical activation that formed a neural association between the two decontextualized events. The accompanying autobiography was then fragmented. However, the body and the associative emotional network had retained the memory.

With the help of Narrative Exposure, the first boat experience was then told to the end during the session, and the experience with the father was worked through in more detail in a separate session. In this way, the two traumatic life events could be separated as distinct but related biographical experiences to be located and historically recorded.

Case of Emma: Claustrophobia in a Frankfurt Elevator, Difficult Situation on a Childhood Sleepover, and a Childhood Cemetery – or Why It Makes Sense to Start a Life-Narration From the Beginning of the Developmental Timeline]

Acknowledgment: The authors would like to thank the Narrative Exposure participant and express their gratitude that she allowed us to share these experiences in this text.

A 43-year-old German psychotherapist volunteered for a live demonstration of NET during a trauma workshop. She hoped to gain insight into her insurmountable *claustrophobia* (fear of enclosed spaces and fear of being trapped) when using elevators. She reported that on several occasions she had panicked upon entering an elevator. "I felt so cramped in such a small space.... I panicked.... I thought I was going to die," she said. Recently, she had developed another problem; she would often isolate herself at lunchtime and spend the hour wandering around the nearby park, often in tears. This sadness could last for days, she said.

Since this was not a real therapy, but just an isolated live demonstration at a conference for mental health professionals, we did not do the step-by-step procedure (i.e., no intake checklists, Lifeline, or processing of earlier stones) as would normally be done in NET. Emma sat down with the facilitator to explore her elevator panic. During this live demonstration of Narrative Exposure, she was asked to recall a specific event in which she had recently been about to enter the elevator at her workplace. She remembered the day, what she was wearing, the stress of the job, and who she wanted to have lunch with as they walked to the elevator that would take them down several floors to the cafeteria.

First Memory: Trapped in the Elevator

After introductory description by the narrator, the therapist slowed down the narrative, using the Narrative Exposure cycle (Figure 17) to stay closely attuned and follow the emotional associations of the memory (sensations, cognitions, emotions, bodily responses, meaning). By going into slow motion and facilitating awareness of these emerging perceptions, the memory associations were activated and memories emerged. Emma explained how she had entered the elevator, which then filled with people until someone closed the door and pushed the button to descend. Emma initially reported that she could not see much, it was dark, it smelled like dust, and the air was bad. The facilitator helped Emma stay with that feeling for a moment. She grimaced, looked pained as if trapped, and gasped. The therapist empathically expressed, "I can see you are having trouble breathing and feeling very constricted!" Visibly more agitated, Emma's sense of panic and helplessness spread. She described her limbs becoming heavy, and she began to sweat. To make sense of this, the therapist invited her to explore this moment in depth, asking: "What do you perceive?"

Emma: "I feel trapped, it's too tight here.... No air!"

Therapist: "What is happening? The people pouring in are leaving you less and less space. There is a sense of narrowness in the cabin?"

Emma moans: "It feels like I can't push, I can't get out. It is terrible. I can't see.... I can't break free!"

Therapist: "I can see you struggling in the chair.... It must be terrible to feel so trapped! Emma?... Can you name it?... Take me with you...."

Second Memor: Stuck Under the Bed

After another moment of describing her experience in the elevator, Emma said: "...It's so tight, the smell of wood, I can't get out.... I'm going to suffocate under the bed...." Then, having said that, she explained how she had found herself under a wooden bed. Soon after, the whole scene came to light: She was about 11 years old, having a sleepover at a friend's house with girls her age. They were all sleeping in the attic of the house, where old furniture was stored. To make more room, they had moved the beds to the side and removed the mattresses. Emma had turned over in the night, slipped off the mattress through the narrow slit, and got trapped under the wooden frame. She woke up under the bed frame and immediately panicked. Staying with these memories, she recalled that the girls had heard her scream, then turned on the light and helped her get out from under the bed.

The therapist helped Emma stay a little longer with the feeling of suffocation, trapped under a wooden frame, in order to allow a more complete narrative and place it in the past context of time and space. The therapist helped Emma to stay with this perception and bring out all of the thoughts, emotions, physical reactions, and meaning. As she began to understand the connection between the situation in the elevator and the experience at the girls' party, Emma immediately felt a sense of exhilaration and relief. After a short time, however, interestingly, the feeling of great sadness returned together with rising tension.

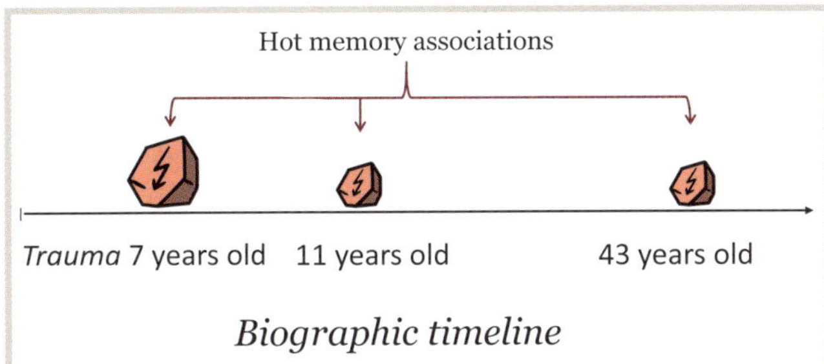

Figure 33. Emma's memory associations were activated and related trauma material emerged.

Third Memory: Friend Buried in a Coffin

Staying with the sadness and exploring it in more detail, another memory arose.

Therapist: "There are tears in your eyes, Emma, you feel so sad...?"

Emma: "My heart is pounding. I am terribly nervous...!"

Therapist: "How can you make sense of this?.... How do you respond to this?..."

Emma: "It feels like I have to do something ... something terrible is happening!"

Therapist sees Emma rocking on the chair moving her legs, and says: "It's hard to keep still! It's so urgent! Focus on this feeling.... Just allow any memory to come to you."

Emma bursts into tears and cries heartrendingly: "She is still alive and desperate! She has to die in that dark coffin!"

Once the memory recall process was stimulated, an even older event came to light (see Figure 33).

By activating the emotional memory associations, event retracing was sparked. The therapist at this point could not know what this is about or who the "she" was in this story. The therapist therefore responded by trying to encourage connection with the feelings to allow the memory to become clearer.

The therapist stayed close to Emma, showing his presence and compassion: "That was a moment of great despair for you...," allowing time for crying and waiting for Emma to calm down for a moment before asking: "Who is dying, Emma?... Let me share this with you.... What 'coffin' do you see?..."

Emma started to begin to tell the whole story now. Her memory associations had finally taken Emma to the original trauma that she had suffered much earlier in childhood, long before the overnight party. She found herself in a situation she had been in 36 years ago, standing in front of a grave with her elementary school classmates. A girl in her class had died in a tragic accident, and the teacher had taken all of the children to the funeral. Standing in the front row, Emma watched as the wooden coffin was lowered into the ground. At that moment, she apparently had had an alarm reaction, had panicked and helplessly imagined that her friend buried in the coffin was still alive and slowly suffocating. The therapist patiently but actively and gently uses the Narrative Exposure cycle to work through the experience, allowing the survivor to understand what had happened and the impact it had had on her, and that the wooden coffin event was connected to the moment under the wooden bed and the fear of being tapped (in an elevator). Once Emma was able to make the connection that the common theme between these three situations was: "a life-threatening feeling of suffocation in a confined space," her elevator panic was alleviated, her nightmares stopped, and she was finally able to grieve the death of her dear friend, and find closure.

Rule: If, during the Narrative Exposure work on a hot spot, memory associations to earlier events arise, the therapist helps the narrator to understand the newly emerging trauma material and to briefly frame this earlier story (time, place, title) in preparation for a more complete exploration and recovery in a separate session. After summarizing the new content, the focus is shifted back to the original stone (the one that involuntarily triggered the older memory associations). The newly recovered memory, however, is dealt with in the next session. It is of utmost importance to conclude all stories properly and not leave any loose ends. Therefore, NET follows the chronological sequence of the life events.

Exploring Specific Events Rather Than Having Abstract Discussions

Storytelling reveals meaning without committing the error of defining it.

Hannah Arendt in "Isak Dinesen: 1885–1963," an essay in the collection *Men in Dark Times*

Sometimes overarching conflicts, problems, and trauma themes emerge in the therapeutic work as part of the narrative of one's life. Discussing a problem in general terms is often not advisable. It is much better to process a real specific event where this issue has arisen. By going through the detailed narrative of a significant, high-impact experience within a larger life context, the individual engages with affect, including thoughts, emotions, bodily memories, and meaning. This often reveals the real underlying themes. For instance, if someone shares that they were subjected to verbal and physical abuse by their family because of new household members, a therapist can guide them in identifying a specific scenario that illustrates this issue (specific event).

During a therapy session, a narrator shared that they "always" felt unwanted while growing up, due to their father favoring their brother over them. This was a recurring issue. The therapist asked the narrator if he could recall a *specific situation* in the past when he had similar feelings because of the father's preference for the brother.

The narrator recounted an incident from their childhood where the brother forgot to close the gate to the animal pasture, but their father punished the narrator instead of the brother. The narrator admits to that experience of being physically assaulted, with a downtrodden expression. The therapist prompts the narrator to provide more details about the situation, including the location, time of day, and categorization of the event on their Lifeline.

Therapist: "Please tell me now how you will label this situation on your Lifeline and then let me take you to the beginning of this event...."

Narrator: "OK, let me think.... This was when I was 6 years old, when we lived in Rajasthan. I would call the story: 'unjust punishment – my dad shouts at me and injures me with a stick.' I recall that Jamal, Vindu, and I were at the neighbor's farm searching for the camels."

The therapist asks for more context and perceptions surrounding the event.

In response, the narrator describes the time of day as afternoon on a hot, dry day, possibly during a government holiday. The narrator also notes that it was getting dark outside...(cont.)

The therapist continues to explore this event to uncover patterns in the individual's experience and behavior with the help of the Narrative Exposure cycle. He writes down the story of the session, just like one of the other trauma stones and helps the participant to fill it in the life-story. After reading the recap at the start of the following session, the narrative progresses to subsequent events on the timeline to examine how these negative experiences have impacted later development in life.

Instead of talking for hours *about* a topic, it is much more productive and effective to dive deeply and in slow motion into the concrete past experiences of adverse, distressing, and sad interpersonal moments (especially during childhood), other life- and integrity-threatening events, as well as strongly positive, happy, and meaningful memories.

However, if the problems and conflicts are not of a traumatic nature and, in addition if there are very few resources available for the number of sessions, due to factors such as ongoing violence during a wa , unsafe treatment conditions, poverty, long distance travel, or lack of therapist human resources, a warning is issued. In such cases, the trauma stones (as listed in the event intake checklist) take priority and become the first order of business.

4 NET for People With Special Needs and Requirements

KIDNET: NET for Children and Adolescents

Trauma Treatment for Children

As we write these lines, there are more than 30 ongoing conflicts in the world, ranging from drug wars, terrorist insurgencies, ethnic conflicts, to civil and interstate wars. The impact of all of these forms of organized violence on children is profound and often long-lasting. Being physically harmed and deprived of physical necessities such as food and medical care often constitutes an ongoing stress. In addition to direct exposure to violence, loss of family members, often with loss of proper caregiving, and displacement contribute to severe traumatic stress in child survivors. War also disrupts normal life, including education, depriving children of the opportunity to develop their full potential. Many children become refugees and are thus uprooted from their homes and communities, creating additional burdens and stresses with a lasting impact on their sense of identity, stability, and overall well-being. In addition, children are often exploited during conflicts, being forcibly recruited, or joining armed groups voluntarily. They may be abused as fighters, spies, or in various support roles. The lack of a protective environment increases the risk of exploitation, sexual and physical abuse, and neglect.

Children, like adults, develop symptoms such as anxiety, depression and PTSD as their exposure to traumatic stressors accumulates. In addition, in their nightmares, children integrate demons, monsters, and witches into their fear network. Nocturnal enuresis and externalizing, as well as internalizing behavioral problems are common. Research from various war zones has reported significant rates of PTSD in children exposed to acts of organized violence and war (see Kinzie et al., 1989, for children from Cambodia; Saigh, 1991, for Lebanese children; Somasundaram, 1993; Elbert et al., 2009; Catani et al., 2010, for Tamil children from Sri Lanka; Dyregrov et al., 2000; Schaal & Elbert, 2006, for Rwandan adolescents; Thabet et al., 2018; Thabet & Vostanis, 1999, for Palestinian children from Gaza; Papageorgiou et al., 2000, for children from Bosnia-Herzegovina; Karunakara et al., 2004; Ertl et al., 2010, 2011, for Sudanese refugee and Ugandan host children; and Catani et al., 2009, for children from Kabul, Afghanistan).

In an epidemiological survey, in which we investigated a representative sample of 420 Tamil school children in the then Liberation Tigers of Tamil Eelam (LTTE)-controlled Vanni Region of Sri Lanka's northeast, we found that 92% of the surveyed children had experienced severely traumatizing war events, such as being caught in a combat situation, being in a situation of bombing and/or shelling, witnessing the violent death of a loved one, among others, and frequently in addition to domestic violence. Of those, about a third of the children suffered from severe and chronic PTSD (Elbert et al., 2009), often comorbid with depression and somatization. we saw a significant relationship between the number of traumatic events reported and the number of difficulties children reported in social and emotional functioning. Factors such as frequent headaches, sleep disturbance, altered memory function, loss of ability to concentrate and pay attention, decline in school performance, loss of trust, and social withdrawal strongly impacted those children diagnosed with PTSD, limiting their chances for future healthy development.

Sri Lanka was also among the countries badly hit by a terrible tsunami in December 2004. A month after the disaster, we assessed symptoms of PTSD in 264 children who lived in severely affected coastal communities, in regions that had been differently affected by the civil war: Manadkadu – northern coast (war zone), Kosgoda – western coast, and Galle – southern coast of Sri Lanka. As expected, the likelihood of PTSD symptoms was not only explained by the severity of the tsunami exposure and related family loss, but essentially depended on previous exposure to traumatic events. The results showed that an individual's trauma history is a key determinant of their risk of developing PTSD in response to a disaster such as the tsunami (Neuner et al., 2006).

Domestic violence can have equally profound and lasting consequences on children, affecting their physical, emotional, and social well-being. The trauma-related suffering frequently promotes behavioral problems, such as aggression, defiance, withdrawal, and difficulties in forming positive relationships with peers. These behaviors can persist into adolescence and adulthood.

Violence in whatever form leads to chronic stress and trauma negatively impacting a child's cognitive development, especially in early years (Schalinski et al., 2019). This may manifest as difficulties in concentration, learning delays, and lower academic achievement. The stress that permanently activates the major defense systems including the HPA axis contributes to physical health problems, producing headaches, stomachaches, insomnia, and other psychosomatic complaints. The risk for long-term health issues increases several times over.

And as if that were not enough, these children are drawn into the cycle of violence (Elbert, Schauer, & Moran, 2018; Elbert, Moran, & Schauer, 2017b; Hinsberger et al., 2016): Without intervention and support, children exposed to violence may be more likely to become, later in life, either victims or perpetrators of violence in their own relationships, but also in their community (Nandi et al., 2017). The risk of engaging in substance abuse as a coping mechanism to deal with the emotional pain and stress also increases. The cycle of violence can be perpetuated through generations. Severe stress during development may leave an indelible imprint on the structure and function of the organism and the brain in particular (McEwen, 2002; Teicher et al., 2002). Ever since the seminal studies by Felitti et al. (1998), Anda et al. (2006), and colleagues, the evidence has become overwhelming that multiple adverse childhood experiences are a major risk factor for many health conditions and others. According to Hughes et al. (2017), these are:

- modest associations, *OR* < 2 for physical inactivity, overweight or obesity, and diabetes (Note: the odds ratio [*OR*] in this case is the ratio of the odds of a health problem occurring in the group who has experienced childhood adversities, to the odds of it occurring in those with a good childhood);
- moderate associations (*OR* = 2–3) for smoking, heavy alcohol use, poor self-rated health, cancer, heart disease, and respiratory disease;
- strong associations (*OR* = 3–6) for sexual risk taking, mental ill health, and problematic alcohol use;
- and strongest (*OR* > 7) for problematic drug use and interpersonal and self-directed violence.

Narratives in Children

Humans form many fundamentally important emotional networks in (early) childhood. These memories will have lasting impacts on the individual's behavior. They may, however, be only implicitly stored, and thus not be verbally accessible. In general, the capacity for autobiographical memory develops with age. Although infants and young children process and retain information (Bauer, 1996), events occurring before the age of 2–3 years cannot be recalled in narrative form. Due to developmental limitations, young children are thought to have problems with explicit memory functions and lack the competence for higher order memories (Williams & Banyard, 1999).

There is no doubt, however, that even very young children will remember traumatic experiences in an implicit way. In very small children, memories for traumatic events may be encoded differently, partly at a somatic and sensory level, and partly at an emotional level, as opposed to the verbally mediated level (Bremner et al., 1995). Due to the presence of threat, traumatic events are usually implicitly remembered, even in early childhood, and the memories can be remarkably accurate (Koss et al., 1995). In very young children (age 2–5 years), who cannot perfectly express themselves in coherent narratives, but who remember fragments, the memory nevertheless has been shown to be accurate and correct (Howe et al., 1994; Jones & Krugman, 1986; Peterson, 1996; Terr, 1988), even when the traumatic event has taken place a long time ago (Widom & Shepard, 1996; Widom & Morris, 1997; Wagenaar & Groeneweg, 1990). Misperception and forgetting significant aspects of the experienced violence and horror are also common.

An active attempt to help children embed the traumatic experiences into their life context is useful in that it helps the child understand and integrate these traumatic experiences (Tessler & Nelson, 1994). In Narrative Exposure, children are asked to describe what happened to them in great detail, paying attention to what they experienced, in terms of what they saw, heard, felt, smelled, the movement they recall, and so on – as well as what they were thinking and feeling at the time.

Although children as young as 7 or 8 years are fully capable of participating in NET, parents and teachers initially report that children are reluctant to talk about the trauma. Experience has shown that many children easily give very graphic accounts of their experiences and are also able to report how distressing it is to live with the related symptoms (Misch et al., 1993; Ruf et al., 2010; Sullivan et al., 1991). Child survivors, like adults, feel the need to discuss their experiences, but often struggle to do so, particularly with their parents and peers. Often, they do not want to upset their caretakers, and so parents may not be aware of the extent of their children's suffering. Peers may hold back from asking what happened, in case they disturb the child further; the survivor feels this as a rejection.

KIDNET – The Evidence

KIDNET refers to Narrative Exposure therapy for children and adolescents. Initial KIDNET studies have been conducted in Uganda with refugee children (Schauer et al., 2004; Onyut et al., 2005) and in Sri Lanka with formerly displaced children in the northeast of the country. Strong evidence for the effect of KIDNET in survivors of organized violence can be derived from subsequent RCTs performed in Germany (Figure 34; see Ruf et al., 2010), Rwanda (Schaal et al., 2009), Uganda (Ertl et al., 2011), Finland (Peltonen & Kangaslampi, 2019), and Korea (Park et al., 2020). A controlled study by Crombach and Elbert (2014), with street children, and by Hermenau et al. (2011), with orphans, all victims of domestic violence, revealed that aggressive and criminal behavior can also be controlled after KIDNET. Interesting case reports have been provided by Fazel et al. (2020) and by Van Es et al. (2023). And finally, Julian et al. (2023) present two case vignettes demonstrating adaptations to meet the specific needs of transgender and gender diverse youth. Currently a multicenter RCT (YOURTREAT; Wittmann et al., 2022; Wilker et al., 2020) is underway to compare KIDNET with other forms of active treatment for young refugees in Germany. There is also a RCT examining the effectiveness of EMDR and KIDNET in refugee children aged 8–18 years, specifically, compared with a waitlist control group (Velu et al., 2022).

In the developing individual, KIDNET enables the repair of attachment wounds and activates emotional networks through therapeutic contact characterized by warmth and empathy during storytelling. KIDNET assists children in confronting their fears from both reality and fantasy worlds. By expressing their thoughts and emotions through storytelling, children gain a sense of perspective and receive restorative support from adults. KIDNET advocates for the rights of survivors and promotes child welfare.

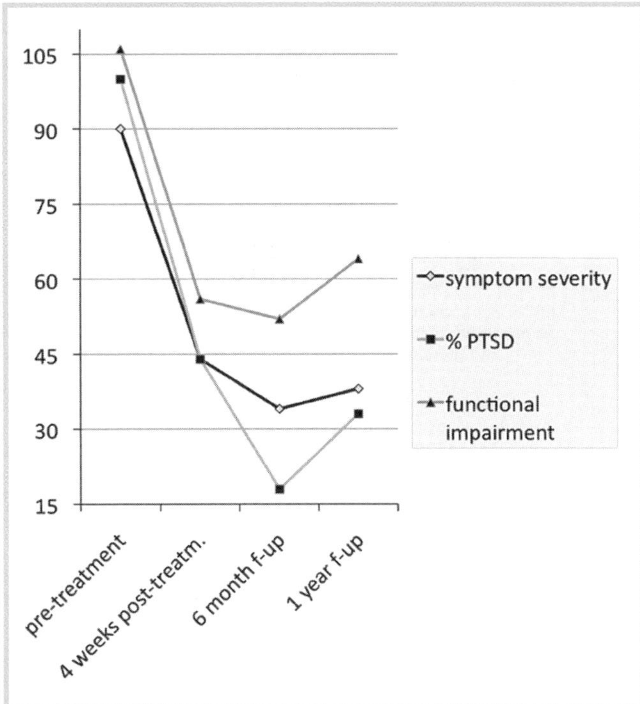

Figure 34. In a randomized controlled trial (RCT), children were randomly assigned to a treatment-as-usual group or a KIDNET group. The latter received therapy delivered over eight sessions. The time course of outcome variables is shown only for the KIDNET group, as the control group received the active treatment after a 6-month waiting period. A marked reduction in symptoms and improvement in functioning in response to the KIDNET treatment continued throughout the first 6 months after treatment. Thereafter, children who continued to live in asylum-seeker accommodation with ongoing threats of violence and actual family violence may not have experienced a further reduction of symptoms. Symptom severity was measured using the UCLA PTSD Index with frequency rating. For illustration purposes, the y axis shows scores ×2. PTSD diagnosis was according to DSM-IV criteria.

General Advice: Utilizing Creative Media With Children

In our research involving children from diverse cultural backgrounds, varying ages, and different cognitive abilities, we have consistently been amazed at the extent to which children can explore and articulate their experiences, emotions, and thoughts associated with trauma. The main objective in child therapy is to establish and maintain trust with the young participant. Building trust

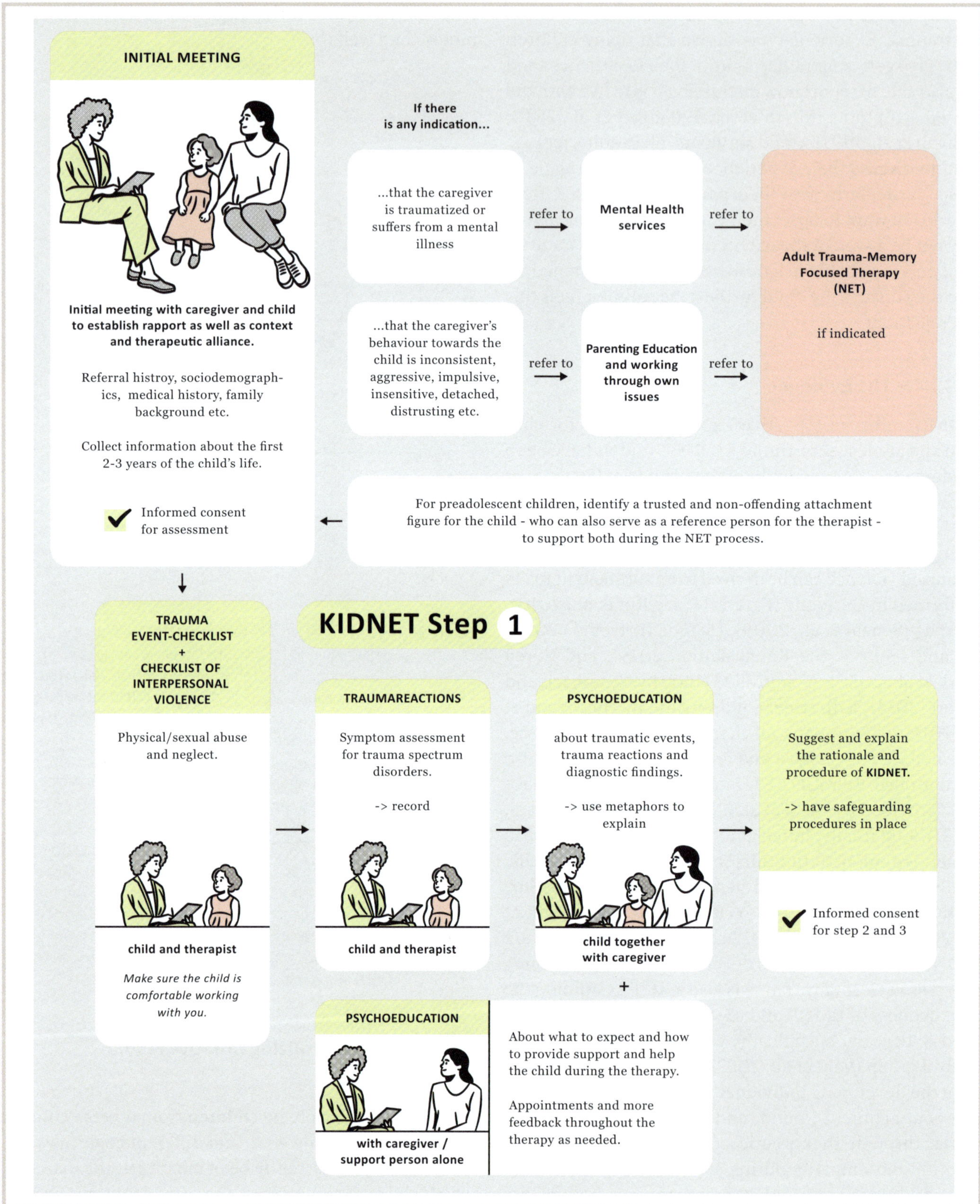

Figure 35. KIDNET Step 1 for prepubertal children who need a supportive caregiver to assist in the treatment of their trauma story. The standard NET methodology and KIDNET both consist of three distinct steps, as outlined in detail in Chapter 3 and for KIDNET in Schauer et al. (2017). Also available as a handout in the online supplementary materials for this book.

through conversation alone can be challenging when working with children, so we frequently incorporate more active displays, props like figurines and drawings, as well as the Lifeline exercise, during therapy sessions. Play and creative media can help children express their experiences (Schauer et al., 2017). For example, we may encourage children to act out their traumatic experiences in role play, by requesting such actions as "show me how your brother sat on the ground when your father came in" or by helping them recall details through painting. The therapist might ask, "Can you draw the expression on the man's face?" "Can you draw a picture for me that shows the house that you lived in and what it looked like?" or "Maybe you could show me in your picture exactly where the soldier was and where you were." Some components, such as reenacting body positions during the narration of the traumatic event, may also be beneficial in psychotherapy with adults, but only when following extensive psychoeducation and appropriate contrast to the past.

For preadolescent children, the therapist identifies a trusted and nonoffending attachment figure for the child who can serve as a reference person for the therapist, to support both during the NET process. Appointments with the adult are scheduled as needed throughout the process. If there are signs that the caregiver has experienced trauma or is affected by a mental illness that is causing concerning behavior toward the child, they should be referred to a mental health service for assessment and trauma-focused treatment, if necessary. Alternatively, refer them to parenting education to work through their own issues.

The first step of KIDNET is illustrated and detailed in Figure 35, including initial assessment steps like an interview and a conversation with the accompanying adult.

Already at the first encounter, it can help to build rapport with the child by asking them to draw a picture (see Figure 36). A traumatized child frequently presents an image of an associative trauma memory (fear network) – that is, the picture fuses elements from various traumatic experiences, sometimes combined with monsters from the fantasy world.

The therapist maintains a close emotional connection with the child and speaks about what is being drawn or shown with images. If the child creates something that appears to be linked to a stressful event, the therapist informs the child that they will speak further about it at a later time. If the child creates something that is not likely to be related to trauma, the therapist acknowledges the child and expresses interest by inquiring about the picture's content. Ideally, the therapist should evaluate the child's personal information, medical history, and family history, including any childhood stressors, with the assistance of a trusted caregiver. Afterwards, the caregiver can fill out questionnaires in a separate room while the therapist records the child's childhood traumatic experiences and other adversities using suitable checklists in a structured interview.

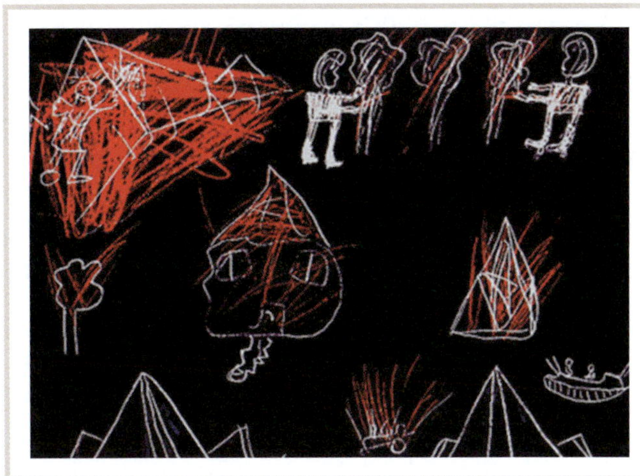

Figure 36. KIDNET Step 0 (recommended component for primary school age children): Build rapport and access their immediate thoughts by grasping implicit, sensory memories (hot memories). One child who was referred to our clinic was given pens and different colored paper. The child was asked to simply paint whatever came to mind.

KIDNET Step 1: Structured Diagnostic Interview Including Event Checklists With the Child

Structured assessment is conducted using the checklist for interpersonal violence, as well as a standard trauma event checklist, followed by assessing trauma reactions. To evaluate potential home-related stressors in children, we suggest using the Pediatric Maltreatment and Abuse Chronology of Exposure (pediMACE; Isele et al., 2014; see Ainamani et al., 2022), available upon request from the authors. This tool is applicable to pupils of all ages. The family constellation and living environment of the child can be recorded, together with the adult as an introduction. Without the parents present, the child is asked to answer yes or no to which stressful social situations they have experienced, ideally when and where (time and place), in the same manner as described above for adult ratings (Chapter 3, Step 1). Taking an allocentric stance, which involves seeking objective facts and contextual information, can empower the child and prevent overwhelming feelings. A complete clinical assessment through a thorough interview is necessary. This will initiate the therapeutic relationship. It is worth noting that preschoolers have trouble with allocentric perspectives, as they tend to retain an egocentric viewpoint, and so we have not tested this procedure on them.

The pediMACE is a list of common adversities that helps normalize a child's experience by making them known to the therapist. It also legitimizes reactions to traumatic stressors. This list is supplemented by the inclusion of exciting, positively worded elements to remind the child that there have been more than just bad moments in life. The pediMACE asks about the following interpersonal events that are relevant to trauma treatment: parental emotional abuse (adults living in the household), parental physical abuse (adults living in the household), emotional abuse by siblings (children living in the household), physical abuse by siblings (children living in the household), emotional neglect, physical neglect, witnessing interparental violence (adults living in the household), witnessing violence against siblings (children living in the household), peer abuse (physical and emotional), sexual violence, and parental loss.

For children who have been exposed to organized or community violence, or other traumatic events such as natural disasters, it is recommended to use appropriate checklists. If the child reports experiencing stress, a diagnostic tool for PTSD, such as the Child and Adolescent Trauma Screen (CATS-2; Sachser et al., 2022) or the Posttraumatic Stress Interview for Children (KID-PIN; Ibrahim et al., 2021) should be used. It is also important to assess depressive symptoms and suicidal tendencies separately. After the informed consent process (depending on the country and community) has been completed, resulting in consent and permission to treat the child, and safety procedures are in place, KIDNET Steps 2 and 3 can begin.

Psychoeducation

After completing the assessment, the therapist explains trauma reactions to both the child and their caregivers in an open and transparent way The use of a trauma checklist is explained to clarify the effects of trauma on the individual, family, and community, and inform the family about the causes of their distressing experience and about the potential remedies. This approach enables the family to regain a sense of control over their symptoms and cultivate hope for improved outcomes. The therapist offers a thorough explanation of the symptoms, utilizing language suitable for the child's age and education level, while avoiding medical terms. Psychoeducation serves in KIDNET as an ongoing complement to treatment, providing a framework for experiences and improving comprehension of symptoms and the reasoning behind treatment. It is typically reiterated briefly and targeted toward the specific problematic area. Adolescents require a comprehensive and objective explanation regarding their traumatic experience and its treatment plan, which may be presented in the presence of their caregivers or alone.

When working with children, therapists can utilize metaphors like "cleaning" the memory to help explain the purpose of therapy ("Have you ever made a mess in your room, and then items fell down that you weren't even searching for, causing you to lose the thing you were trying to find?"). The therapist can also utilize the comparison of an infected wound that is painful and in need of disinfection before it can heal. Such analogies may aid children in grasping the goals of therapy (Schauer et al., 2011) and can aid in psychoeducation by illustrating the interconnectedness of sensory elements (i.e., seeing, hearing, touch), thoughts, feelings, bodily reactions, and meanings. This will provide an informative explanation of their medical condition, a concise overview of the treatment process, and an invitation for voluntary participation. Any remaining questions the child may have regarding the treatment will also be answered. It is vital to explain to older children the significant role of discussing the traumatic event, in alleviating their suffering. Moreover, giving testimony is a crucial step toward documenting the violation of children's human rights and asserting their dignity.

KIDNET Step 2: Lifeline With Children – Make It a Game!

The Lifeline approach for children and adolescents follows the same guidelines as that of adults. It plays an important role in KIDNET and fosters quick connections by incorporating creative methods that allow the child's life story to develop in an entertaining way. Provide the line to the child and clarify that it symbolizes their life, with the start indicating birth. Instruct the child to place the rope on the ground, representing their future. Mark the point of birth and current location (Figure 37).

Offer an assortment of rocks and flowers in varying colors, sizes, and shapes to symbolize significant and less

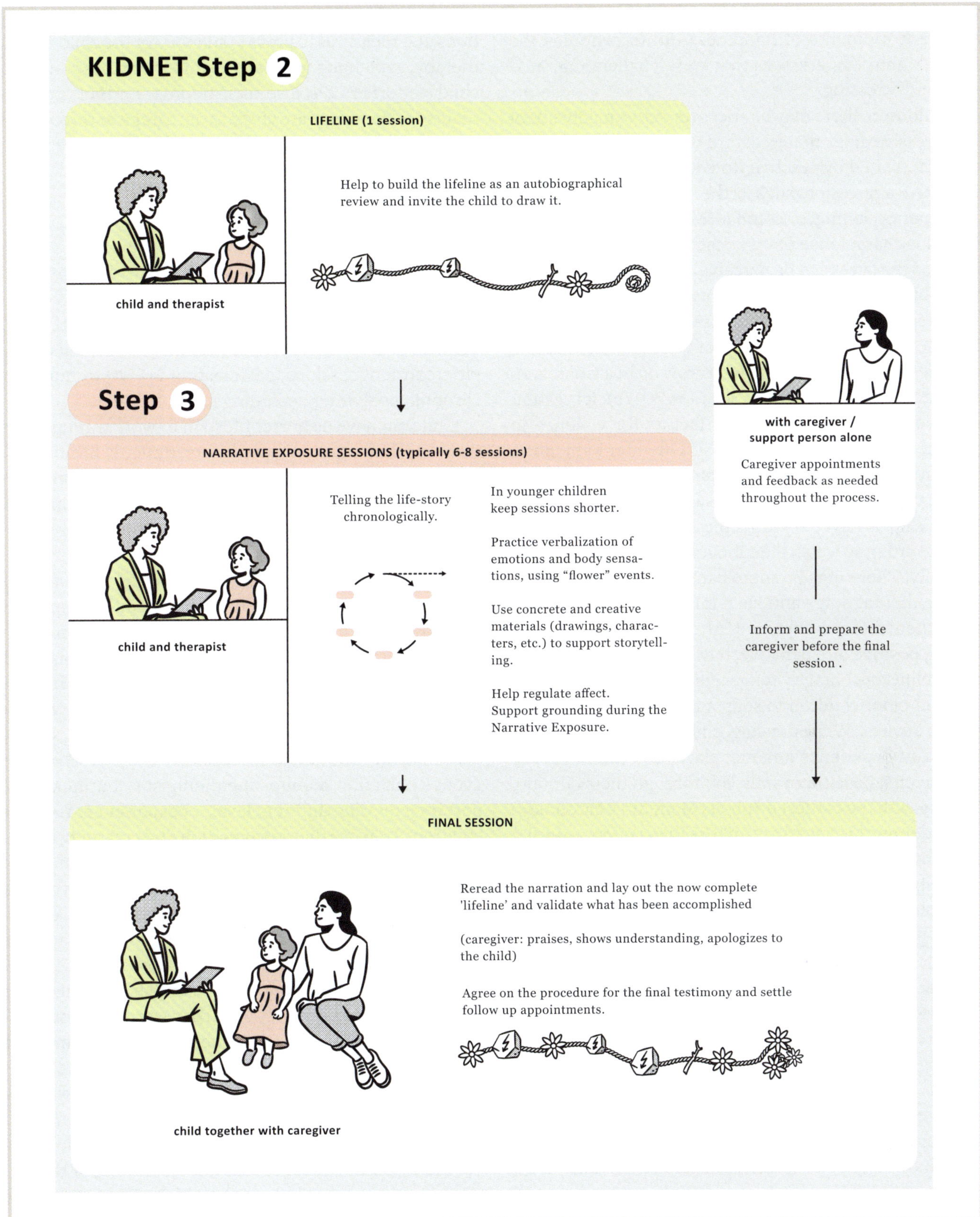

Figure 37. KIDNET Step 2 (Lifeline) and Step 3 (Narrative Exposure) for prepubertal children who need a caregiver to assist the trauma treatment. Also available as a handout in the online supplementary materials for this book.

significant life events. Instruct the child that the flowers represent moments of happiness in life, whereas the stones signify experiences that were challenging, anxious, or distressing.

In addition, there may be sticks for active involvement in aggressive acts – that is, acts of violence that may have been motivated by reactive (to counter a threat) and/or appetitive aggression, such as the enjoyment of fighting, delinquency, killing, or combat (Elbert et al., 2018). The former is characterised by a negative emotional valence, whereas the latter can be perceived as positive. This suggests that aggressive acts may be motivated not only by the intention to counter a threat or to obtain a reward, but also by intrinsic enjoyment of violence. This state is particularly fostered in boys who grow up in a violent environment (Elbert, Moran, & Schauer, 2017b). It is essential to address all motivational factors for violence in treatment (see the section Forensic Offender Rehabilitation and NET for Ex-Combatants, below).

Ask the child to arrange the symbols along the Lifeline. It is not always easy to get the child to follow a chronological order, so watch their movements and placements carefully. There may be some back and forth of objects, so take mental notes and keep talking with the child to make them feel accompanied. After all of the significant events, positive and negative, have been represented on the Lifeline, encourage younger children to draw the Lifeline and older children to snap a picture of it with their mobile devices. While drawing, children should give each important experience a name, place, and their age. For adolescents, have them walk you through their Lifeline, starting with the earliest symbols. Maintain a chronological order and, if necessary, adjust the sequence until a clear timeline is established. This drawing will function as a helpful tool for having the significant events in the chronology of the child's life readily available to look at. As you progress along the timeline, both positive and negative occurrences may surface. Such additions are welcome and can be incorporated by prompting the child to add them to the Lifeline drawing.

The Lifeline session is conducted without the presence of caregivers, older siblings, or other adults in the household, as are the Narrative Exposure sessions. Information that the child discloses should be shared also with the adult only with caution and care (and in accordance with the minor's right to confidentiality). For instance, if an 11-year-old girl reports being sexually abused by her uncle. When confronted with this, the mother (sister of the uncle) may express doubt and show clear disapproval toward the child's actions.

The therapist invites the caregivers to discuss expectations and measures to provide support for the child during therapy, explaining in detail the importance of praising a child's efforts to disclose their trauma. Further appointments and feedback are given to the caregiver throughout the therapy as needed. Sometimes a person close to the child may require their own counselor to unburden, express, and ventilate their thoughts and emotions.

KIDNET Step 3: Narrative Exposure

This next step involves the primary process of KIDNET. The child survivor narrates their entire life during multiple treatment sessions, each lasting 60–90 minutes, in chronological order according to the Lifeline.

Children have a shorter lifespan to work through, but they can have quite a number of difficult life events. Younger children may initially struggle with imaginal exposure, because they typically view events from an egocentric perspective, which they are just beginning to become aware of.

The narration procedure adheres to the same principles as that for adults, including the Narrative Exposure cycle (Figure 17). The narrative sessions may commence with a short psychoeducation, then the therapist and child look together at the Lifeline illustration. As children narrate experiences differently from adults, due to differences in cognitive and linguistic development, socialization, and emotional expression, a highly arousing event's narration requires the therapist's continual support for exploring different levels of experience. Younger children often use their imagination and creativity in stories, sometimes including fantastical elements and less focus on facts. Adolescents have more concise narratives as their attention span develops. Watching the child's body and emotions can help the therapist understand the story better.

Younger children may utilize simpler language and sentence structures than adults. They possess a more limited depth of comprehension and perspective compared with adults. Their interpretations of events are often centered around immediate sensory experiences, whereas adults consider broader contexts and abstract concepts. To construct meaning, mentalization and insights into life are essential, as well as an understanding of the potential motivations of offenders, which children may not possess as readily. For instance, an 8-year-old may struggle to comprehend the implications of sexual abuse and its aftermaths. It is the therapist's responsibility to address the youth's stage of emotional growth and conveying information in a clear and straightforward manner, without any avoidance (Ruf & Schauer, 2012; Schauer et al., 2017, 2024). A 17-year-old may seek justice and retaliation without fully understanding the consequences of taking legal action against a family member. Consequently, it is imperative for the young person to undergo counseling before testifying.

Moreover, further counseling sessions can address the adolescent's experiences of victimization, such as gender-based violence, marginalization, or hate crimes, which may be beyond their comprehension.

Here are some practical tips for younger children:

- Help by verbalizing body sensations and emotions.
- Keep summarizing what you understand.
- Give a lot of affirmation – for example, "Wow, you are a really good storyteller; I understand so well when you explain things to me ..."
- Remember that attention spans are short – do not get too ambitious with the story! The main thing is to get through it!
- When listening to the story, always think of the child at the age when the incident occurred. This will help you adjust your language and processing speed.
- If available, for younger children have *helpers* sit with the child to tell the stories (toys, stuffed animals, etc.) and a play area or corner to which the child can retreat or where they can cover up while talking.
- Make retelling fun! Include some small mistakes when reading the story back at the beginning of the next session so that the children can correct you. For example, "The door opened just as you were sitting on the yellow sofa" (in fact, the child told you the sofa was blue). Children love to correct adults!
- With younger children play a game at the end of the session! "You're doing great! If we continue like this, there will be a good time to play a nice game."
- As you go along, don't forget to work some of the "flowers" into the chronological storytelling. Those stories are great for making the child feel happy, proud, and loved!

The therapist informs the supporting adult in time about the situation in the last KIDNET session, where they are to both be present together with the child. The caregiver is provided with information on how the session will proceed, on the rereading of the narration, and on the presentation of the final Lifeline. The adult should be prepared for that upcoming session and understand how to react. The therapist confirms that they are ready to work together with the caregiver during the final session and are willing to gain an understanding of the child's traumas. Adolescents, however, often prefer to be without an adult in the final session.

During the last session, the entire testimony is reread in the past tense and first person. Sometimes, children may choose to read their stories to the therapist (and parent) themselves. This is certainly encouraged. The therapist and attachment figure attentively listen and respond with empathy, warmth, and understanding, providing supportive validation. The caregiver explains and apologizes to the child for any wrongdoing or neglectful behavior.

At the end of the last KIDNET session, the child is invited to showcase their completed Lifeline, which includes specific plans and aspirations for the future depicted as flowers. The child may also draw their future plans and aspirations, such as "When I finish school" "When I return home" or "When I learn how to ..." Prevent any negative stones for future worries or concerns.

In conclusion, KIDNET is an empirically supported intervention that therapists can tailor to the needs of both child victims and offenders who have suffered from trauma. Combining KIDNET with other treatment approaches simultaneously is not recommended. Moreover, relying solely on isolated components like the Lifeline as a singular approach lacks justification from both the evidence and theoretical framework. Instead, we propose that individual treatment should be guided by the theoretical objective of linking trauma-associated memory to its context and significance. The child and adolescent can have valuable learning experiences in self-awareness and mentalization when aided by an attentive, empathic, and responsive listener to their life stories. This ally can assist in verbalizing feelings, comprehending relational events, and offering corrective relationship experiences.

FORNET: (Forensic) Offender Rehabilitation & NET for Ex-Combatants

Offender rehabilitation (FORNET) is an integral part of NET and involves empathic listening and understanding of the person's inner universe as they report both victim and perpetrating experiences in their lives, when emotional and physiological arousal reached extreme levels. The affective valence of adverse situations in the past was negative for the most part. However, studies suggest that individuals may experience positive emotions, including the desire to hunt not only animals but also humans, when stimulated by threat and aggression ("lust for hunting"; Elbert et al., 2010). To symbolize such events on the Lifeline, a stone might not accurately represent the achievements of a fighter, nor would a flower adequately acknowledge the injuries and deaths occurring during the fight. Stenmark and colleagues (2014) demonstrated that without fully addressing the wealth of emotions experienced during interpersonal violence, NET is unable to reduce symptom levels in offenders. This leads to the option of additional symbols on the Lifeline, and it requires that the therapist fully understands the emotions called into play during perpetration and fighting. As most readers may not have been engaged in aggressive and violent acts, we present here a world of affects that has been revealed to us in surprisingly similar ways by forensic offenders, gang members, street children, and members of regular and irregular armed groups.

Violence Breeds Violence – How and Why?

Aggression refers to hostile and attacking behavior that threatens the physical or emotional integrity of another human or animal. Motivation can be categorized as follows:(1) *Reactive aggression* is the struggle to escape from a perceived threat. This mobilizes anger; that is, an emotion in defense, or as a counterattack or revenge after suffering injustice (such as loss of resources, loss of status, or severe frustration). When it serves as a defense, reactive aggression is morally justifiable and marked by arousal with a negative valence. It subsides when the fight is successful, and the danger is over. This facilitation can be perceived as a rewarding response. (2) *Instrumental aggression* means that an extrinsic reward drives the aggressive and violent behavior. It can be driven not only by the endeavor to acquire material goods, but also by a desire for social status.

> **Example for appetitive aggression**
>
> "I can honestly say that I've experienced this mental state, or at least I think I have. You tell me.
>
> "When I was young (and stupid) I used to get in fights. Not a lot, but it happened. When I was in a fight, it was as if all I could do was fight more and harder. I can't even say that I was thinking at all. There was no sense of right or wrong; there was no sense of time passing; all I could see was the guy I was fighting. There was just the immersive flow, and it carried me forward.
>
> "I've also experienced this feeling in competitive athletics (basketball, which I played for decades). I was utterly unconscious of the things I was doing (and they were pretty complicated because I was, if I don't say so myself, pretty good). It was as if the game was playing me. Very strange, and somewhat addictive. It was a good feeling."
>
> (From a report by a highly educated scholar)

(3) *Appetitive aggression* reprensts an underappreciated factor that is often tabooed. It refers to the intrinsically rewarding experience of aggressive action. Indeed, we reluctantly accept that the desire to hunt, including the thrill of hunting humans, is part of human nature (Elbert et al., 2010; Elbert, Moran, & Schauer, 2017a; Elbert, Moran, & Schauer, 2017b; Köbach et al., 2021). However, the prospect of capturing prey is often too distant to motivate hunters to expend the considerable effort required. Consequently, evolution has shaped both human and animal hunters alike to engage in a self-rewarding chain of action: The thrill of the chase, the rushing hunt, and the killing of the prey is always a great experience, whether or not you succeed in consuming your prey (Elbert et al., 2010). It's amazing how much motivation a prey animal or an incentive can provide! Even when there's no material benefit to be gained, the cat will chase the ball, just like people on a soccer team. Humans love to hunt in groups, whether it's in games or even while watching a sporting or war-like event on a screen. The resulting intrinsic reward can condition aggressive behaviour to the point of addiction. If you don't think that this is cool you have not understood what it means to be an addicitive hunter! (Elbert et al., 2017a, 2017b).

The latent passion for battle and dominance can be evoked in almost all men and in some women. The snowballing outcome of groups, tribes, or communities that enact this aggression is war and destruction, to the point of trying to extinguish entire ethnic groups. It is often covered by the morally more acceptable other forms of aggression (e.g., "God commands us to kill those who do not believe," or "We have to kill the cockroaches to save our people," or like a kind of James Bond, one is granted the "license to kill" to save the world – and this does not necessarily elicit negative emotions in viewers of the films.

Reactive and appetitive aggression drive two cycles of violence (see Figure 38). The *reactive cycle* with negative

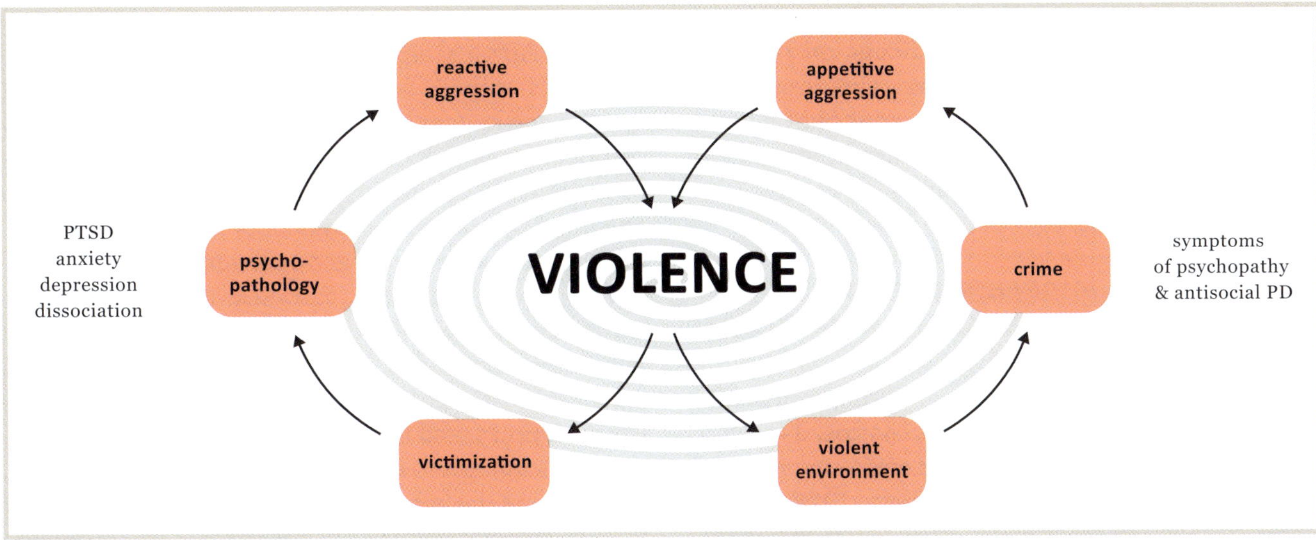

Figure 38. Bi-cycle of violence: The reactive (negative valent – left) and the appetitive (positive valent – right) cycles of violence interact to produce aggressive and violent behavior. The reactive cycle serves to reduce negative emotional arousal (e.g., fear) while the appetitive one fosters positive affect. PD = personality disorder. Drugs and propaganda are two means to lower the moral barriers and thus fuel both sides of this dynamic.

emotional valence is driven by threat and victimization, also any humiliation experience, which then lead to trauma-related disorders such as anxiety, PTSD, depression, dissociation, and eventually anger and fight, in the form of reactive-impulsive aggression. The *appetitive cycle*, with its positive emotional valence loop, is fueled by an environment that hijacks our reward system via the desire to hunt, thus positively reinforcing violent and criminal behavior, culminating in symptoms of antisocial personality disorder and psychopathy. Such an appetite for aggressive behavior is part of our human nature, and it is likely that testosterone boosts its rewarding properties (Elbert et al., 2018).

Both sides then include a secondary instrumental element, such as successfully eliminating threat or gaining safety, social status, or prey. All of these factors may favor, but are not required for, the motivation of violent behavior. While it is clinically and scientifically helpful to differentiate the forms of aggression, violence usually results from a mixture of the respective motivational drivers.

During development, especially at school age, children learn to set their moral barriers to regulate aggressive behavior. Under alcohol or other drugs, these barriers break down, and aggressive actions become more likely. Accordingly, substance abuse can fuel cycles of violence and drive individuals further into mental illness, both through the reactive trauma cycle and through appetitive aggression and desire for violence (Sommer et al., 2017).

Who becomes a perpetrator of violence? The available research indicates that individuals who use violence against their partner, children, or in the community, or belong to a violent group, are typically survivors of interpersonal trauma experienced during sensitive periods of their own psychological development. This evidence suggests a clear and overwhelming pattern (e.g., Capaldi et al., 2012; Vagi et al., 2013). Thus, the experience of severe interpersonal violence in childhood and adolescence is an important driver of later criminal behavior. Even in combatants in war-torn regions, childhood maltreatment may predict appetitive aggression which increases with combat exposure (Nandi et al., 2015, 2017). The link between childhood maltreatment and later violence has been demonstrated in many studies, such as in peaceful civil societies (e.g., Hawkins et al., 2000), refugee populations (e.g., Müller-Bamouh et al., 2016), and crisis regions (Augsburger et al., 2015; Hermenau et al., 2011; Nandi et al., 2015).

In numerous studies, gender-specific pathways have been identified that lead to the development of appetitive aggression and the use of force. Differences between male and female aggression can be observed as early as 17 months of age, with boys displaying more physical aggression than girls (Tremblay et al., 1999). Therefore, childhood maltreatment may result in impulsive-aggressive behavior, particularly in boys, while impulsive-self-injurious behavior may be more prevalent among female victims of interpersonal violence (Webb et al., 2017). The developers of violent video games are effectively capitalizing on the male urge to hunt and the allure of combat. They are exploiting the gratifying and prosocial experience of fighting and hunting in a group, for commercial purposes, which can potentially result in addiction for players.

Torn Between Victory and Defeat – Associative Memory Network of the Fighter

We interviewed members of armed groups, including child soldiers from various war scenarios, as well as young people who grew up in violent environments, such as street children (Crombach & Elbert, 2014) or gang members (e.g., Sommer et al., 2016, 2017; Hinsberger et al., 2016; Hermenau et al., 2013; Hecker et al., 2015). Moreover, we evaluated inmates in prisons across Europe and Africa. Corresponding to the NET logic, we inquired about their thoughts and emotions when a fight approached and during such a violent encounter. To our surprise, many individuals with significant exposure to potentially traumatizing events were resilient to the *building block effect* (see the section Survivors of Organized Violence) and did not experience trauma symptoms. They reported being carried away by the desire for combat and forgetting their own vulnerability. A skilled fighter may deny the possibility of defeat, avoiding fear, and pursuing the goal like a hunter. However, danger exists at all times, and fear remains in the background, ultimately surging to the forefront and impacting thoughts, feelings, and the individual as a whole. Soldiers exposed to such difficulties may become at risk of developing trauma-related disorders and subsequently search for an

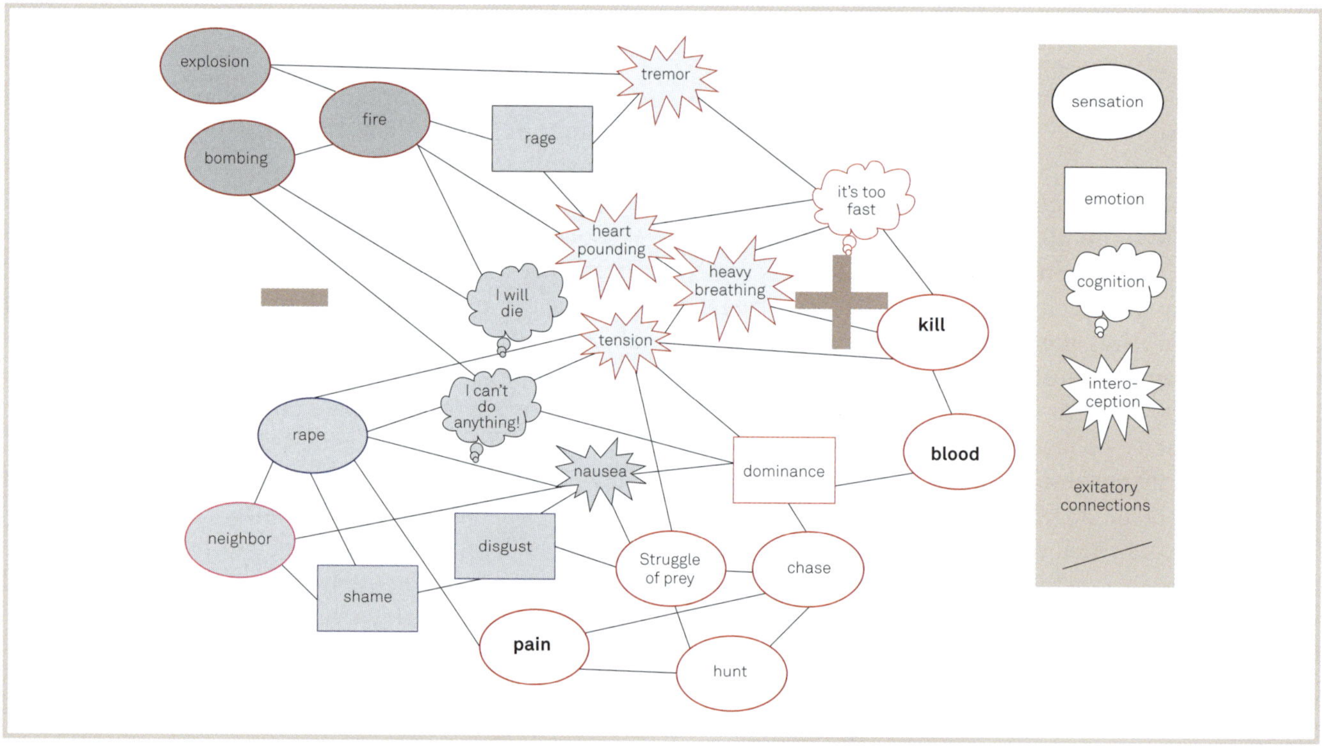

Figure 39. Emotionally salient experiences form an associative memory in which activation of individual representational elements lowers the threshold of activation of other elements. While a fear network (dark ovals) represents aversive experiences (minus sign), the hunting network (white shapes) is characterized by positive affective valence (symbolized by the plus sign in the sketch). Both networks feature many overlapping representational elements and are therefore highly interconnected, competing for cues indicating either positive or negative emotional valence. For example, blood can elicit fear and cause physical shutdown accompanied by nausea and trembling, or it can serve as a significant cue for aggression stimulating a lust for hunting, nourishment, and heroism, depending on factors such as context, age, gender, and prior experience. Experienced combatants exhibit resilience to trauma sequelae, but they may develop PTSD and depression *after* leaving an armed group, if the receiving society negatively attributes their mission and experiences. This negative attribution can transform a hero to a traumatized victim and vice versa. Social acknowledgment and inclusion can decrease the likelihood of developing PTSD in combatants returning home. (e.g., Sommer et al., 2017).

exit from their armed group. Posttraumatic stress, characterized by fear and horror, becomes more dominant with each experience of traumatic stressors, creating an increasing trauma load. Those who commit acts of interpersonal violence, either organized or individual, find themselves in a conflicting situation between the rewarding feelings associated with their actions and the perceived threats that activate the fear-centered part of their associative memory network. Figure 39 illustrates this situation.

The goal of NET is to reorganize the associations in the fear network by connecting the individual representational elements to the place and time of the experience and thus not allowing a set of cues to massively activate the whole network. In FORNET, the very same procedure is used to reorganize the "hunting network" - that is, the positive valence side. Additionally, social acceptance and inclusion are leveraged to control aggressive or competitive behaviors, ideally within group settings.

The Steps of FORNET

Individuals exposed to violent acts, including those who have committed violence themselves, are at risk of developing symptoms of PTSD, depression, and even dissociation, instead of aggression. It is important to objectively recognize the mental health risks associated with exposure to violence as well as perpetration of violence (as a consequence) and provide necessary support. However, current treatment for these trauma-related consequences often only addresses one aspect of this distressing issue. Untreated tendencies toward extreme aggression can perpetuate ongoing violence and cause suffering for both the victim and offender. FORNET (Elbert et al., 2012; Elbert & Schauer, 2021) addresses the valence-tension in associative memory and aims to influence both appetitive aggression and PTSD symptoms in individuals who have experienced and perpetrated interpersonal violence (Figure 40). After successful implementation in the DRC (Hermenau et al., 2013; Köbach et al., 2017; Köbach et al., 2021; Robjant et al., 2019), treatment studies have been conducted in Burundi with street children (Crombach & Elbert, 2014) and in South Africa among members of criminal gangs (Hinsberger et al., 2020). In these treatment studies, FORNET significantly reduced PTSD symptoms both statistically and clinically, as well as decreasing aggressive behavior, violence, and criminal acts. However, there has yet to be an RCT conducted on prison inmates. The tendency to commit violent acts can be inhibited if one can work through one's own traumatic experience of violence as well as the actual positive experience of committing violence. Perceptions, cognitions, emotions, arousal, and meaning should be recognized in both victim and perpetrator situations. Remembering experiences of threatening, injuring, and killing can be consciously sorted into past memories, put into perspective through complementary, ambivalent, and negatively arousing areas of experience, such as feelings of fear or disgust, negative arousal, and unpleasant social emotions and thus more fully understood.

As in NET, the first step of FORNET involves checklists. However, in this case, the checklists include not only information about traumatic and negatively stressful experiences but also about negatively or positively arousing violent behavior. Box 2 provides an example of such a checklist. The adapted psychoeducation by the therapist then needs to give information about traumatization, appetitive violence, and the human tendency to engage in fighting and hunting as a prosocial activity which can generate intrinsically motivated pleasure. It is crucial to explain the interplay between reactive and appetitive aggression (Figure 38).

Step 2 in FORNET involves the construction of a Lifeline in which, in addition to the typical stones and flowers, the individual's symbols (sticks) indicating their own acts of violence and coexperience of acts of violence (see Box 2 Checklist of violent acts) are presented in chronological order and placed in the context of the individual's lifetime, as well as in the broader systemic and sociopolitical context of that time. A treatment plan is created according to the individual's idiosyncratic experiences and traumatic events.

In Step 3, the Narrative Exposure, the life-threatening and violent events are selected to be worked through in chronological order in successive exposure sessions. Typically, exposure sessions occur on a weekly basis, but not more than twice a week. Especially for combatants, the number of traumatic events and acts of violence usually far exceeds the number of possible sessions for the time-consuming work of exposure. Events that should be worked through in depth can then be selected and prioritized for imaginative exposure according to those that meet the following criteria:

- The offender experienced physical, sexual, and emotional violence (Egeland, 2009) in their own childhood, especially by caregivers.

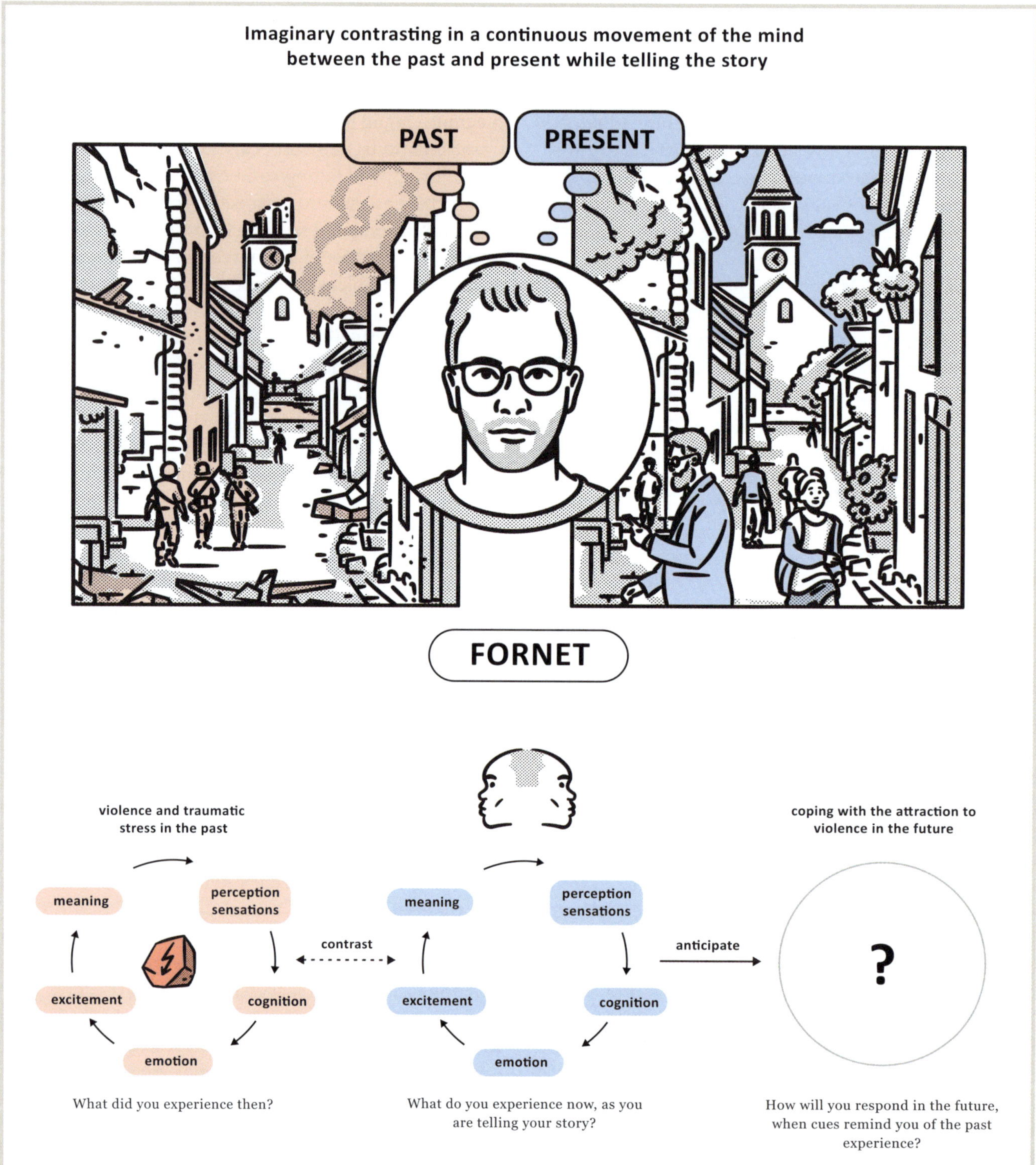

Figure 40. The Janus face of FORNET. In the exposure sessions of NET, the Narrative Exposure focuses on the perception at that time, reflects the thoughts and feelings accompanying them, and partially reactivates the physical arousal. Contrasting it with today's experience, FORNET puts special emphasis on the moral classification of the experiences. Ambivalent feelings during the violent acts are fully addressed. FORNET then emphasizes which influences these experiences might have on future behavior. The goal is to be able to better control aggression in the future and to consciously recognize positive experiences of fighting and hunting, as well as to learn to decouple impulses from actual behavior. Even in the case of heinous acts, the therapist unconditionally accepts the emotions that have occurred.

Box 2. Checklist of violent acts

Violent acts in which the person has actively engaged in aggressive and violent behavior include fighting, hitting, rape, and other threats to human life events (see THL checklist in Appendix 1; and see as well Weierstall & Elbert, 2011).

Have you ...

- Verbally threatened someone, such as calling them "fat," "ugly," "stupid," or similar names?
- Yelled at someone? Intentionally frightened someone by threatening injury to organs, tissues, or the central nervous system, such as physical violence, burns, strangulation, submerging someone under water; preventing someone from breathing; threatening to use animals, drugs, weapons or knives, or pointed, sharp, or blunt (impact) objects; confining someone; administering something by force that could harm the person; etc.?
- Aggressively socially excluded (ostracized) or belittled someone – for example, kicked them out of your home or from your group, insulted, humiliated, deliberately shamed, bullied ... them?
- Thrown an object at someone – for example, a shoe, a tool, etc.?
- Hit someone with your hand or fist, or knocked them down?
- Ever followed and chased someone to threaten or hurt them?
- Inflicted injury, pain, or torture (animal or human – any sentient being)? In other words, have you ever behaved in a way that caused injury to others? Including as part of your job?
- Were there bruises, bleeding, broken bones or any serious injuries?
- Did you experience any kind of (blood) frenzy while doing this?
- What increased the desire to go on?
- Did you touch another person in a sexual way without their permission?
- Did you force someone to have sex against their will?
- Have you robbed or stolen from someone?

- There were other significant traumatic events that occurred early in life, which can be sequenced chronologically.
- Some events were associated with the greatest stress (distress or eustress) – that is, high emotional and physiological arousal.
- Events of different types can be prioritized, over a second exposure of the same event type.
- Events associated with violent acts are included in balance with the experience of traumatic threat.
- Exposure to interpersonal violence outside the context of participation in an armed or criminal group is also included.

Events that occurred in close temporal proximity are worked through within the same session (e.g., kidnapping, rape, and forced torture and/or killing as initiation events that occurred within a 24-hr period are worked through in a longer session). Exposure sessions never conclude until any perceived pleasure in the aggression and accompanying physiological and emotional arousal have subsided and/or been neutralized. The excitement must have calmed down; been contrasted with other, more ambivalent sensations (that have also been present but suppressed), thoughts, and moral classification in the here and now; and been accompanied by good grounding in the present.

FORNET not only focuses on the past, but also imagines future scenarios, FORNET has, so to say, a *Janus face* (see Figure 40): In addition to the individual Narrative Exposure of highly arousing experiences from the past, the future-oriented component was added in FORNET to allow survivors to become aware of cues that may trigger or attract them to future violent behavior in the community and at home.

When possible, FORNET includes soliciting support in group sessions from comrades with similar experiences. Because ex-combatants are often a stigmatized population whose emotional world of combat experience cannot be readily accessed by civilians, the group format facilitates social entry into a peaceful community. This forward-looking component includes skills training in recognizing negative affect and basic anger management, conflict avoidance, and problem solving in stressful situations. Special emphasis is placed on increasing motivation to behave in a nonviolent manner and to take on a constructive role in the community.

- The narrator is encouraged to talk about positive and negative perceptions, thoughts, emotions and bodily sensations, and meaning content – even with memories of horrific acts of violence and assault.
- The participant is encouraged to verbalize all perceptions, emotions, thoughts, and body feelings, as well as the interpretations related to the violent act, and to describe and contrast the *current* experience when these memories are recalled.
- The therapist guides the narrator and contrasts then with now.

- The goal for violent acts is understanding and attributing meaning.
  - Under what circumstances did the violent act occur?
  - How do you feel about the violent act today?
  - What will determine your options for action in the future?

In addition to constructing the individual narrative of past formative experiences, the thoughts and feelings that may arise in future situations are discussed during several sessions, likewise at weekly intervals. Where possible, this can be implemented in a group format in addition; The group sessions aim to develop skills and motivation to avoid engaging in violence within the community. The first session focuses on role reversal from member of an armed group or gang to a civilian, as suggested by Hermenau et al. (2013). The second and third sessions include psychoeducation and basic anger recognition, emotion regulation, and behavior change skills to avoid violence-provoking conditions. When possible, Session two introduces a *buddy system* in which clients are encouraged to form pairs to help each other cope with frustrations. Sessions three through six focus on deconstructing experiences of violence and violence avoidance in the previous week. Group members are encouraged to support each other's attempts to avoid violence, suggest alternative methods of conflict resolution, and problem solve practical difficulties. The therapist reduces their own involvement in the group over the course of the six sessions, and clients are encouraged to meet without the therapist and to discuss ways of successful occupational development (Robjant et al., 2019; Köbach et al., 2021). This last stage is necessary to obtain social status, to escape from poverty, and to limit frustration.

Although the link between past interpersonal trauma experience and future violent behavior has long been clearly established (see Delsol & Margolin, 2004, for a review), to date both public health and rehabilitation programs and violence prevention programs have overlooked the need to heal the underlying trauma of perpetrators and failed to recognize and honor their emotional and mental turmoil in receiving and perpetrating violence. Extinguishing the resurgence of past violence is required to bring aggression into its acceptable bounds. The studies on FORNET have developed an evidence-based psychotherapeutic solution supported by evidence from half a dozen controlled clinical trials.

Dealing with aggressive and violent actions during Narrative Exposure

Killing or injuring

- Reactivate and verbalize all perceptions, feelings, thoughts, body sensations, and meanings.
- Reactivate and verbalize then; that is, explicitly put into words and a narrative.
- Be as specific as possible about the first killing or injury, since ambivalence, fear, and hesitation can be experienced (hesitation can be experienced even more clearly).
- Besides the basic emotions (disgust, fear, or joy et cetera) also the social emotions (pride, envy, shame, contempt, revenge) are named
- Specify how the victim was perceived (how did the victim look? Did they scream? How were the victim's reactions experienced – at what moments did inhibitions appear and how were they overcome? How was the victim hurt, made to bleed, ...?
- Work out which justifications helped in the killing or injuring of another person (e.g., "outgroup," "enemy," or "subhuman").
- Feel and verbalize what emotional reactions (basic emotions like fear and social ones like revenge, hatred, or envy) supported the act.
- Put into words current and present thoughts and feelings about the first killing or injury, and discuss the meaning of this event for them and in their life, together with the therapist and discuss.

Rape

- During the detailed recollection and autobiographical reconstruction of a rape, the client names positive (pleasure, positive arousal, dominance) and negative (fear, disgust, shame) feelings.
- Especially during gang rape; that is, rape in groups of usually two to six men, perpetrators report feelings of disgust, fear of failure, and loss of control.
- After autobiographical processing and a change of perspective to the present day, the therapist and client discuss sexual desires of the client and compare their expected pleasures with the experiences from the rape.

Robbery and looting

- Again, the first such act is given a special meaning, along with its positive (reward, feelings of power) and negative (fear of injury, defeat, and punishment) feelings.
- In general, acts of violence are discussed, especially when they were accompanied by high levels of excitement and thus unforgettably contributed to the formation of a hunting network.
- In the context of attributing meaning, it is not forgotten that many of the perpetrators were also victims of such acts.

Double Avoidance in Veterans

The fear network contains painful memories, so any activation is avoided. In most civilian settings, however, fighters may also avoid reporting the positive valence side of the associative network of fighting and warlike actions. Those who are not involved in combat, nonfighters, and nonhunters are unlikely to comprehend and accept the appetitive side of wanting to fight and kill. As a result, the soldier avoids recalling not only fearful but also positive memories in therapy. Even though young people are sent into battle, society often does not accept acts of war. This also leads those affected to morally question their actions, resulting in feelings of shame and guilt. It impairs the ability to engage in restorative (recuperative) behaviors for emotional or physical injuries. In this situation, the therapist may need to have a discussion with the client to educate them that it is not their job to portray the client as a heroic figure or point fingers of blame at them. Rather, the goal is to comprehend the survivor's emotional and cognitive experiences fully by working in depth during Narrative Exposure (while also taking into account shame and guilt, see Chapter 5). The deep value of comradeship, the unwavering sense of purpose that military service and group unity impart, must be addressed in the narratives as much as the grief of its loss in order to fully integrate the past.

The NETfacts Health System: Healing Traumatized Communities

As wounded, people may be cared for, but as storytellers, they care for others [...] all those who suffer, can also be healers. Their injuries become the source of the potency of their stories [...] Because stories can heal, the wounded healer and wounded storyteller are not separate [...] When any person recovers her voice, many people begin to speak through that story...

Arthur A. Frank (2013, p. 90)

NET is a treatment aimed at helping individuals who have experienced trauma. Nevertheless, entire communities may find themselves subjected to recurrent trauma stemming from organized violence, natural disasters, ideological terror, or marginalization. Such events have impacts beyond those directly affected. Hence, the dynamics within the community may lead to a break down at the societal level, ultimately amplifying the individual's distress. Repeated air strikes, a tsunami, or ongoing state-sponsored violence such as persecution and torture can have a psychological impact on those within and beyond the group. All community members can be left scared by these events, which may affect them for the remainder of their lives. The longer and more frequently the threats and stressors persist, the more challenging it can be to build up and maintain a normal life thereafter.

To support traumatized communities, a team of psychologists and conflict researchers have developed the NETfacts health system in cooperation with the aid organization vivo international (Robjant et al., 2020, 2022; Schmitt et al., 2022). Complementing NET, which focuses on the individual, NETfacts combines individual treatment with a collective process.

<NETfacts in a nutshell (Figure 41): A representative sample of individuals in the community are first screened for signs of PTSD and significant aggressive behavior. Affected individuals are each offered individual treatment with typical NET. The individual trauma narratives are then combined to shed light on major events. In sessions offered to all community members, the community works through the history of their shared traumatic events.

For example, after a (para)military raid on their village, the first community session uses the symbolic objects flowers and stones (for positive and negative experiences), sticks (for combat), and a symbol for loss (e.g., candle) to visualize the community's Lifeline and develop a unified understanding with a focus on the traumatic events (Figure 42) In subsequent sessions, the *collective memory* of the community is supplemented with the personal experiences of its members. Major stones are considered from the different perspectives obtained from the set of individual (but anonymized) narrations. On the one hand, this helps everyone in the community to come to terms with the traumatic event and acknowledge it as part of the community's history. On the other hand, it challenges harmful narratives such as stigmatization and rape myths (Schmitt et al., 2022).

Not only are traumatized individuals afraid of their own memories, but also communities show collective avoidance that may prevail. Survivors are socially silenced, and often blamed for their experience of traumatic stressors. They are looked down upon for what they have been through and for not being able to hide their mental pain. We can only help lessen trauma and harm

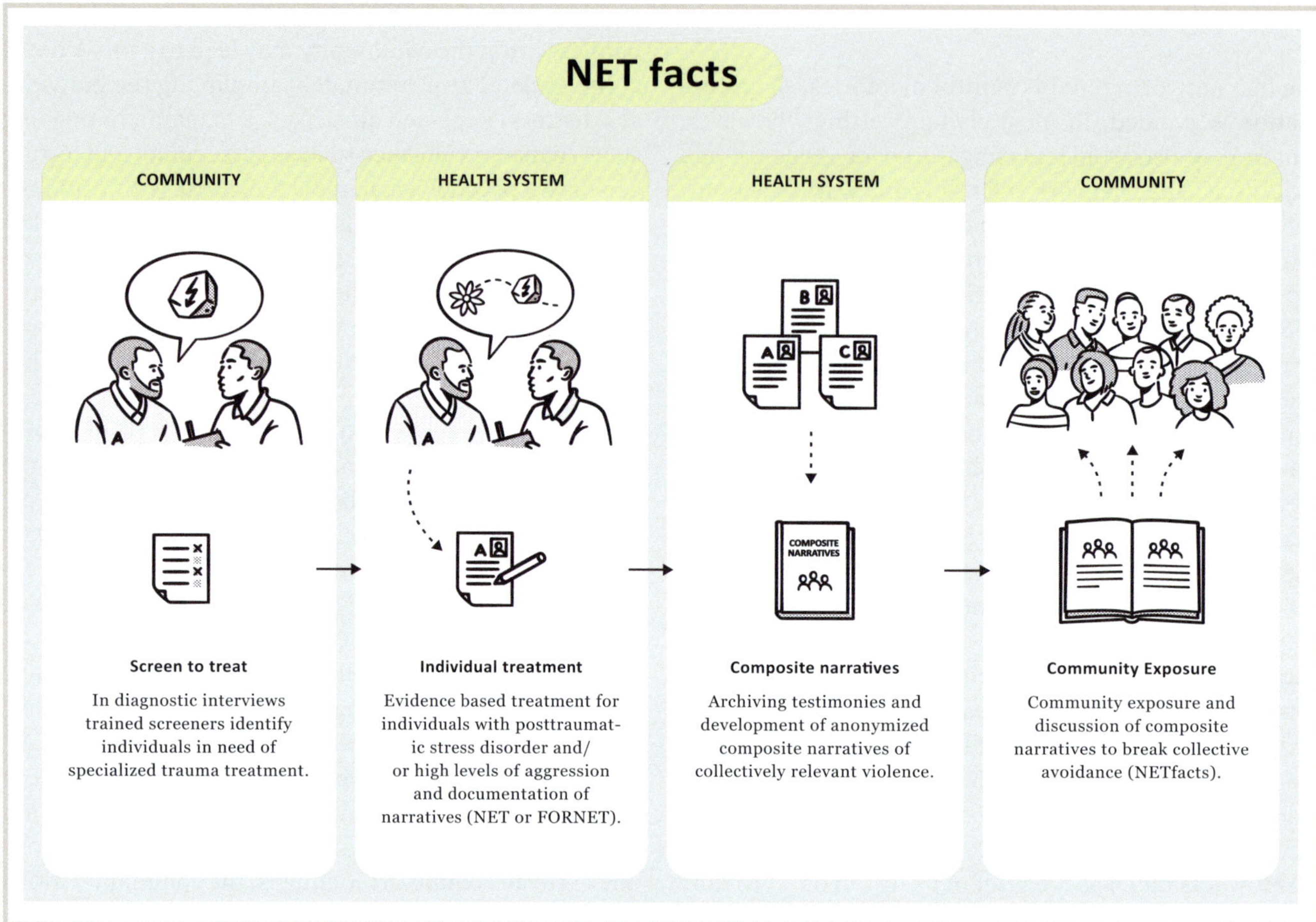

Figure 41. The procedure of the NETfacts health system. During NETfacts, the community is confronted with composite narratives constructed from narrations of individual NET. These include the following: (1) Collective awareness of trauma survivors' peritraumatic and posttraumatic experiences increase social support, but survivors often do not disclose them. (2) Not knowing the details may cause misinterpretation and maintain prejudices, stigmatization, and social exclusion. (3) Public discourse based on first-hand testimonies facilitates perspective taking and fosters social cohesion (Figure composed with advice from A. Köbach, personal communication, 2024). Also available as a handout in the online supplementary materials for this book.

caused by violence, by creating a place for those affected to speak out. This should be accessible not only during one-to-one therapy with a counselor, but also to the broader community. This insight motivated us to develop the NETfacts health system (Robjant, Schmitt, et al., 2020, 2022; Schmitt et al., 2022). It gathers facts from personal treatments and promotes the handling of natural disasters and of violations of human rights by and within neighborhoods. Accounts from individual witnesses differ from a historian's record. They stick to the NET approach, meaning they do not just report on the basic facts of what happened, when and where it took place. Instead, they highlight the emotions, thoughts, and reactions felt by the survivors when the unthinkable occurred, as well as their efforts to make sense of it all.

The theory has been explored in Africa's war-torn Great Lakes regions and also in camps with criminal groups in South Africa. In most cases, the number of people suffering from trauma in these conflict-ridden areas is too great and resources too scarce to provide tailored treatment to all who require it. Current findings suggest that those with milder symptoms of trauma may be capable of integrating into the community. Stigma and exclusion can be reduced, and suffering can be acknowledged by society (Sommer et al., 2016).

NETfacts uses a stepped-care model with three parts (Robjant, Schmitt et al., 2022). Firstly, severely traumatized survivors are given NET. Secondly, FORNET provides NET for Forensic Offender Rehabilitation, acknowledging that perpetrators are often also victims,

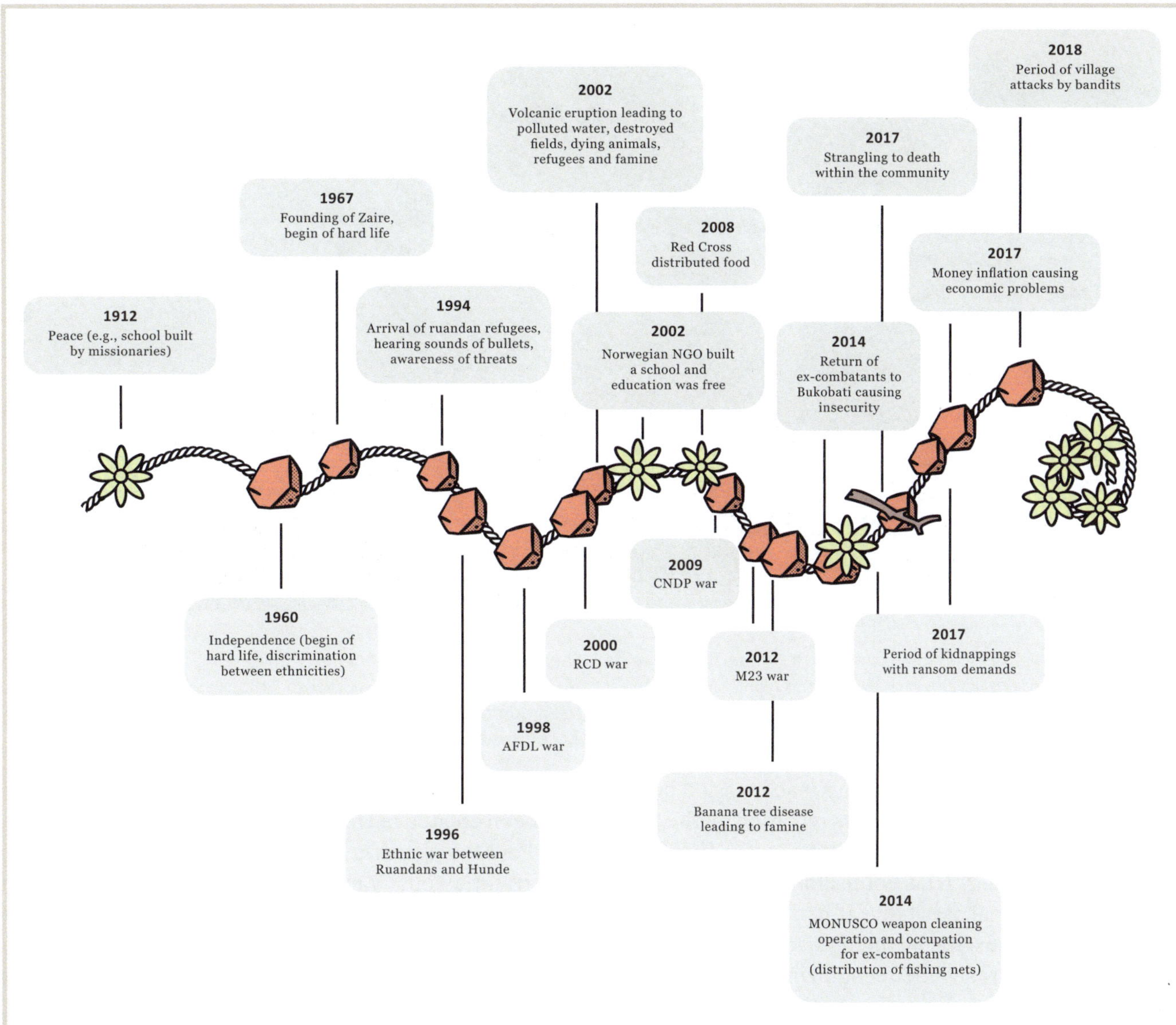

Figure 42. Lifeline of a community that had to suffer violence and trauma repeatedly. The various abbreviations refer to irregular armed groups (based on data from Schmitt et al., 2022).

helping them cope with trauma, and reduce their aggression and attraction to violence. Finally, Step 3 entails a community intervention, sharing and discussing facts focused on vivid memories from NET. Community leaders and a NETfacts facilitator work together to address avoidance of traumatic events and aid the community in dealing with significant and highly problematic issues.

Robjant et al. (2022) used NETfacts in six war-ridden communities in the DRC and compared results with those from the classic NET program, with a total of 1,066 persons. The results showed that both NET and NETfacts significantly reduced the severity of PTSD and depression in all cases. Additionally, after NETfacts, fewer rape myths and stigmatizations of victims were accepted, resulting in a decrease in emotional and physical violence in the community and beyond.

A village attack, for instance, as noted by Schmitt et al. (2022), represented a collective traumatic event but could also contain diverse individual experiences, such as running for one's life, witnessing torture, being raped, being abducted into an armed group, or, especially in the case of combatants, being forced to kill, or willingly killing, another person. Community members without PTSD were given the opportunity to narrate a meaningful personal event during an exposure session before the second community session, which took place 2 weeks

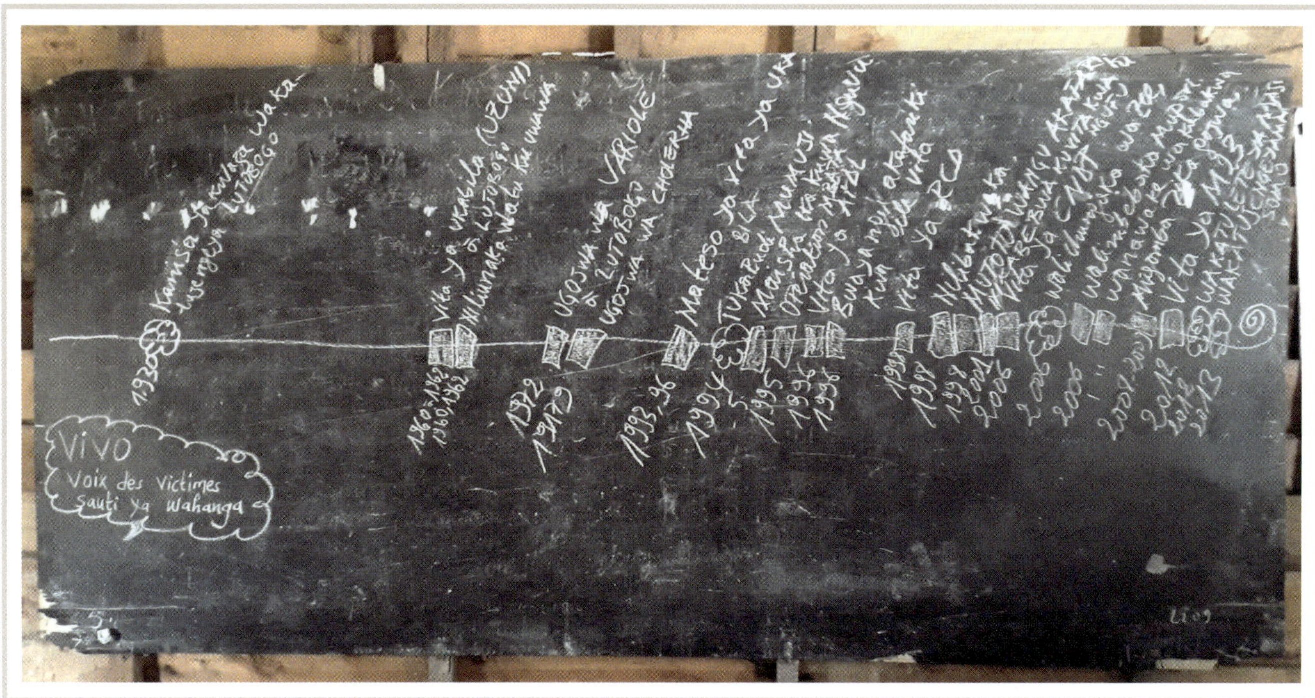

Figure 43. In a NETfacts session conducted by Amani Chibashimba, villagers created their community's Lifeline. Amani now heads the follow-up project in which several thousand people benefit from NET and NETfacts every month. Photo by Katy Robjant (available at https://www.uni-konstanz.de/fileadmin/pi/fileserver/2022/Traumatisierte_Gemeinschaften_1.jpg).

later. In three subsequent meetings, each session began with a brief reminder of the events recorded on the Lifeline. The chosen composite narratives were then read aloud and discussed. NET counselors were present to provide professional assistance if necessary. Attendees were prompted to exchange their personal thoughts and emotional responses while recognizing and predicting the various needs of the main character following the event. Each conversation was concluded by harmonizing the protagonist's traumatized requirements with those of the community. The final meeting was terminated by gathering aspirations for the community's future, symbolized by flowers placed on the coiled section of the Lifeline.

In the trials by Schmitt et al. (2022, Figure 42) and Robjant et al. (2022, Figure 43), NETfacts demonstrated immediate beneficial effects for trauma-related suffering. The rejection of rape myths was also supported in the eastern DRC region, where organized and individual violence has led to endemic rates of rape. Additionally, attitudes toward ex-combatants improved, and their experiences were more socially acknowledged. It is widely accepted that this lowers mental symptoms and supports integration into society. However, the long-term consequences of this intervention remain to be examined.

A brilliant example in the form of a captivating theater has been created in Umeå, Sweden by Susanne Axelsson and Per Mossegård, in collaboration with Resurscentrum för traumastöd, Vårsta diakoni, and Skuggteatern (https://www.skuggteatern.com/barrikad). In the production titled *Barrikad*, a play was crafted from composite narratives drawn from local female FORNET clients who actively contributed to the development of the script, with their narrations thoughtfully anonymized. After each performance, the artists engaged in meaningful discussions with the audience to assess the play's impact.

ElderNET: NET as Trauma-Memory Focused Treatment for Older Adults

Older individuals are especially vulnerable to suffering after traumatic events – particularly older individuals with physical or cognitive disabilities, and especially in complex humanitarian crises (van Boetzelaer et al., 2023). Although they traditionally hold a position of respect in their communities and have knowledge and experience from which we can learn, their voices are too often unheard and not taken into account. While it is possible to find something positive in a negative experience, it is important to note that this does not mean that the traumatic stress was positive or that it can outweigh the suffering and challenges associated with the trauma. However, through narrative biography work, it is possible to reduce suffering and develop a positive perspective that can be helpful in healing from trauma. "ElderNET" aims not only to provide relief from trauma-related symptoms, but also to enable older people to reflect on their lives, to give them a voice to share their experiences and insights, and to help those who have experienced human rights violations discover their inner strengths and gain a deeper understanding of their relationships with others.

Obstacles and Specifics of Trauma Treatment in Old and Very Old Age

Older people typically make little use of psychotherapy. This has to do in part with a lack of openness on the part of those affected, who were not brought up to express or talk about their feelings, especially not to strangers. Furthermore, there are not enough opportunities for older people to share and disclose, which can lead to silence and an increased risk of developing cognitive deficits and PTSD (Burri et al., 2013). Effective interventions can also prevent or slow the decline of memory function and the development of dementia in later life.

To better serve older individuals, interventions such as life reviewing or life resolution seeking may be more appropriate than attempting to modify their cognitive structures or behaviors, including addressing "wrong" beliefs or sticking points. Therefore, we are committed to promoting a narrative lifespan approach called ElderNET as an age-appropriate, life-affirming adaptation of NET that emphasizes self-reflection and review of the life lived. Respect for the wisdom and experience of older individuals (Jeste et al., 2020, 2021) but also considerations of age-related cognitive and physical challenges, both confirm the appropriateness of a Life Narration. However, they also suggest an adaptation of the three pillars of NET (intake checklist, Lifeline, and Narrative Exposure) to a long life with a limited lifetime ahead and a senescent mind and body. Insight and gaining wisdom with its features of prosocial behaviors, self-reflection, and emotional awareness, may reduce loneliness and improve well-being especially its compassion component (Lee et al., 2021; Ekwonye, 2022).

Reemerging of mental disorders in individuals who had seemed to control problems after previous difficult periods in their past might pose an additional challenge in older age. Anxiety or depression may return or worsen as a result of loss of health or ability. Cognitive aging occurs gradually, whereby episodic memory especially may be affected (Greene & Naveh-Benjamin, 2023; Blazer & Wallace, 2016). With NET, it is possible to successfully treat individuals with cognitive decline, up to the extent of intellectual disability (Marlow et al., 2022; Mayer et al., 2023; Mayer & Needham, 2011; Mayer, 2020). And while typical trauma reactions, such as depression, substance use, obesity, etc., aggravate cognitive decline, trauma memory-focused therapy can counteract this process (Mauritz et al., 2016, 2021, 2022).

Using NET, we had, already 2 decades ago, together with Dana Bichescu, focused on the stories of older survivors by continuously verbalizing and contrasting sensations, emotions, behaviors, and details of the now and the then. The therapist's attitude was empathic and nonjudgmental, while the participating older men were guided to confront their fears along with their chronological narrative. The men, living in Romania, who were aged around 70 years at the time of treatment, had been imprisoned and tortured while spending half a dozen years in detention, some 40 years ago.

As organized violence usually involves prolonged, severe, and/or multiple exposures to trauma, in most cases it is difficult and unreasonable to identify a "worst" event. Moreover, trying to approach a traumatic scene using a ready-made "technique" may be inappropriate or even immoral, as in the case of severe abuses of human rights. The goal of NET is more holistic. The life of the person as a whole is examined, from birth to the present day, with the purpose of gradually identifying all positive and negative emotional moments.... Emotional memories are put into words and contrasted with the emotional experience elicited during the recall.... The act of reliving one's own life, by seeing, hearing, smelling, etc. scenes from the past, allows one not only to understand the meaning and the development of the person but also to recognize coherences, life-patterns, coincidences, and not least of all who the survivor was when encountering the first (second, third etc.) trauma.... The way of writing down the whole life of the person, ... the way of writing down the whole life of the survivor, and the distribution of the document in a ritualized manner to be signed by all witnesses present during the narration.... The narratives serve not only therapeutic but also social and political purposes by the documentation of human rights violations.

Bichescu et al. (2007, p. 2213)

The survivors received ElderNET treatment in five 2-hr sessions once or twice a week. PTSD symptoms and depression decreased substantially, and avoidance and arousal symptoms especially started to disappear, which improved sleep and cardiovascular conditions in the older men.

In 2018, Mørkved and Thorp presented a case study on NET with a 70-year-old Norwegian woman whose intake checklist revealed that she had suffered emotional and sexual childhood abuse, as well as multiple other traumatic events during childhood, adolescence, and adulthood. She had attempted suicide in her youth but had been rescued. At the time of assessment, the survivor presented with hyperarousal, anxiety, physical dissociation, severe nightmares, sleep and fatigue disturbances, decreased social functioning, and deep-seated feelings of shame and guilt. The woman reported severe avoidance, depression, and reduced hope for the future. She expressed dysfunctional assumptions about her value as a human being and difficulties regulating her emotions. Additionally, she suffered from several physical and neurological problems, which had caused her health to deteriorate over the years. She had been living on prescribed antidepressants for years. Results after 16 NET sessions showed that her PTSD and depressive symptoms had decreased to mild levels, a process that continued into follow-up. Treatment could be administered safely and effectively to this woman with her complex trauma history and PTSD. She did not experience any suicidal thoughts, and there was no noticeable cognitive decline (Mørkved & Thorp, 2018).

ElderNET highlights the benefits for older adults in reviewing their major important and arousing experiences across the whole lifespan, while supporting an autobiographical testimony that addresses existential themes and meaning making. Reviewing their life can significantly improve the quality of life in older adults (Lely et al., 2017, 2022; Lely, De la Rie, et al., 2019; Lely, Knipscheer, et al., 2019; Mørkved & Thorp, 2018; Sharif et al., 2018, Bichescu et al., 2007). PTSD treatments for older adults have raised questions about the safety of trauma processing for vulnerable individuals and the need for trauma exposure to effectively treat them. Lely, Knipscheer, et al. (2019) demonstrated that directly targeting traumatic memories with NET did not harm these vulnerable participants. Treatment dropout rates were low in comparison. Lely states that "many older adults prefer to share their experiences, with the aim of re-appraising maladaptive meanings and with the hope to break the cycles of re-experience and avoidance, which frequently maintain exhaustion and despair" (p. 375). Looking more closely at participants' narratives, Lely et al. describe many "ghosts from the past" that haunt people into old age, especially after childhood abuse, neglect, and violence (Lely, De la Rie, et al., 2019). Therapists who allow their patients to revisit their past experiences can help them make positive changes that will impact their lives for years to come (Bisson et al., 2013; Maercker & Zöllner, 2002; Maercker & Bachem, 2013).

The Past as a Resource – Reminiscence Through ElderNET

Personal narratives in the lives of older people often focus more on the past. They repeatedly describe how the world was "back then" – the seasons, their hometown, and routine activities, as well as activities with loved ones when they were alive. The personal past is a critical aspect of identity in adulthood, especially in the later phases of life (Westerhof et al., 2020). During conversations, older adults frequently recall past experiences in the context of the present, which provides them with a shared sense of meaning. This feature of talk is far less salient among young adults (Boden & Bielby, 1983). The natural tendency to reminisce in old age (Coleman, 1989), embracing the memories and *storying* of one's experience in the present, has healing potential even in the face of loss and a limited future (Harvey et al., 2001). Memorizing times of self-efficacy and strengthening hope can be an effective method to enhance the quality of life of older people (Nikdel et al., 2016). Many older people feel a sense of loss as they age, and reminiscing about their past can help them relive fond memories and feel a sense of comfort. In addition, sharing stories from the past can help in old age to bond with their loved ones and pass on family history to future generations.

Sharing memories in the presence of an empathic, mindful, and nonjudgmental listener, and later sitting back and listening to one's own life stories, is a uniquely fascinating and validating experience (Schauer et al., 2005). In contrast, secrecy can be experienced as burdensome and stressful, especially since every life has secrets that cannot be shared with anyone, often for that entire lifetime. Revealing secrets helps to gain new insights and release emotions, which in turn leads to better mental and physical health (Pennebaker & Seagal, 1999; Kelly, 2002).

Traumatic childhood experiences, especially those that cannot be discussed openly with others, put individuals at higher risk for disease, especially those who have experienced trauma that they have not discussed with others (Pennebaker & Stone, 2004). Translating distressing experiences into words can significantly impact one's health. Storytelling is a natural human process that helps individuals understand their experiences and themselves, especially when accompanied by the written word. This process allows for the organization and coherent remembrance of events while integrating thoughts and feelings, providing individuals with a sense of predictability and control over their lives. Seeing through biographical situations can allow a new perspective and give structure and meaning to experiences, making their emotional impact more manageable. This promotes a sense of resolution, reducing rumination and allowing troubling experiences to gradually fade from conscious thought.

As early as 40 years ago, Carlson's interviews with older community residents supported the view that reminiscing promotes the maintenance of self-esteem and continuity of identity in the last stage of the life cycle. The interviews demonstrated the quality and content of positive reminiscing (Carlson, 1984). Other studies have shown a direct positive relationship between self-positive reminiscence functions (identity, death preparation, and problem solving) and psychological well-being (life satisfaction, and fewer depressive and anxiety symptoms). Prosocial reminiscence and advocacy (conversation, teaching or informing others) also appear to be associated with well-being (O'Rourke et al., 2016).

Reminiscence involves sharing thoughts and feelings about one's experiences to recall and reflect on important events. The stories of the past provide a source of affirmation, hope, and belief that one's heritage will be preserved. In addition to enhancing self-identity, reminiscing may also protect against depression and loneliness (Bjornestad et al., 2019). In a study of 47 nursing home residents, a reminiscence group showed improvements in depression and loneliness after sharing memories, life events, family history, and personal achievements (Franck et al., 2016).

Trauma memory therapy in old age can help to process the trauma, and promote social inclusion and resilience. It can also promote a healthier way of dealing with one's own body and thereby counteract negative physical consequences. In this sense, psychotherapy in older people is not only indicated for the treatment of mental disorders, but also serves to maintain activity thus to prevent the deterioration of mental and social functions. It has been shown that depression and nightmares decrease at the end of NET, and that in the month afterwards, psychological and physical health increases as well as gratitude. On the other hand, there is less lamentation and more pride and a sense of strength in having made it through life and shown perseverance (Lely, De la Rie, et al., 2019). Participants selected for these NET studies showed no signs of mental disability.

For ElderNET, which focuses on advanced age, it is also important to consider the needs of vulnerable individuals. Marlow and colleagues (2022) have developed useful suggestions, which we have incorporated in the emerging ElderNET concept.

Adjustments of NET Steps for ElderNET Protocol

Introductory Phase and Event Checklists

During the introductory phase, the following steps are important: Get to know each other and find out about the special needs of the older person (how can they sit well – e.g., positioning of legs, arms, back; what are their requirements for medical breaks and for needing to drink, etc.).

- Ask about their abilities in the area of sensory perceptions such as sight and hearing. Explain that you will speak slowly and clearly with patience to ensure understanding and predictability. Sometimes it may be helpful to reduce the amount and level of vocabulary and abstraction.
- Organize transportation: In order to ease the situation in case of (multiple) chronic diseases and to compensate for reduced mobility, perhaps a driving escort should be organized for the journey to and from the session, or with appropriate digital assistance, the eNET format (see the section eNET – Delivering NET via the Internet) could be considered.
- Improve the structure and predictability of the treatment procedure by clearly announcing each subsequent step.
- Completing event checklists may take longer due to the increased number of events and the need to recall times from the distant past.

Lifeline Session

When moving on to Step 2, the following considerations need to be taken into account: Repetition of the rationale for the Lifeline exercise should be considered: Recall that quite different traumatic stressors can result in similar cognitions and emotions, fusing them into a general memory of stressful experiences.

- Use the language of the survivor, when explaining the cause of symptoms and the procedure of the Lifeline.
- Persons with older age (and their therapists) may want or need to stay seated during the Lifeline procedure: The materials can be placed on a table or a paper-and-pencil version can be provided, particularly if placing materials on a line on the floor is physically challenging.
- Stones and flowers maybe supplemented with visual aids, such as emoticons (emotion icons) to support the client's understanding of the meaning of the symbols.
- Directive questioning is recommended to keep the client focused on the Lifeline.

Narrative Exposure

When moving on to Step 3, further considerations may need to be taken into account: Increased prompting and direction from the therapist are recommended to support the client's narration during Narrative Exposure. Be aware that older individuals may have age-related changes in memory and cognition. Adjust the pace of therapy and use memory aids or prompts if needed.

- Repetition of the rationale for narration, including psychoeducation about exposure as well as the use of historical documentation, is recommended. Personal narratives mean learning from and understanding of the past.
- Shortening of session duration or breaks maybe necessary for older participants.
- Survivors are encouraged to bring along documents such as photos or souvenirs to support their expression and recall. This includes the use of drawings, letters, cherished small items, etc. to inform the listener and guide the client through narrating different aspects of their experience. This approach increases predictability for the narrator and supports the testimonial reality.
- Older people may require additional time in sessions to process information and progress at a slower pace, if necessary. It is important to note that particularly surprising discoveries about the meaning of stressful experiences and their interconnections may take time to be fully comprehended.
- Older individuals may have a political agenda that is intertwined with their experiences. The narration acknowledges this, but clients are informed that they should avoid using the narration for societal or political purposes. Survivors are advised to carefully consider and plan before making any part of their testimony public. Ideally, several months should be allowed for trauma symptoms to subside before engaging in confrontational activities.

Therapists want to be aware that there are areas that require great sensitivity to people of advanced age. Older individuals often experience loneliness due to the loss of loved ones, their own illnesses, or unresolved stress. This can be especially difficult when their ability to persevere or maintain independence decreases. To establish a meaningful personal connection, it is important to have an honest and open dialogue with the older person and to listen to their life story. Furthermore, like ethnocentric views, racism, or gender bias, generational bias can arise: a younger therapist may have difficulty with the morals and values of an older storyteller. Therapists' age stereotypes can also contribute, as they may underestimate older people's potential for change through psychotherapy. And vice versa, older people may deny the competence of a younger therapist. They may seem preachy and condescending. Therapists should be mindful of their own emotions. When working with survivors, it is important to recognize transference phenomena and understand that the survivor may be trying to regain control that was lost during the traumatic event. To maintain structure and focus on specific events, therapists may use the Narrative Exposure cycle rather than engaging the participant in discussion. Remember that sometimes turmoil occurs because avoidance gets in the way.

General Considerations for Implementing ElderNET

When working with older individuals, some modifications and considerations may be necessary to tailor the therapy to their unique needs:

1. **Assessment and diagnosis**: Ensure a comprehensive assessment is conducted to confirm the diagnosis of a trauma-related cause of the suffering and rule out any other medical or psychological conditions that may present similar symptoms, since chronic diseases, multiple chronic diseases, and unrecognized problems can impair communication and memory skills.
2. **Medical history**: Gather a detailed medical history, including any preexisting medical conditions and medications, as these can influence the communication and expectations for healing.

3. **Trauma history**: Understand the specific traumatic events the older person experienced, as well as their coping mechanisms and past attempts at treatment.
4. **Cultural and generational sensitivity**: Be mindful of the person's cultural background and beliefs, as these can influence their perception of trauma and willingness to engage in treatment. Be aware that values and moral guidelines vary greatly across a lifetime.
5. **Physical health**: Take into account the person's physical health, mobility limitations, and any chronic illnesses that might impact treatment planning and implementation. Ensure that the therapy environment is comfortable and accessible.
6. **Social support**: Assess the person's social support system, as older individuals may face increased isolation and may benefit from involving social others in the treatment process. Engage family members, caregivers, or eligible friends in the therapy process, as they can provide valuable support and understanding.
7. **Medication management and other professionals:** If medication is prescribed or the client is seeing other professionals, consider contacting the treating doctor, psychiatrist, or other professionals to work hand in hand with them. Typically, the survivor can help with suggestions, and who to get in touch with. Collaborate with other health care professionals, such as geriatric specialists, social workers, and caregivers, to ensure a comprehensive and integrated treatment plan.
8. **Resilience**: Survivors of old age have managed to live for a long time. Show your validation and respect when discussing their Lifeline and listening to their narrations.
9. **Fear of death and dying**: Traumatized individuals have survived near death situations and/or existential threats to life and integrity in their personal past. Now, at old age or very old age, they are confronted again with the end of their lifetime and with fear of having to endure suffering and pain. Our experience is that trauma survivors self-avoid addressing one particular issue that the therapist needs to carefully inquire about – namely, their concern that the moment of dying will feel like the horror and helplessness already experienced peritraumatically. Here, explanation and psychoeducation help to understand the distinction, but also trauma processing, so that individuals do not have to endure additional pathological fears and trauma triggers (e.g., feeling of futility originating from past trauma moments of desperation). Timely and detailed planning of trauma-informed support that guarantees self-determined decisions helps empower the survivor, as well as caretakers knowledgeable of trauma reactions and dissociation.
10. **Ongoing trauma**: Participants presenting with acute or chronic trauma symptoms may be suffering from current and ongoing trauma. Be aware that abuse of and aggression toward older people is not uncommon. It may include physical, sexual, psychological, and emotional abuse; financial and material abuse; abandonment; neglect; and serious loss of dignity and respect.
11. **Personalize the treatment:** It is important to personalize the treatment approach for each person based on their specific needs and circumstances. Involving the older individual in the decision-making process can empower them and enhance treatment outcomes.

NET in the Face of Foreseeable End of Life

Who wants to live is condemned to hope.
Claude Lanzmann, *Shoah*

If anything can, it is memory that will save humanity.
For me, hope without memory is like
memory without hope.
Just as man cannot live without dreams,
he cannot live without hope.
If dreams reflect the past, hope summons the future.
Elie Wiesel

Mental health thrives on hope, on the prospect that things will get better, that the body will heal, and that suffering will end. What does hope look like at a very advanced age? Is there hope at the end of life? And how important is that?

The life story is a valuable tool for reflecting on important questions. Additionally, certain aspects of the NET process can promote a positive outlook. Above all, it is important to allow participants to ask themselves: "What is my life priority for my last years? ... for the last part of my life? What do I want to focus on?" (Jeannette Lely, personal communication, 2024). The *flowers* of hopes and wishes for the coming time can be symbolized on the *future* part of the Lifeline, and the therapist invites the narrator to name and place them.

A meaningful activity can also be the completed Lifeline on the theme of "what mark I have left on the world," like the concentric circles of influence of the famous stone thrown into the water (the survivor can symbolize and name situations, people, activities, etc.).

Next, specific positive events (flowers) can be explored in-depth using the Narrative Exposure cycle. Examples include moments of pride, love, spiritual experiences, accomplishments, moments of happiness, activities that left a mark, and people we could teach and inspire, "what I have passed on to the world, where I can place my life in a larger context," etc. Again, the therapist makes sure to revisit and explore concrete, specific events.

After processing traumatic experiences, individuals may discover previously hidden strengths and resources. To identify them, questions can be asked about how they managed to survive, what actions they took, and how they coped with the aftermath. It is important to consider who provided support during this time. The therapist may ask, "What helped you in the days, weeks, months and years that followed? When did you first feel a sense of hope or relief?" To survive and endure one or more traumatic experiences, whether short term or long term, requires extraordinary skills. We can be sure that individuals who still have expectations and want to engage in storytelling must possess resilience and a sense of gratitude and hope. It is important to recognize the hidden resilience factors that may seem accidental or insignificant. These qualities can be seen as flowers on the Lifeline of a survivor. Again, the therapist provides in-depth Narrative Exposure work with these specific events, focusing on sensory perceptions, thoughts, emotions, bodily reactions, and the meaning behind these moments. After the session, the positive emotions and physical sensations can be kept as a memory. The experience is described in detail (narrative) so that it can be remembered for a lifetime, including the final stages of life.

Finally, let us learn from the voice of an 87-year-old female survivor of World War II, reflecting on the narrative process during ElderNET:

It is often difficult to speak at first. I'm always afraid that no one will understand me! Without the foundation of complete trust and the hope that whatever I say will be accepted, I could not talk about these stressful experiences. This requires a safe space. I find working on these past experiences surprisingly demanding. Again and again, I am drawn to look closely – at myself, at the fact itself, and at the circumstances. These meticulous, careful narratives of the hurtful events are constantly in danger of being denied and broken off. But if I persevere, the fear of it dissolves, the event itself loses its overwhelming importance and fits into the series of other memories, becomes more or less "normal."

The events do not disappear from my consciousness, they remain scars, but it is no longer an open wound. I can integrate it and live with it. (Pause) ... After the therapy I had a dream: (pause) .... I am with a restorer in the middle of nowhere. He is putting together old broken vessels. Many hundreds of pieces, an amphora of precious old Israel glass, of mythical Davidic origin, made of sand from the Canaan desert. It is blue and shines. He repairs the cracks with a golden brush stroke. It looks beautiful. Finally, he gives it to me and says, "From now on, take good care of 'her'!" Then he leaves. I am deeply shaken and yet blessed ... still. (K. E.)

eNET: Delivering NET via the Internet

This chapter is a summary from Elisa Kaltenbach, Katy Robjant, Maggie Schauer, Elisabeth Kaiser, and Patrick McGrath, *Online Narrative Exposure Therapy: A Practical Guide for eNET,* Hogrefe (in preparation).

Introduction

Consistent with NET principles, NET via the Internet (eNET) seeks to uncover and bear witness to survivors' subjective experiences. The therapist assists the participant in this journey toward emotional processing and meaning making. Further, the therapist aids in the survivor's transformation of their traumatic memory into present reality through contrasting with the past.

The major benefits and risks of eNET are shared by other e-health interventions. The most obvious advantage of eNET is that it overcomes geographic barriers to health care. Treatment and supervision has become possible even across continents. Earlier research on various types of e-health using video and telephone clearly established that a wide range of therapy was possible without in-person contact. For example, Olthuis et al. (2016) systematically reviewed 19 RCTs with 1,491 participants and found that substantial improvement in PTSD, depression, and quality of life were the norm. The comparison with face-to-face treatments, with a smaller sample, was more nuanced, and there was a difference in follow-up favoring face-to-face treatments. First investigations using eNET are in progress and show promising results (Kaltenbach, Patrick, et al., 2021; Kaltenbach,

Chisholm, et al., 2021; Robjant et al., 2021; Olthuis et al., 2023; Olavarrieta & Benuto, 2022). Similarly, McGrath and colleagues successfully conducted telephone-assisted parent training, with participants showing strong outcomes in several trials (McGrath et al., 2011; Sourander et al., 2016). Individuals' comfort and privacy can also be enhanced by eNET. People with mobility problems or serious physical or mental illness may be able to attend for therapy with less difficulty and less reliance on others with eNET rather than with in-person therapy.

Most of the risks associated with eNET, in comparison with in-person NET, can be mitigated. The biggest concern with using eNET seems to be the risk of dissociation. It may be possible to control some of these risks by recruiting a therapy assistant (a professional, friend or family member, depending on the individual case) to be present or nearby, in case the survivor were to dissociate. Less severe dissociation can be managed by including antidissociation protocols that the participant becomes proficient in before beginning therapy, that can then be introduced during the *stone* exposures when needed (following Schauer & Elbert, 2010; Schauer & Schalinski, 2022).

Some survivors may not have the computer literacy or comfort to receive eNET interventions. However, individuals may use their smartphones also for video connections. The costs of the data transmission must be considered.

Structure of eNET

Like NET, eNET is a structured therapeutic approach that comprises various interrelated components. It involves 8–12 weekly sessions ranging from 90 to 120 minutes each. For survivors with complex trauma, the number of sessions may be doubled. Scheduling the number of sessions before the narration begins is crucial to avoid difficulties in overcoming avoidance, since both the participant and therapist assume that there will always be later sessions for disclosure, as in NET.

The different sessions are structured as follows:

Session 1: Symptom Assessment – Finding Right Treatment Approach for Trauma Survivor

Identifying the mental health disorders that a person is experiencing is crucial to determining an appropriate treatment plan. It is necessary to determine if the person suffers from a trauma-spectrum disorder. Are comorbid disorders present? Structured questionnaires are used to evaluate an individual's traumatic experiences, PTSD, and other mental health concerns. It is crucial to assess additional factors like dissociation, somatic health issues, life circumstances, and current stressors to determine if eNET is ideal for the participant. After a thorough symptom assessment, provide the psychoeducation and perspective before ending the first double session (as in NET, the session length in eNET is approximately 90 minutes). Depending on the individual, the symptom assessment can sometimes take more than one such session. On the other hand, depending on their skills, survivors can provide some information on their tablet or computer by themselves. However, we strongly recommend that the checklist of *traumatic experiences* (threats to life and integrity) is administered by the therapist. This information is essential to the NET process. It is also important for establishing a therapeutic alliance.

Session 2: Psychoeducation and Introduction of the Toolkit

Additionally, for consent to eNET, preparation for eNET, and challenges during and between sessions, this extra eNET session (compared to NET) requires information regarding trauma, trauma-related disorders, and their development. Participants must comprehend the proposed treatment normalization, legitimization of mental health disorders, and treatment possibilities, to stay motivated and committed to the treatment. The therapist will explain their responsibilities in creating a therapeutic alliance.

The psychoeducational session holds greater significance in eNET than in NET, as it prepares participants to take on their responsibilities and understand the underlying symptoms and mechanisms. A crucial element of this session involves detailing the procedure, including its pros and cons, to enable participants to make an informed decision on pursuing this treatment. The final segment of the psychoeducation session will cover planning for video-related obstacles. This section is more detailed than what was covered in NET due to the narrator having additional tasks as compared with in-person NET. This is also a good opportunity to get to know each other and get to know how to respond.

This session will also include information about dissociation, introduce a toolkit that will be used when there is a risk of dissociative responding, and the instructions about potential help in case the need arises.

Session 3: Lifeline

The Lifeline session is essential to create an overview of the different events in the individual's life and their chronological order. It helps the therapist and the survivor to create a road map regarding which experiences you will want to focus on in eNET. (See the Chapter 3: Building the Lifeline.) In eNET, the Lifeline can be done with different digital tools (specific app, white board, etc.). After the Lifeline session, a therapy plan is created that includes the events that will be discussed in detail during the exposure sessions, as well as the total number of sessions (to be communicated with the participant prior to the first exposure).

From Session 4 Onward: Narrative Exposure Sessions

As in NET, the exposure sessions are the core of eNET. The aim is to become fully aware when and where hot memories have been built. This will allow the reevaluation of traumatic events and their meaning. As with in-person NET, structured exposure of traumatic events in chronological order will be achieved by detailed narration (usually one traumatic event per session). Repeated exploration of sensations, cognitions, emotions, body sensations, and meaning for past events, as well as the present moment, are of utmost importance in eNET. Toward the end of the session, the exploration of the meaning of the event helps to reduce the arousal. The session should not be ended before normal arousal levels and a sense of relief have been reached by the narrator.

After the session, the therapist writes down the narration of the exposed event. However, in eNET, it may be possible to record the session and use – if available – AI tools to construct a first version of the narrated content, which then, of course, will need editing by the therapist. The therapist will then read the narration to the narrator at the beginning of the following session. Subsequently, the life narration continues with the next story being told in-depth.

Last Session

The aim of the last session is to summarize and reflect on the survivor's life and their experiences with eNET. It will shift the focus from past experiences to the present and future. If necessary, further treatments modules are recommended – for example, for strong appetitive aggression or drug addiction and craving.

In this last session, the therapist and the narrator take time to reflect on the life story as a whole. There are different options for this: (a) laying out the Lifeline again, (b) going through the initial Lifeline and adding new elements (if necessary), or (c) rereading the entire narration. Questions about meaning are then explored. Along with this, the eNET treatment, the narrative process, and changes in symptoms are reflected upon, and feedback is provided. Ultimately, the focus shifts from the past to the present and future. The flower elements from the Lifeline will be used to represent the survivor's wishes for the future Subsequently, the survivor selects the format in which they desire to receive their Lifeline and narration. A brief conversation on their preference for using their life story can facilitate appropriate utilization of their testimony, such as for human rights purposes. Allow for a few moments at the conclusion of the session to chat and bid farewell. Staying connected via Internet options is a viable option for follow-up communication.

General Elements for eNET Sessions

Greeting and Readiness Check

Greet the person and welcome them to the session.

Before starting with the content, ensure that the participant is ready.

Example of a readiness check:

Hi [name]. Great to see you today. I am looking forward to our session about [name topic] today. As usual, let's do a quick check-in to make sure you're all set to start this session:

Can you hear and see me well?

Do you have a glass of water ready?

Do you have your narration tool kit next to you? [e.g., touch stimulator, smell]

Did you eat and drink enough in the last few hours?

Do you have your phone close by in case we lose the connection on the video link? Is it still the same number?

Do you have 1.5 hrs for our call today?

Where are you right now? [check address]

Is there anyone who might disturb you in the next 1.5 hrs? [if yes:] Can you please tell them or ensure that they shouldn't interrupt you?

Please let me know if someone comes in the room or you are distracted during our session.

The therapist ensures that all of these issues are crossed off on their own side as well – for example, the participant may be told to adjust the camera if they cannot be seen well.

Example of a check-in at the beginning of the session:

How did you feel after our last session? Did you notice any changes? What were contents of any intrusions or nightmares you had?

How do you feel right now?

Did you experience any stressful or traumatic events since our last session?

Are you ready to start our session?

Body Scan

The body scan in eNET deserves particular attention, because of the restrictions in observing the body reactions of the narrators. Here is an example:

Let's assess your physical sensations at the moment. How are your hands? How are your arms? Can you identify any sensations in your shoulders? What is your neck feeling like? How are you feeling in your head? How is your chest? Any tension? Are you experiencing any difficulty breathing? How is your abdominal area? How is your back? Can you feel sitting on a chair? ... How do your legs feel? ... How do your feet feel? ... Great. Let's keep a good awareness on how your body feels. If you notice any changes, please let me know....

Examples of Deeper Questions About the Body Scan:

- Hands:
  Do your hands feel warm or cold? Do your hands feel sweaty? Do your hands feel tense? Are your hands clenched right now?
- Arms:
  Do your arms feel heavy or light? Are your arms tense?
- Shoulders:
  Are your shoulders tense? Are you pulling up your shoulders right now? Do your shoulders feel heavy? How is your posture right now?
- Neck/throat:
  Does your neck feel stiff or soft? Can you swallow well?
- Head:
  Do you feel some tension in your head? Where in your head do you feel some tension? Are you clenching your jaw?
- Chest:
  Does it feel like there is some pressure on your chest?
- Breathing:
  Is your breathing calm or fast? Is it superficial or deep? Are you breathing evenly?
- Belly:
  Do you feel some tension in your belly?
- Back:
  Is your back tense? How does the chair feel on your back?
- Buttocks:
  Are your buttocks tense right now? Does it feel comfortable to sit on the chair?
- Legs:
  Is there tension in your legs? Which parts of your legs feel tense?
- Feet:
  Do you have your feet on the ground? How do they feel on the ground? Are your feet warm or cold?

In general, check-ins during and at the end of each session correspond to those in NET.

Establish Therapeutic Alliance and Address Important Information Regarding Video Calls

In eNET, building a therapeutic rapport can be even more challenging than in in-person NET, because the therapist will not be in the same room, and the use of remote video platforms can convey a sense of distance between people, even when it is clearly possible to see each other's faces. Via video platforms, individuals do not have access to as many cues about the other person; their movements, their body expression, even their dress sense, the way they smell, their overall persona – all of which help individuals get a sense of the other person and contribute to building trust and rapport. Conversely, some may feel less anxious about the possibility of meeting someone via a video connection, where they may feel more in control (not having to travel and to go into an unknown building) and more able to "escape" or avoid elements of the interaction and their own presentation to the therapist. The therapist therefore needs to make even greater efforts to convey trust and empathy, build rapport, acknowledge the person, be responsive, and emotionally attuned – and this may be more difficult to achieve for therapists too.

How to Address Important Information Regarding Video Calls

As an example of how to address some important features of video calls, the following text can be presented:

The eNET sessions will take place via video calls. Doing the sessions via video has beneficial as well as challenging sides. A lot of people appreciate that they can do the sessions from the comfort of their home. We intend to give you the highest amount of privacy and confidentiality; however, we cannot guarantee that there will not be safety breaches. This is especially the case when writing emails; please consider the information you include in emails. An email or a WhatsApp message, by mistake, can easily be sent to the wrong address. Another topic is the privacy you have in your room. This is your responsibility. It is very important that there is no other person present in the same room and that you make sure that nobody can understand what you say. This will allow you to speak freely. Interruptions happen more easily when we are at home; please make sure that you inform the people around you that you cannot be disturbed during the sessions.

Explain Dissociation and Introduce Dissociation Exercises

Preparing a participant for potential dissociative symptoms is essential in the preparation process during eNET. This preparation will also be done for those who do not report dissociation symptoms. Preceding this session, dissociation symptoms have to be assessed in detail, and the suitability of eNET for the individual and any necessary adjustments (e.g., having a therapy assistant) should be discussed (see Session 1: Symptom Assessment). During psychoeducation, it is important to explain what dissociation is, to introduce tools and exercises to address it in the sessions, and to practice them. Since the person is physically out of reach, we ask them to bring a *narration toolkit* that can help them stay grounded in the present during their sessions. The therapist has a similar kit during the sessions; this way they can show the participant what kind of tools to bring to the psychoeducation session, and in later sessions you can remind them to use these tools more easily by mirroring their use.

Content of the narration toolkit:

- Glass of water or other non-alcoholic drink
- Touch stimulator (e.g., massage ball, children's toy that make a noise)
- Strong smell (e.g., lemongrass, mint, spice; this should not include ammonia, and it should be different to the smells present during the trauma!)

Example of How to Explain Dissociation and Introduce Dissociation Exercises

Sometimes when we remember traumatic experiences, we feel dizzy or like we're losing awareness of our surroundings ("going away a little bit"). This happens when our mind and body feel like the past events are happening again. It is a reaction that the body initiates to keep us safe in situations of threat. We call this dissociation. It might have protected you during your traumatic experience in the past, but today you are safe, and your body can learn again that it doesn't need to initiate this defensive reaction any more. Commonly people who experience such a reaction in a session also experience this in their daily life. Do you sometimes experience this?... [also refer to the dissociation questionnaire conducted during Session 1: Symptom Assessment]. It is not dangerous, it is just important that we make sure that you don't hurt yourself if, for example, you fall.

We will go through some exercises and tools that show you what to do in case you start feeling dizzy in a session. They are all very easy and might seem very simple at first, but they support you in distinguishing past and present experiences from each other. You can use these tools together with me in a session, or you can also do them alone.

Example of How to Introduce the Narration Tool Kit

There are some tools that you should bring along to each session. They can help you to stay present. Some people also find them helpful in other situations where they are reminded of their past.

[Glass of water or soft drink] I highly recommend you bring a drink – for example, a glass of water or a soda for each session. It is good to have a sip of water when you talk a lot, but it is also helpful when feelings get stronger. In such a case I might ask you to take a sip of water.

[Touch stimulator] Another thing I recommend you to bring along is a touch stimulator. It can be any small object that has a rough surface and that you can easily take into your hand. Maybe a toy or simply an open zipper of your jacket that you can rub your fingers on? It is important that it is nothing you could potentially hurt yourself with. Such a touch stimulator can help you to feel your hands, to move it in your hands while we talk and to stay present this way.

[Strong smell] A strong smell is something very powerful when you feel disoriented. There are different smells that are suitable – for example, mint, lemon, lemongrass. It can also be another smell, but it should not have ammonia or be a perfume. Do you have such a smell?... If not, would you be able to get one? You can also see if you can find a strong smell in your spice cabinet; just make sure it is catching your attention when you smell it.

Let's quickly repeat and write these down so you remember these three things for the next session: a glass of water or soda, a touch stimulator, and a strong smell.

Additional sensory stimulants such as utilizing cold packs and sour drops can heighten awareness of the present surroundings. Additionally, while engaging with the subject, the therapist can shift the individual's attention focus every now and then to the present by inquiring about their surroundings, such as what they see from their chair, the texture of the desk, pictures at the wall, or if not in a room, what nature looks like where they can see it, and describe other identifiable objects.

Example of How to Explain the Response to Dissociation Symptoms in a Session

When you feel like you perceive your surroundings in a different way – for example, you can't hear me as well, you start seeing blurry, or you feel dizzy – please let me know right away. You should interrupt me whatever we are talking about and tell me how you feel. If you feel like you can't talk, try to lift up your hand to show me that you are not feeling well. This is very important; the earlier you tell me, the easier it will be.

Example of How to Explain the Procedure if the Narrator Starts to Dissociate

In the rare event that you become disoriented and are unable to respond effectively, I will remain on the call with you until we can reconnect. While doing so, I will continue to address you by your first name and suggest some movements to perform while seated in your chair. It may take some time for you to regain your full awareness. Physical movement will have a positive effect on your blood pressure and may counteract the effects of immobility.

If you do not respond after a period of time, I will attempt to reach you on your mobile phone or landline. Sometimes, hearing a familiar voice can help bring you back. Let's try this now. When I call you, please see how it feels for you [therapist initiates phone call and engages in a brief conversation while maintaining eye contact through the screen].

If there is still no response, I will contact your emergency contact to enter the room and address you directly.

Emergency Contact and Support Person

The participant's social support system is more crucial in eNET than with in-person treatments. Involving those around them can help keep the participant motivated, especially when avoidance is a factor or if they need to discuss the session afterward. It is also imperative for the therapist to have an emergency contact, particularly in cases of dissociation.

Preparation of the Lifeline

Depending on how the therapist plans to conduct the Lifeline, the procedure needs to be introduced (see the section Step 2: Building the Lifeline in Chapter 3, for the exact instructions).

In face-to-face NET, an actual line, stones, flowers, candles, and sticks are used. In eNET, a proper visual presentation can be technically challenging. There are different approaches to conducting the Lifeline online. The following options are currently frequently used; alternative approaches adapted to the technical possibilities and the needs of the survivor are feasible as well.

1. **Lifeline software application:** There are software applications in development that contain the symbols of the Lifeline. The app should allow that the therapist and the survivor can work on the Lifeline simultaneously. Each symbol can be named in the application. The application can be reentered at a later time (e.g., in the subsequent sessions), and the participant can add symbols to the existing Lifeline.
2. **Online whiteboard:** You can use the whiteboard function that is available in most video platforms. The person draws the timeline and symbols, and the therapist writes down the name of the events. The limited space available on the whiteboard should be addressed at the beginning to ensure that the space is structured in a way that gives enough room for all time periods of the participant's life.
3. **Flipchart whiteboard:** A flipchart whiteboard is set up, and the Lifeline is drawn on it. The camera should capture the flipchart whiteboard as well as the person.
4. **Real-life symbols:** The therapist may hold the Lifeline materials (actual string, stones, flowers, candles, and sticks) and lay them down for the Lifeline. The camera should focus on the Lifeline as well as the person.

These approaches can be modified as needed. The therapist makes a special effort to keep the survivor fully engaged and to prevent avoidance. It is critical that both parties can see the Lifeline and each other's video image throughout the session. This ensures that reactions to the identification of life events can be observed, which provides an initial indication of emotional significance and can help to identify if the person is having difficulty or wants to avoid naming events.

After completing the entire Lifeline, participants are given time to reflect on the course of their life. An overview of creating meaning can be provided, but a deeper understanding can only be achieved through the narration of the entire story (Step 3: Narrative Exposure). At the end of the Lifeline session, it is essential to document the content, which can be accomplished by capturing a screenshot or photograph. The name, time, and location of each event must be clearly visible in the picture or documented separately to establish the therapy plan after this session. The entire Lifeline procedure should be completed in one session lasting approximately 90 minutes. It is recommended to inform the participant of this at the outset and avoid splitting the session to minimize discussion of emotionally charged event details. Even when multiple events need addressing, it is possible to stay in the cold memory (allocentric view) and complete the Lifeline within a single session.

Important Considerations for the Narrative Exposure Sessions via Video

There is a risk of connection interruption in eNET. The therapist will guide the narrator through the presented tools in the psychoeducation session to ensure their readiness and ability to complete the narration in case they get disconnected (e.g., by writing down the last part). Alternatively, the emergency contact person can come in and listen to the end of the story. This individual must receive a briefing beforehand on how to do so.

Unexpected events, such as emergencies, suicidal behavior, harm to others, nonsuicidal self-harm, increasing symptoms, and adverse events may occur during any therapy. Adequate preparation for these incidents can help to mitigate any negative outcomes and reduce stress associated with handling them. Many of these concerns are applicable to eNET therapy in the same way as for other therapeutic methods.

Suicidality includes a wide variety of behavior including passing thoughts of suicide, intentions to commit suicide, plans to commit suicide, attempted suicide, and completed suicide. Passing thoughts of suicide are common, especially in persons with disorders from the trauma spectrum. Suicide attempts are much less frequent, and completed suicide is rare. The risk of suicidal behavior is causally related to adverse childhood experiences. Our observations suggest that suicidal tendencies typically subside once the narration is successfully completed.

5 Challenging Moments in the Therapeutic Process

There are some typical problems that we face when conducting exposure therapy with survivors of trauma. Others have already tried to highlight some of these critical issues (Bisbey & Bisbey, 1998). The following description may serve as an opportunity for a deeper understanding into how to accomplish the NET procedure.

Avoidance

Even after careful and sound psychoeducation, it is very likely that a narrator may at times want to avoid revisiting distressing and sorrowful memories. Avoidance strategies vary from person to person. Some individuals may speed up their narration to complete the task quickly, while others may detach themselves from the present moment. Furthermore, some people may refuse to talk about a particular event type or try to change the subject to avoid the discussion. If avoidance is present, the therapist may need to empathically assess the situation and explain the mechanisms again, even if they were previously discussed during the psychoeducation phase. There are two steps to dealing with avoidance: First, openly acknowledge the narrator's attempt to avoid, confirming that you understand the desire to avoid. Second, explain that as a therapist, you have an obligation to notice and point out when the survivor is avoiding. You can then explain that as a team, the two of you will work closely together to prevent avoidance. In some treatments it may be necessary to boost motivation in this way several times.

Another reason for avoidance may be that the victim or perpetrator is not sure that you will be able to handle hearing their story. Most survivors have never had the opportunity to tell their story or have never felt comfortable talking about their experiences in full. This is true for adults as well as children or teenagers. In addition to telling the person about your credentials as a counselor (e.g., that you have worked as a researcher, therapist, social worker, nurse, or teacher in the field of counseling, human rights abuses, or organized violence – as applicable to you), share the facts about the populations you have worked with. Assure the narrator that you have the expertise to aid individuals in their journey to overcome personal challenges. Display your proficiency in handling any potential challenges that may arise. Your main purpose is to provide support to the person as they revisit the most distressing moments of their past. Those who struggle with hearing trauma stories may not possess the necessary skills to become effective therapists in this position. Therapists should have addressed their own personal trauma-related issues and ensure proper self-care and mental hygiene before administering trauma memory–focused therapy, as tension and anxiety are transferred.

Etiology and Treatment of Trauma-Induced Dissociation

General Characteristics of Dissociation

Dissociation serves as a protective mechanism for our body against potential threats to our social (rejection, abandonment, etc.) and physical integrity (such as tissue, central nervous system, or organ damage, or loss of oxygen). It achieves this by distorting our sense of self and deactivating our mental awareness, emotions, and conscious bodily perception, resulting in a state of disembodiment where we do not feel or perceive our surroundings and are not able to react to internal or environmental stimuli anymore. Dissociation is a mental process of disconnecting from one's thoughts, feelings, memories, or sense of identity. Dealing with dissociative individuals poses a major challenge in the acute care and treatment of trauma-spectrum disorders. Dissociation is not a singular behavior, but rather a complex orchestrated adaptation of functions in the areas of consciousness, perception, sensation, emotion, behavior, memory, and as a result, personal identity – the essential unity of the self. The goal of a dissociative response is to override the active response (flight, fight) and to ensure survival when faced with a serious, inescapable threat.

"Shutdown": Biological Meaning of Dissociative Experience and Its Clinical Consequences

In a threatening situation, the organism can respond with either an alarm reaction (flight or fight) or a shutdown, a "playing dead" in shock and syncope (Schauer & Elbert, 2010; Bracha, 2004; Chessell et al., 2019; McKinnon et al., 2016; see Chapter 2: Stress and the Defense Cascade and see Table 4). Central to a shut-down is the closing of the thalamic gates. This will dampen and blur the input from all senses (except olfactation) to the cortex, and with it the sensory perceptions (see Shut-D scale available at https://doi.org/10.23668/psycharchives.4596). Active behavior will be inhibited to disable flight or fight. This response set is an evolutionarily ancient, automatic program that is likely to be activated in the event of massive danger. In particular, stressors that are classified as immediately threatening, as painful, or that may cause severe injury activate the shutdown arm of the defense cascade (Figure 1). *Peritraumatic* dissociation dominates this descending edge. Once massively threatened, victims are increasingly stunned, mute, and immobile, and there is hardly any indication of their activity. Victims survive by no longer emitting any prompting signals (cues) that could activate aggression or hunting instincts in predators and perpetrators (Elbert et al., 2018), or any attention-grabbing vocalizations (mutism). The skin surface and mucous membranes cannot be damaged by involuntary defense reflexes if the aggressor has made skin contact, penetrated body orifices (in the case of sexual violence), or invaded the body (also applies to medical measures). However, for a threatened organism to actually no longer react at all or only weakly in the face of life-threatening situations, it is (evolutionarily) necessary that not only the motoric apparatus is restricted, but also the perception and with it the cognitive and emotional possibilities that would drive detrimental and ultimately fatal behavior. In this way, destructive behaviors that would lead to injury or violation of social integrity, especially in attachment-dependent individuals, are effectively restricted (Schauer & Schalinski, 2022).

What survivors say about dissociation

"Dissociation can appear any time."

"Generally, when I read something traumatizing, or something that reminds me of the traumatic event, I feel dissociated."

"It's like a dream."

"Most of the time, I fly."

"There's nothing in my head anymore."

"I realize I've spent two hours doing the same thing, while I thought it took 10 minutes."

"Pain is too strong, and my body can't take it, so it protects me."

"I don't know how people cope without dissociation."

"When I'm in class, I realize I switched off for 10 minutes, and I have to catch up."

"I have the feeling of being completely mad."

Sara Danböck (personal communication, 2022)

The more often a person has to confront traumatic stressors in a state of helplessness, the greater the tendency to dissociative symptoms will become (Schauer & Elbert, 2010; Schalinski, Schauer et al., 2016; McKinnon et al., 2016; Lanius et al., 2018). This applies in particular to individuals who have experienced interpersonal violence, especially sexual violence and neglect, during their childhood. As a result, when painful events are recalled, dissociation may also manifest posttraumatically with its disorder-specific symptoms, particularly when the individual is already experiencing high levels of physiological arousal or psychological tension (Schauer & Elbert, 2010).

The general characteristic of dissociative disorders is the partial or complete loss of the normally integrative functions of consciousness. Repeated severe threats to life and biological fitness (see Appendix 1 for THL checklist; Köbach et al., 2016) can lead to dissociative psychopathology with dramatic consequences for the possibility of integrity, self-control, mentalization, and the general occupational and social functionality of the personality. With the DSM-5, individuals suffering from PTSD who also exhibit dissociative symptoms can now be classified as having a dissociative subtype of PTSD (APA, 2013). The ICD-11 accordingly introduces complex PTSD as a separate category from PTSD. It is worthwhile for practitioners to assess this symptomatology (e.g., with the Shut-D scale; Schalinski, Schauer, & Elbert, 2015,

Table 4. Threat factors that play a role in the development of dissociative symptoms (adapted from Schauer & Schalinski, 2022, p. 63)

Threat characteristics	Mobilization *versus* Shutdown	
Type of context	Positive arousing pleasurable aggression, or reactive anger arousing	Dark, threatening environment, negative arousing, fear arousing, or disgust arousing
Immediacy of threat	Slow, predictable	Fast rising intensity of a stimulus, loud, very close
Possibility of counter-attack	Yes, physically defensive	Physically helplessness, fixation
Physical contact with the aggressor	Own aggressive behavior reactive or appetitive, pain associated with *anger* (appetitive aggression, i.e., bloodlust or fighting is mentally protective)	Physical contact, invasion, penetration, pain associated with fear, injury by sharp objects, by acids, electricity, fire, strangulation, suffocation, etc., penetration or invasion of body orifices under fear, body fluids of other people such as blood, urine, or semen, or corpses and decomposition
Threat to social integrity, exclusion from group or loss of status	Impulsive aggression, dominance or defending status, retaliation after humiliation	Submission, shame, traumatic loss or grief

2016; Schalinski, Teicher, et al., 2016), diagnose it accordingly, and intervene in a targeted manner during trauma treatment.

During a shutdown, the person subsequently becomes paralyzed, appears weak, is tired, feels heavy, and can no longer act. Anxiety and tension decrease noticeably as a result, but so does the ability to perceive, remember, and react. Factors that increase the likelihood of a person experiencing a shutdown response are as follows: (a) sudden threat with total helplessness, rapid arousal peak, often with startle; (b) when the feared perpetrator or object is in close proximity and has physical superiority through skin contact; (c) the presence of bodily fluids like fresh blood, urine, excrement, semen, or disfigured corpses pose contamination risks; and (d) situations involving the risk of injury, penetration of the body, or penetration of body orifices, that elicit negative feelings of fear and/or disgust (Table 3).

From this list of factors, one can easily see that the experience of sexual abuse, where strong disgust reactions are often involved, clearly fulfills criteria for eliciting dissociative shutdown reactions. While threat heightens information processing and physiological arousal, it has been shown that, contrary to stimuli that elicit arousal and fear, disgust information is processed in the brain in a suppressed sensory perceptual and attentional way. This is akin to the central ecological function of disgust to minimize contact with contagious objects to avoid contamination and disease. At the physiological level, disgust tends to activate parasympathetic responses, reducing heart rate, blood pressure, and respiration, thereby suppressing action (see Krusemark & Li, 2011). Conversely, fear swings these systems in the opposite direction by stimulating sympathetic pathways, prompting fight or flight. Despite both being threat related, fear and disgust engage opposite mechanisms with contrasting behavioral consequences.

Posttraumatic Reexperiencing of Fright, Flag, and Faint

Dissociation is subject to conditioning mechanisms. A repeatedly traumatized child, for example, learns to suppress emotions through dissociation. Emotions prepare the person for responses. Fear for instance is intended to mobilize the body for flight, anger, or fight reactions. As these behaviors could pose dangerous consequences during childhood, the child learns to dissociate when emotionally tense. Then, in later life, individuals may experience feelings of immobility or fainting in situations of intense emotional or physical arousal caused by conflict (such as anger, sadness, frustration, etc.). Insufficient or distressing care of infants with limited sensitivity, minimal comforting touch, and inadequate physical contact, plus a lack of cerebellar developmental stimulation through carrying and rocking, result in excessive stress and heightened likelihood of dissociation in later years, due to unreliable arousal regulation. This is particularly true when attachment figures fail to offer comfort, support, or reassurance, but rather induce anxiety, pain, and ongoing negative arousal in the child. Long-term studies have demonstrated that attachment disorders and emotionally unavailable attachment figures during the first 2 years of life are strong predictors of dissociative disorders in later life (Dhossche et al., 2012; Thekkumthala et al., 2019). Macfie et al. (2001) investigated 198 preschool-aged children (average age 5 years) from low-income families and found that dissociation scores (on a 10-point scale) were very high in those with physical (8.9) and sexual (7.3) abuse, but also substantial in the neglected group (5.5).

The behavior that was exhibited during the threat can subsequently be triggered again by internal and external cues – for example, when similar internal or external stimulus configurations activate the unprocessed trauma memory associations in the present (such as a similar smell, similar environment, a similar-looking person, or a similar physiological reaction, similar emotion, or body position). Dissociative reactions can be triggered in everyday life by emotional proximity to the trauma subject, by high internal tension and arousal, or by intrusions that impose themselves, typically during physiological changes, for example when the person wants to relax or before falling asleep.

The Shut-D scale was developed to assess the intensity and frequency of dissociative symptoms, taking into account the described biological basis for these responses (Schalinski, Schauer, & Elbert, 2015, 2016). It is thus based on an etiological model rather than mere observation of responses. Figure 44 presents a typical distribution of the scores in trauma survivors who also present with PTSD, and in healthy control subjects.

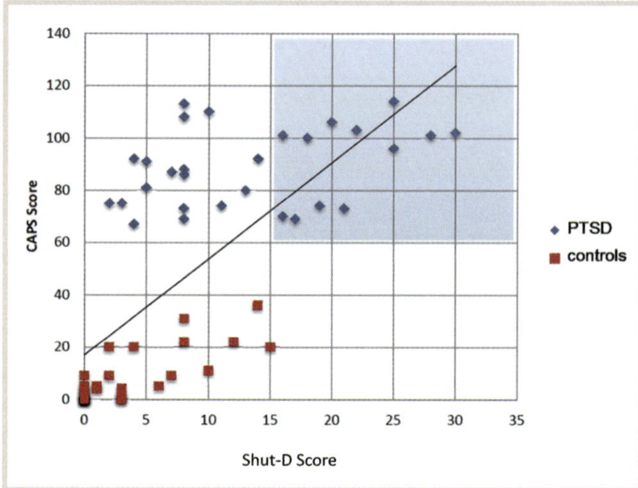

Figure 44. A high load of PTSD symptoms (measured with the Clincian Adminstered PTSD score, [CAPS], x-axis) may or may not be associated with high dissociative symptoms (Shut-D score, y-axis). The correlation would not appear in the PTSD group alone, i.e., the intensity of dissociative symptoms cannot be predicted from the PTSD symptom intensity. Moreover, the distribution of dissociative symptoms is continuous, questioning a categorization into two groups. Nevertheless, in individuals who fall into the shaded area, the dissociative subtype can be diagnosed according to DSM-5. (Data from our outpatient clinic.)

Trauma Dissociation and Self-Harm

If memory cues from traumatic experiences are not connected explicitly to their historical context, they can unpredictably elicit reactions and behaviors in everyday life, impeding the remission of trauma symptoms. Individuals experiencing high levels of internal tension may engage in self-injury, specifically causing tissue damage using sharp or pointed objects, as a means of regulating their emotions through the biologically prepared relaxation response. It is a maladaptive coping mechanism that can lead to serious physical and psychological consequences (Schauer & Elbert, 2010). Pain becomes increasingly altered by the release of endogenous opioids and by altered regulation of cannabinoids (Wilker et al., 2016). This leads to blunted emotional responses, weakened episodic memory, and impaired working memory, as well as reduced cognitive and verbal performance, depersonalization (McKinnon et al., 2016), changes in perceptual and interoceptive awareness and a detached awareness of the self and the environment, as described by the shutdown reactions of the defense cascade. The endogenous opioid system plays a central role in the emotional

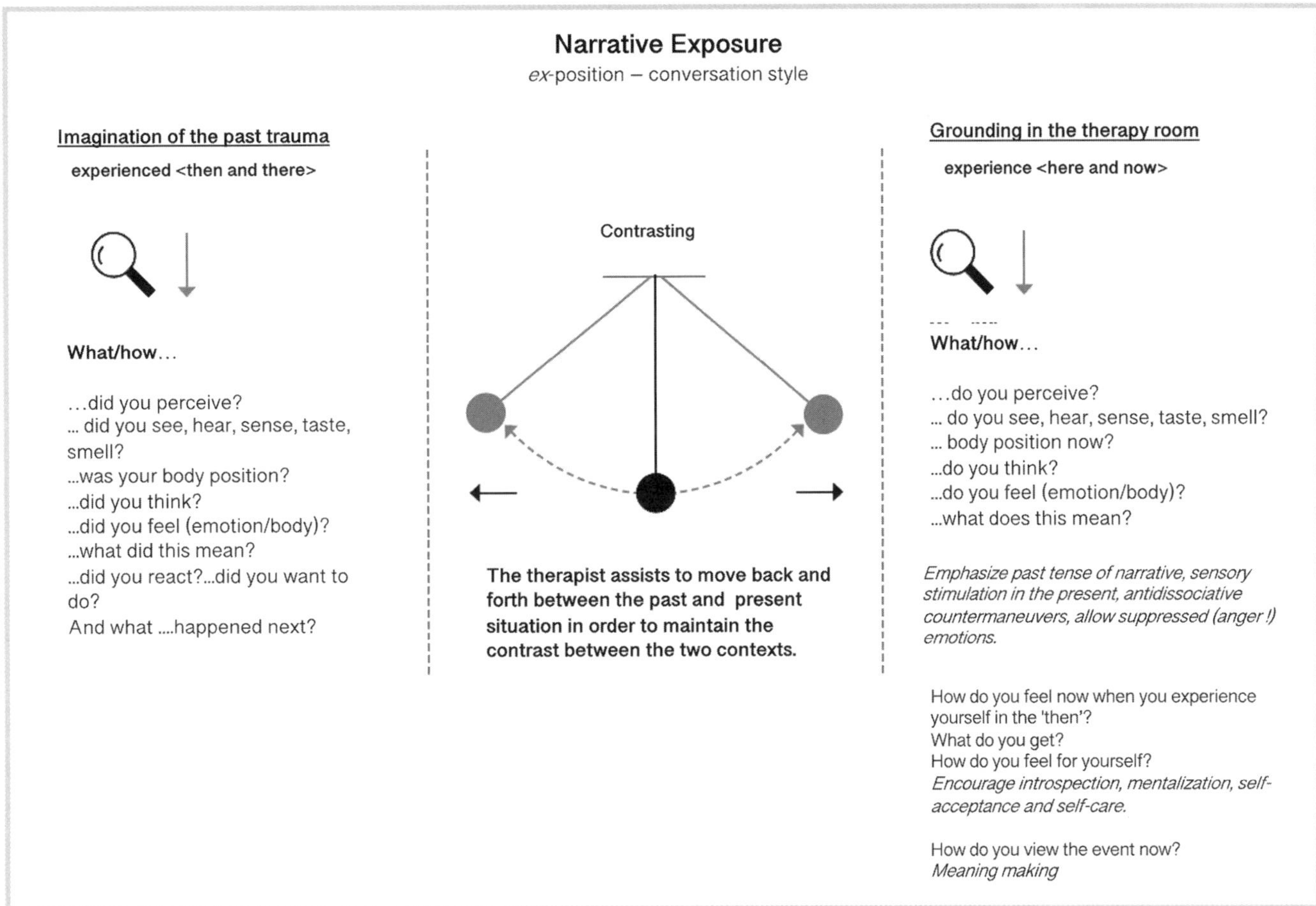

Figure 45. Counteracting dissociation: The therapist helps move the narrator's attention more frequently than usual (!) between imagining the past event and being grounded in the present. Translated with permission from Schauer, M., & Schalinski, I. (2022). Zur Biologie des Überlebens – Ätiologie und Behandlung traumainduzierter Dissoziation [The biology of survival: Etiology and treatment of trauma-induced dissociation]. In J. Müller, M. Ruf-Leuschner, B. Grimmer, C. Knaevelsrud, & B. Dammann (Eds.). Traumafolgen: Forschung und therapeutische Praxis, p. 71. Kohlhammer. Also available as a handout in the online supplementary materials for this book.

shutdown (Lanius et al., 2018; Kozlowska et al., 2015). As the skin tissues get numb, the individual feels little pain when self-harming by cutting or stabbing with sharp objects, burning, hitting, or biting, etc. At the same time a parasympathetic decline sets in and with it the desired relief, relaxation, drop in blood pressure, and decreased heart rate (principle of negative reinforcement).

Remission of such trauma-related dissociation symptoms can best be achieved through Narrative Exposure of trauma material, while at the same time actively counteracting any psychological, physical, and intellectual dissociative shutdown (Schalinski et al., 2015; Schauer & Elbert, 2010).

Trauma therapists view dissociation as a notable impediment to the successful implementation of trauma-focused exposure therapy. Dissociation's biological purpose is to decrease intense emotions, hindering emotional processing while disrupting information processing and mentalizing abilities. As a result of dissociation, individuals are unable to respond adequately to speech and other interventions, which can lead to frustration for the helper. Attempting to prevent or discourage this intense behavior by isolating the trauma survivor or withholding positive attention is unlikely to be effective in cases of dissociation, as it is precisely the evolutionary purpose to ignore the "attacker" and the surroundings, refrain from exhibiting any behavioral reaction, and shut down sensory, cognitive, emotional, and physiological response systems. Background knowledge of the biological significance of this behavior can be helpful in guiding therapeutic approaches and care situations by allowing for selective intervention.

Recognize and Treat Dissociation

If there was a chance to escape from the threat in the past traumatic situation, the mobilization to flee (fear) or to fight (aggression) begins again as soon as the trauma material is remembered: cardiac activity increases (palpitations), blood pressure rises, and there is vasoconstriction in the periphery (cold hands), which is intended to reduce blood loss in the event of injury. If these signs predominate, the narrative xposure takes place as described in Figure 17.

However, if there is a strong parasympathetic shutdown reaction accompanied by weakness and fainting, a drop in blood pressure, progressive emotional numbness, and a decline in cognitive function, countermeasures are indicated to prevent the person from becoming flaccid, unable to move, and possibly completely dissociated. This reaction may occur if the peritraumatic situations were characterized by extreme helplessness. This is particularly the case if there has been penetration of a body orifice or tissue damage, exposure to bodily fluids – for example, blood or semen (i.e., disgust as a leitmotif; Krusemark & Li, 2011), or severe pain – for example, in torture.

The therapist should therefore be aware of the client's physiological arousal during the session in order to intervene antidissociatively in time (Table 5). In general, when dissociation sets in, reorientation of consciousness (grounding) and contrasting the contexts of then (trauma) versus now are the best approach. This is done by consciously contrasting on all levels of the hot memory (perception, thinking, feelings, body, and behavior). It is also very important to stimulate sensory perception in the present, in order to prevent the perceptual channels from closing and thus a gradual dissociative splitting off occurring. Narrators can thus be reorientated in the present again and again when reliving the past: Consciousness should oscillate like a pendulum between then and now (dual consciousness) to give the trauma survivor control and the opportunity to process. Contrasting the past event with the present is crucial for overcoming dissociation. This includes contrasting contextual information regarding time and place (e.g., war scene vs. treatment room), the allocentric versus the trauma egocentric position (mapping of the space and elements of the trauma scene, e.g., in drawing), differences in sensory information (auditory, visual, tactile, gustatory, olfactory, etc.), and the different kinesthetic and physical positions.

In children, adolescents, and adults with dissociative symptoms, these symptoms should be assessed at the beginning of the clinical diagnosis: For trauma-focused therapy, it is important to be able to predict the tendency to dissociate, in order to intervene directly and effectively. It is worthwhile to use a specific symptom checklist for diagnosis (e.g., Shut-D scale, Schalinski, Schauer, & Elbert, 2015, 2016). In the Shut-D scale, the frequency of dissociation symptoms occurring in everyday life is assessed by 13 items. Individuals with significant dissociations should learn the biology of survival through psychoeducation and understand these reactions to be an adaptive strategy. On the one hand, this contributes to normalization, and on the other hand, it can reduce existing fears (e.g., the fear of dying if one faints).

The three main areas of behavioral changes that characterize a shutdown reaction peritraumatically can also be observed later, when recalling the traumatic experiences (Schauer & Elbert, 2010):

1. **Functional sensory deafferentation:** Incoming stimuli seem not to reach beyond the gates in the thalamus, and stimuli are perceived as weak, distant, and unreal. During treatment, the affected person may become unresponsive, with unfocused gaze.
2. **Reversible palsy**: Stiffening because of heightened muscle tonus leads to visible decrease of bodily movements and immobility, posturing, and finally waxy flexibility also during treatment.
3. **Inhibition or disconnection**: Areas responsible for language processing and production of speech are inhibited or disconnected (unclear vs. confused speech, fragmentation of sentences, inability to speak, almost no, or belated, response to acoustic stimuli).

Summary: Dissociation keeps our body from being potentially injured (damage to the tissue, CNS, or organs or loss of oxygen) by deactivating our mental awareness, emotion, and conscious bodily perception (not feeling it, not being there – *disembodiment*) that drives and motivates our behavioural action and response, leading to disruption in memory function and a distorted sense of self. *Do not react, move, or respond even if you are experiencing physical or emotional pain and life-threatening situations!*

Preparations Before Imagery Exposure

Before implementing imaginal exposure, a therapist ought to establish the individual's early warning signs of dissociation and practice antidissociative techniques together with the survivor to become acquainted with the methods. It is advisable to discuss with the person who occasionally faints, how to handle such a situation during therapy sessions. For narrators who have a tendency to shut down during a trauma narrative, these measures should be used concurrently with Narrative Exposure, post psychoeducation. In general, the three "S"s rule (see Step 3: Narrative Exposure in Chapter 3) applies, especially in contact with dissociating people: S (settle in), S (speak slowly), and S (say first name); as well as orient in the here and now.

Changes in Speech Comprehension and Production

Use acoustic stimuli that are not threatening and sensory stimuli to stay in contact with the affected person whose "senses are fading" (sensory deafferentation, see the section Recognize and Treat Dissociation, above). Help to counteract disorientation. Explain what you are doing in simple language. If the person can still speak a little, encourage them to perform simple tasks, and ask: "Can you hear me? Who am I? Where are we?" to get speech production going. Give immediate, practical, short answers and reinforce and reward each verbal utterance and physical response from the dissociated person. First names are particularly effective, as they can still be recognized even if the person is otherwise severely impaired. Sometimes victims have had to say certain things during the abuse. So be careful with requests for speech and behavior and always explain why you are asking them to speak.

Loss of Perception of Internal and External Stimuli

What to do when the organism of the narrator has initiated the shutdown: Initially, stimulating the afferent pathways to the brain is helpful to end dissociation. Depending on the person's tolerance, stimulate the experience in the here and now with sensory stimuli such as touch (e.g., massage ball), cold stimuli (cold pack wrapped in a cloth), auditory stimuli (addressing by first name, clapping after announcement, and pointing out sounds in the environment), or olfactory stimuli (e.g., essential oils, note that olfaction is not gated by the thalamus). A stimulus in the other sensory categories should be clear enough to overcome the gates, but should not cause pain or negative sensations, as this would further increase dissociation. Consciousness should be positively motivated to return to reality, to the safe and pleasant therapy room.

Stimulation of the olfactory system is particularly helpful, as the olfactory pathways do not run through the thalamus and therefore cannot be blocked by the thalamic gates during dissociation. Accordingly, there is no need for an intense or even pungent scent. Fresh ginger, mint, fruit scent, etc. are suitable after consultation in order to create clear stimuli contrasting the past situation. Make sure that your olfactory stimulation material is safe for the person's health and is not associated with the trauma. Sensory anchors to the here and now, directing attention to the place associated with safety and reassurance, can also be therapeutically conditioned and then used during exposure. A different sensory environment (contrast!) to the trauma environment is favorable here; that is, different smell or taste. Offer scents and olfactory stimuli that are strong enough, positive and refreshing, and bear no resemblance to the smells at the time of the traumatic event.

However, refrain from using ammonia as an odor stimulus. The pungent smell of ammonia compounds is unsuitable for the purpose of stimulation in trauma survivors during dissociation with a tendency to shut down, as it provokes disgust. Disgust information, in fact, leads to suppressed sensory-perceptual processing and averted attention in the brain; that is, the opposite of grounding in the here and now. In addition, disgust physiologically leads to a drop in heart rate, blood pressure, and respiration, which intensifies rerealization and presyncope. Although ammonia is able to stimulate the trigeminal nerve through its pungency, the odor component is biologically linked to bodily excretions and the genital area, which can trigger associations. Disgust can increase dissociation and makes habituation more difficult, therefore prolonged imaginative exposure to odors, tastes, and sensory stimuli of high disgust quality should not be induced (saliva, sweat, semen, putridity, decay, blood, corpses, etc.).

It is better to concentrate therapeutically on understanding the internal processes that took place at the time of the trauma during the disgust situation by asking the narrator: "When you felt very disgusted during the (trauma situation), what did you think (cognition) and what did you do next (behavior)?" As soon as consciousness returns, ventilate the experience and give a profound psychoeducation. It is important to invite them to talk about inner processes to facilitate understanding. Only return to the trauma narrative when the narrator is safely oriented in the present.

Procedure for Tonic Immobility

If the person freezes muscularly, the arousal will have reached the maximum level on the curve. It is then important to calm the physiological arousal so that the person can move and speak again – that is, has control. Even in an acute case (if you are called to an accident, etc.), remain calm and speak slowly and clearly to the survivors. Explain in simple terms and loudly enough what is happening and can be perceived in the present. Orient the person in the here and now, using friendly sensory stimuli for grounding. The presence of familiar (reference) persons can also have a calming effect. Encourage the sensory perception of the surroundings, the feeling of body (parts), and guide the affected person to move fingers, legs, arms etc. until the person is fully oriented again, heart rate and blood pressure have returned to normal, you can make eye contact, and the survivors can speak. Give them the opportunity to ventilate the experience.

Procedure for Flaccid, Collapsed Immobility

To stabilize blood pressure and heart rate in this state, immediate stimulation of the physiological activity level and motor skills through countermaneuvers, such as tensing the voluntary muscles and clearly stimulating perception in the here and now, is recommended. Involve the affected person in active body movement. Processes such as vasovagal (pre-) syncope can be counteracted by applied tension (Öst, 2002) – for example, crossing legs and tensing calf muscles, clenching fists, and tightening arm muscles. Physical counterpressure maneuvers (e.g., squeezing a ball, pushing hands against each other, arms against the wall) are also suitable for achieving a short-term increase in blood pressure. Or use the muscle-venous pump (the toes and heels of both feet are pressed into the ground synchronously or in opposite directions to support the return transportation of blood). You can also use a balance board to stimulate large parts of the muscles and cerebellar activity. All of this can be used during imaginative exposure in trauma treatment if posttraumatic dissociation is present.

Procedure for Shutdown With Short-Term Unconsciousness

If you observe vasovagal syncope in a trauma survivor and a fall occurs, make sure that the person is not injured. Remain calm, use simple language, and call the person by their first name. Even if the individual appears unresponsive, explain the procedure, which should ideally be based on the person's previously discussed wishes (e.g., if the person does not want to be left alone or for unknown male persons to be brought into the room). Make sure that you always announce all of your actions in advance, such as "I will now put your legs up and touch your lower legs. This will allow your circulation to recover." Continue with grounding exercises and invite sensory awareness and orientation of consciousness into the here and now, where there is safety and support. Stay with the person until they are reoriented. Discuss the situation together later and learn more about their reactions and their early recognition features. But also note that the probability of such an incident is quite low.

Table 5. Practical examples for countering dissociation (adapted from Schauer & Elbert, 2010)

Levels of therapeutic intervention	Therapeutic intervention when uproar is dominant during the exposure session	Therapeutic intervention when shutdown is dominant during the exposure session
Differentiated approach during exposure	Therapist safely moderates the optimal (arousal) activation of the associative memory (event) structure in relation to its autobiographical context. They facilitate the narration of the event, taking caution to avoid overengagement and overwhelming.	Therapist frequently inquires about (identifies) indications of dissociative shutdown during the exposure. In the event of such indications, the exposure is interrupted by continuous reality testing, re-evaluation of the patient's state, and the implementation of countermeasures such as: • cardiovascular activation • sensory stimulation • encouragement of speech production until trauma material can be processed without shutdown

Table 5. Continued

Sensory-afferent	Emphasize the exploration of sensory details of the *past* traumatic event, comparing or contrasting with sensations and emotions in the present during recall	Emphasize the exploration of sensory details of the past traumatic event, comparing or contrasting with sensations and emotions in the present during recall + stimulation of the senses in the *here and now* – for example, present positive fragrances (e.g., lemon), offer tasting probes (peppermint oil or chilli gum), switch on bright light, present tactile information (e.g., texture, icepacks), direct attention to auditory stimuli in the here and now
Motor-efferent	Compare and contrast past sensations and bodily reactions from present during recall	Emphasize activation of the skeletal muscles, enhance blood pressure and muscle tonus (above all, use applied tension, physical exercises, leg crossing, physical counterpressure maneuvers), and use body balancing tasks
Language processing	Emphasize the narration of the *past* traumatic scene	Emphasize the narration of the *past* traumatic scene, supported by the facilitation of continuous narrative engagement in the *here and now* (e.g., active communication and enhanced speech production)
Emotional processing	Support full emotional expression	Support full emotional expression allowing and promoting specifically anger affect that has been inhibited peritraumatically
Nutritional demands		Pay attention to adequate nutrition (caution for malnutrition or eating disorders); increase dietary salt and fluid intake in daily life; advise to drink half a liter of water, if tolerated, before exposure to trauma material
Counteract and abstain from:		
Dont's during exposure treatment	Termination of exposure before contextualization and integration can take place (i.e., giving in to avoidance) Allowing extreme fear, that is, sympathetic arousal, to reach an excessive level without effectively calming the patient Isolating or leaving the survivor alone in a state of tonic immobility (or collapsed immobility)	• Termination of exposure before contextualization and integration can take place • Disengagement from the here and now • Relaxation (instead of activation) • Sensory similarities between the trauma context and the therapeutic setting • Stimuli that are associated with disgust or similar to body fluids and feces (i.e., ammoniac) • Threat cues in the here and now (instead: present safety signals) • Semidarkness in the room and objects for hiding (e.g., large plants, sitting behind furniture)

Other Helpful Considerations to Manage the Tendency to Dissociate

Punishment Increases the Tendency to Dissociate

Punishments for dissociative behavior, such as aversive stimuli – for example, sudden loud noises, inflicting pain through a cold stimulus, or rubber snapping on the skin, etc. – can increase the tendency to dissociate, because if the present is unfriendly or threatening, consciousness will not return to it. Great care should also be taken with physical touch, as this can trigger trauma memories and increase dissociation. In addition, announce all actions and remain at eye level – that is, do not stand physically above the person. Do not leave dissociated people alone or punish them by isolating them. Shutdown is a powerful, biologically determined mechanism designed to ensure survival by "playing dead" and maintaining a stable circulatory position. Trauma survivors can learn to fight against the occurrence if they understand what is happening to them, and how the body reacts and why. However, this process cannot always be influenced or stopped at will, at least not until a form of exposure therapy has been carried out.

Anger as a Direct Counterpart of Dissociation

Anger counteracts dissociation and successfully combats shutdown. Remember: You cannot be angry and dissociate at the same time! Allow suppressed feelings of opposition or defense, invite them to be named and verbalized. Emotions are okay. It is safe to experience them in the therapy room without having to dissociate. Allow outrage toward the attacker from back then, encourage feelings that were peritraumatically repressed; however, make sure that the feelings are tiedto the spatiotemporal context of back then and are not directed toward the therapist or helpers.

Physical Condition Can Be Crucial

Ensure the participant is well nourished (blood sugar) and hydrated: for example, a glass of water, juice, or tea before the session and sipped during the session in an upright position. (Caution: Never try to give fluids at the same time as when people are in tonic or flaccid immobility; risk of aspiration!) Underweight and starving persons dissociate very quickly.

Be aware of feelings of disgust toward certain foods after sexual violence and check for comorbid eating disorder symptoms.

Pay Attention to Lighting and Room Conditions

Good lighting and brightness in the therapy room is important for successful trauma processing for individuals with a tendency to dissociate. Shutdown occurs much more quickly in dim light and in semidark, hidden niches, than in an open, well-lit room. Therefore, have the survivor sit in the middle of the therapy room and work with good activation and muscle-tensing exercises (applied tension) while narrating.

Allocentric Instead of Egocentric

If reality threatens to become blurred, take an allocentric position together with the survivor, have the narrator look at the trauma scene and themselves from the outside – for example, as if you were both standing at the door and looking into the room, or from above from a bird's eye view. If appropriate, sketch the situation on a piece of paper (context) to look at it from the outside. Make sure that there is always a feeling of safety and control for the person in the therapy situation.

Corrective Relationship Experience and Mentalization

Dissociation not only changes the perception of and reaction to external stimuli, but also the processing of internal processes. The perception, thinking, and understanding and feeling of physical, emotional, and mental processes are then distorted. The experience of the self can also be lost. To stimulate the perception of inner experience, ask the person direct questions about how they perceive themselves in the here and now. Encourage explicit observation and verbalization of the inner states, as the conscious "ex-centric" position has an antidissociative effect: to see myself in the traumatic situation from the inside, and at the same time to see myself in the past from the outside.

Recognizing and verbalizing thoughts and feelings in others and in oneself in an undistorted and sensitive way requires successful parent–child interactions in development (Gergely et al., 2002; Bateman & Fonagy, 2013). Ideally, parents react to the child's emotional expressions in a specific way, which can leads to the child becoming aware of their own emotions through the caregiver's reaction. As survivors of childhood traumatization, which is often accompanied by a tendency to dissociate, have often not been able to experience a reliable mirroring of emotions by adults those affected often have an undifferentiated awareness and understanding of their emotional states. Here, the corrective relational experience can become effective precisely during and at the moment of imaginative exposure, to see oneself from the outside (allocentric) and inside (egocentric); a process that can have an antidissociative effect with the support of the therapist. Help dissociative people to find words for their states and their experiences (naming, attributing meaning), and switch back and forth between now and then. Explicitly support the narrator in observing their own experience, understanding it, and relating it to their own behavior and that of other people. The more explicitly the person concerned learns to recognize and describe the inner processes and their physical behavioral response, the less helpless and overwhelmed they will feel, and the more contrast there will be with the past.

Summary of How to Handle Dissociation During NET

Prevention

- Assess dissociative symptoms and triggers beforehand (use the Shut-D scale; Schalinski, Schauer, & Elbert, 2015, 2016).
- If dissociation symptoms are reported, discuss procedure in case of dissociation during the trauma work.
- Check if client ate and drank prior to the session.
- Check the suitability of the room (enough light, window, alone in room, etc.).
- Encourage a comfortable and upright seated position that enables bodily movements for activation, if necessary.
- Ask to be allowed to use the client's first name (given name) in case of dissociation.
- Have the dissociation tool kit handy (massage ball, olfactory stimuli, etc.) and use its items without stopping the narration.
- Additional tools for online sessions:
  - Practice dissociation exercises
  - Introduce dissociation tool kit to client
  - Use of cellphone
  - Get contact information of emergency contact close by or have a treatment assistant nearby.

In Exposure Sessions

- Repeatedly assess the circle for past and present.
- Address when a client becomes very emotionally aroused (e.g., by saying, "I can see you getting fearful now").
- Ask the client to change their bodily posture.
- Ask the client to drink something.
- Keep addressing the different senses of the client.

Possible Signs of Dissociation

- Client cannot distinguish between past and present, gets drawn into the past as if it is the here and now.
- Change in physiological arousal.
- Skin turns pale.
- Warm instead of cold hands.
- Numbing of body parts.
- Drop of heart rate and blood pressure.
- Nausea.
- Change in language comprehension and production.
- Client talks in fragmented fashion, is unclear, or stops talking.
- Tunnel hearing.
- Client reports that their surrounding looks blurred or different – tunnel vision.
- Reduced awareness of surroundings and loss of reality.
- Client does not react, hear, or notice you.
- Client startles when you address them.
- Client seems confused.

Antidissociation Strategies During NET

Movement

- Change the survivor's body posture to a posture that is not connected with the event.
- Have the survivor start with small movements and increase the movements slowly.
- Have the survivor stretch.
- Have them tense their muscles.
- Open a window and feel the breeze.

Hearing

- Continuously talk with the client.
- Talk calm and clearly.
- Contrast past and present.

- Repeatedly name the client's first name and your name.
- Name time and place.
- Name reason for being here.
- Label the experience.
- Emphasize that the client is safe.
- Name characteristics of the present that differ from the event.
- Ask the client to listen to their surroundings.
- Use a sound that is distinct from the experience during the event.

Seeing

- Encourage the client to look around and notice their surroundings.
- Encourage the client to look at their body.
- Encourage the client to look around.

Speaking

- Encourage the client to talk to you.
- Anchor the conversation in the here and now for a few minutes, but return as soon as possible to finish the story being told. Do not leave event narratives that have been started open-ended. This can cause great distress to the survivor in the days to come; at least retell the narrative in a more summarizing way until the experience has ended in the past and there is significant relief in the present.
- Ask simple questions (not emotionally charged).
- Ask the client to describe their surroundings for better grounding.

Touching – Invite the Participant to Do the Following:

- Rub hands.
- Clap their hands.
- Touch and feel the chair below them.
- Touch different fabrics and textures.
- Massage their muscles, neck, arms, etc.
- Use a massage ball.
- Touch a distinct object.

Smelling and Tasting

- Smell natural scents like mint, lemon, lemongrass, orange, etc.
- You can also have candies, lemon wedges, a piece of ginger or similar ready.
- Drink a cold (nonalcoholic) beverage.
- If necessary: positioning in shock; legs 20–30 degrees up.

After the Dissociative State

- Dissociation is very exhausting for the affected person; it is important to give them enough time to recover.
- Provide psychoeducation.
- Continue at least roughly with the narration until you reach a safe moment!!
- Make sure you meet again soon and do a good reading back, and again go into Narrative Exposure at the most emotionally and physically arousing moments.
- Remember – once you have managed to bring a client through an event and they manage to narrate all parts (especially the most shameful and difficult ones), dissociation is over!

With an antidissociation intervention, you will overcome dissociation and master the completion of the narrative. This will markedly and soon diminish, if not completely abolish, the dissociative behavior.

Shame and Guilt and the Threat to Human Life

Alors, c'est ça l'enfer. Je n'aurais jamais cru.... Vous vous rappelez: le soufre, le bûcher, le gril....
Ah ! Quelle plaisanterie. Pas de besoin de gril: l'enfer c'est les autres!

J.-P. Sartre, *Huis Clos*

There is substantial evidence that social threat causes and contributes to a broad array of mental pathologies, as well as amplifying symptom responses in individuals suffering from trauma spectrum disorders. Events that involve social threats resulting from violations of core social motives (such as the pursuit of status and belonging) and that bring about intense affective reactions (including despair and defeat) have harmful effects. Therefore, expanding memory theories of psychological trauma to encompass threats to social integrity is a crucial advancement. These theories include PAST Physical and Social Trauma framework (Neuner, 2023) and Threats to

Human Life (see THL checklist in Appendix 1; Schauer et al., 2011; Köbach et al., 2016). Within associative fear networks, these emotions are tied to the stimulus characteristics of the traumatic experiences and can be reactivated in social situations.

Social emotions are contingent on the thoughts, feelings, or actions of others as we experience, remember, anticipate, or imagine them, and involve mirroring ourselves in the eyes of others. From an evolutionary perspective, self-conscious emotions elevate us from *social animals* into humans. There is a high emotional cost to our human nature in this. Painful, crushing feelings are fundamentally stressful, but effectively motivating. They help us to continuously monitor social responses which feeds back into our emotion and behavior, especially to quickly identify social threats, and foresee rejection and aggression. This existential dependence on our *(internalized) assumptions of how others view us* for the sake of self-regulation via the experience of stress in the pursuit of social recognition and status, is a typical trait of the human species (Schauer, 2018).

Throughout our lifespan we remain vigilant for potential challenges, whether to our existence from harm to our *physical well-being* (such as exposure to extreme temperatures, contaminants, suffocation, or tissue damage), or to our *reproductive success* (such as through rape or harm to offspring), or in the form of threats to *social integrity* (such as social rejection, isolation, deprivation, exclusion, and loss of important bonds, family members, and status). Social threats are harmful to our innate social nature (please refer to the THL checklist in Appendix 1). Human beings are inclined to strive for stable social interaction and inclusion, a particular status in the community, autonomy, dependable bonds, and high reproductive value. Threats to social integrity that impact *affiliation* and *social rank*, which are fundamental social motives, can constitute an existential threat – a well-established fact that has long been known to be integral by mental health professionals and scientists. Charles Darwin set out in his writings, that we fear devaluation and we long for validation and praise (Darwin, 1872/1998).

Starting with congenital, culturally independent basic emotions when we are infants (primary emotions, including fear, anger, and happiness; Ekman, 1999), the ontogenetically later social emotions are also inborn, but shaped by the social-interactional learning of our cultures. The development of social emotions necessitates cognitive *representation of the self* as self-reflective awareness. We are aware of our own self-awareness, and acknowledge that we relate to ourselves and that we are perceived by others – and this realization holds significant value and judgment for us. This ability, and our need to constantly monitor the state of our social integrity, and to respond to this introspection and improve our actions accordingly so that we can optimize them for social success, is crucial to our mental and physical thriving – indeed, to leading a successful life.

Guilt and shame both work toward this primary goal in different ways, as we will explore in the next section.

Difference Between Guilt and Shame

Guilt, the state of being responsible for carrying out or not carrying out an appropriate behavior, has often been called the emotion of choice when it comes to rehabilitating an individual (Tangney et al., 2007; 2011; Tangney, Stuewig, & Hafez, 2011; Tangney & Dearing, 2003; Gilligan, 2003). Guilt proneness assessed in childhood predicted fewer sexual partners, less use of illegal drugs and alcohol, and less involvement with the criminal justice system. Shame proneness, negative self-evaluation, in contrast, was a risk factor for later deviant behavior. Shame-prone children were more likely to have unprotected sex and use illegal drugs in young adulthood (Stuewig et al., 2015). There is empirical evidence in favor of guilt feelings among the social emotions of guilt, shame, and pride when compared with each other in children and adolescents and their relationship to experiencing certain psychopathology (depression, anger, aggression, and delinquency; Muris & Meesters, 2014).

Studies in adolescents and adults report that guilt and shame are related to depression and suicidality, with shame having the stronger association; this may occur because shame, especially after emotional abuse (Kealy et al., 2018; Holmes, 2018), is a severe experience of inferiority and rejection that is difficult to repair or expiate (Sekowski et al., 2020; Neuner, 2023; Webb et al., 2007; Campos et al., 2013). We react with strong emotional, behavioral, and physiological responses to threats to our social status, such as humiliations and degradations.

When social integrity is threatened, it can lead to a series of defense mechanisms that resemble those found in bodily attacks. These can include both an increase in physiological and psychological arousal (up-regulation), as well as a decrease in arousal and functioning (shutdown). When encountering conflict and aggression, a submissive response may be helpful to reduce the likelihood of being attacked, though de-escalation. However, repeated experiences of defeat in ongoing aggressive social contexts can lead to lasting consequences for the individual, such as persistent feelings of inferiority and inadequacy.

Research has identified social stress responses, including despair and defeat, as key experiences that can lead to depression and suicidal thoughts (Shanahan et al., 2019; Copeland et al., 2020). Moreover, during childhood development, threats to social integrity typically result in pathological changes in mood and cognition. Victims of emotional abuse may experience a tendency toward internalized shame, resulting from heightened self-awareness of humiliation and negative messaging and criticism. Such messages are often related to the self. Adolescents who have undergone emotional and verbal abuse tend to experience shame more than guilt (Sekowski et al., 2020). While pride is a response to social validation (e.g., success, power, high reproductive fitness, mastery of body functions), shame is a response to social defeat – a display of extreme compliance and obsequiousness – trying to stop social aggression. Our inbuilt *social barometer* informs us about our social status, thereby ensuring that we behave in ways that maintain our status and others' acceptance, and enable us to avoid group rejection (Leary et al., 1995).

As described, shame is defined as an unpleasant feeling that involves a global negative self-evaluation. Thus, the essential difference is that shame involves the anticipated social devaluation of the self, whereas guilt involves the disapproval of specific behaviors, actions, or thoughts. There is substantial evidence that intense feelings of guilt in response to actions taken or not taken immediately before or during the event are highly correlated with the severity of posttrauma symptoms (Stotz et al., 2015). Feelings of guilt and shame, as well as trauma symptoms, were all associated with the number of traumatic event types experienced by the subjects in that study. The more types of traumatic events experienced, the more likely we are to feel guilt, shame, and trauma symptoms (Stotz et al., 2015). Shame-proneness has been found to be positively correlated with symptom severity across the trauma spectrum (Stotz et al., 2015; Leskela et al., 2002) and is associated with negative cognitions about the self (Badour et al., 2020). Thus, shame and guilt are both highly sensitive areas arising from developmental issues, and both have significant implications for trauma therapy and research.

Guilt

If an individual had control over their actions, then they bore moral responsibility when having violated norms and values with poor justification for personal choice of behaviors (Kubany et al., 1996). The social emotions of shame and guilt were evolutionarily selected as psychological mechanisms that support group living. The wrongdoing of an individual can lead to collective stress and jeopardize the group's cohesiveness or even survival. Guilt serves as a warning system for safer future behavior, as well as a means to induce visible and observable emotional discomfort such as social pain and rumination. In addition, visible suffering is essential for reintegration into the social community after a potential violation of values or wrongdoing. Survivor guilt exemplifies what biologists refer to as "the downside of winning" (O'Connor et al., 2000). In order to be well-received back into the social group, it is important to signal emotional distress to convince others of our submission through insight and learning ("How could I have done (or not done) *that*?") and our visible purification and willingness to take responsibility (e.g., by offering to make amends, thinking about reparation, confessing, and/or apologizing). Feelings of guilt, however painful, have been shown to make us better people. In contrast to shame, where the person feels bad about themselves, guilt means feeling bad about one's *specific behavior*, meaning there is something wrong with what I did, not with who I am.

But why do many survivors of trauma, including victims of interpersonal violence, war, crime, physical and sexual abuse, and others, feel intense guilt and shame that are closely linked to their traumatic experiences? What have they done wrong as individuals who have been victimized? It may seem counterintuitive, but feelings of guilt and the behavior of rumination reveal our search for control, suggesting that we could have influenced the outcome of a situation through different behavior – for instance, thinking, "It's my fault I was raped," and then deciding to wear, for example, different clothes that cover more of the body in the future, provides a false sense (illusion) of control.

Similarly, other community members may also engage in victim blaming as a means to reassure themselves that they will not experience such an event (as per NETfacts). While strategic options may have been limited in that particular situation, a sense of control remains crucial when we feel helpless. It can enhance awareness and preparedness for future scenarios. The distress and emotional pain in guilt is caused by the tendency for knowledge about event outcomes to bias our recollections of what we knew *before*.

Furthermore, false beliefs that unforeseeable outcomes were foreseeable and therefore preventable, and beliefs that one was capable of knowing that an unforeseeable negative outcome was going to occur and one could have acted to prevent this outcome, can strongly emerge (Kubany et al., 1996; Kubany & Ralston, 2008). Survivors may amplify or misrepresent their roles in traumatic events. Therefore, therapists often work with clients to rectify flawed beliefs and identify cognitive errors that contribute to these specific distortions (Leach, 2017).

The fact that victims regularly feel guilty when they have been helplessly violated is disturbing. Nevertheless, the function of these "distorted cognitions" in survivors of traumatic stress is noteworthy. In the realm of survival, not responding to the ubiquity of threats to life and integrity ("No matter what, it would have happened anyway") would be emotionally unbearable, behaviorally stupid, and lead to evolutionary extinction.

To recognize and avoid the massive negative consequences next time, we are well advised to link the "punishment" to our own actions. This way we signal obligation and hope to appease aggression. Survivor guilt and remorseful behavior promotes compassion from the group and helps engage altruistic behavior (O'Connor et al., 2000). Guilt feelings motivate behavior to address problems, to repair and to manage anger proactively (Furukawa et al., 2012; Tangney, Stuewig, & Hafez, 2011).

Treating Trauma-Related Guilt NETwise

In Narrative Exposure Therapy, the treatment of guilt is embedded in the core procedure (Schaal et al., 2009; Schauer et al., 2020), and is addressed with consideration for its significant social role, taking on the task that the person suffering from guilt feelings should strive to show remorse and take reparative action to prepare for future social threats and ensure group inclusion and cohesion. Reasons for one's past behavior become more easily apparent with thorough narrating, including sorting out the occurrences and decisions, fostering self-acceptance, and enabling understanding of one's actions *in context*, including emotional and physiological states – for instance, that it is understandable that poor decisions may have been made under exceptional circumstances and under intense pressure. Trauma therapy often involves a complementary exercise aimed at objectively assessing one's own wrongdoing or failure, relative to those of others involved and the circumstances surrounding the incident. Survivor guilt, a fear of rejection by the social group after surviving while others did not, can be alleviated by the group's welcoming reception and the sharing of one's narrative.

Psychoeducation Regarding Understanding and Function of Guilt Feelings and Display of Guilt

Based on evolutionary principles, trauma-induced guilt serves a purpose in communities, despite its disturbing emotional nature that has led some to describe it as involving "dysfunctional" thought patterns and "distorted" thinking (Beck & Clark, 2015). However, recognizing that these deep-seated feelings of pain and remorse have a vital biological function, such as taking behavioral consequences seriously and securing social norms in groups, and the recognition of that may contribute to a more complete understanding of this gripping social emotion. Thinking in hindsight ("How could I have foreseen and prevented this outcome at the time?"), or weighing the merits of actions taken against ideal options ("I wish this option had existed," "I wish this solution had occurred to me at the time," "If only I had had more time to think about it"), and ruminating about causal relationships ("It feels like I caused the outcome, since I couldn't do anything about it") are justifiable social ways of signaling that we *care* about the outcome, that we take the *outcome seriously*, and this calms the group's anger. It is a plea to be taken back into the *social group*, to be loved and seen as worthy.

Carry Out Narrative Exposure With Past Events That Have Evoked Guilt

The next step in NET, when high level ofguilt are present, is to create a perfectly detailed narrative of the event(s) during the exposure – for example, using the Narrative Exposure cycle (Figure 17). In addition, other prior events, moods, health status, relationship dynamics, etc., play into each incident. Only then can we have an informed reflection on how the younger self's actions or inactions in that very hour should be judged. Comparing the emotional and physical experiences with the NET-typical moving back and forth in time "past versus present" (Figure 20 and Figure 45) of imagining and talking about the past and then returning to the present from time to time, allows the survivor to relive what happened then. Exploring the hotspot with awareness and conscious consideration of social emotional moments helps to shed light on the process.

In the following example, the therapist assists a woman with feelings of guilt in recounting an experience in which she witnessed another girl's rape after having been attacked herself:

When you were lying in the corner of the room after being assaulted by the attacker, you reported feeling extreme fear.... From that position, could you observe any actions the rapist was taking toward the little girl?... How far away were you from the little girl? .... Did you hear her screams? Additionally, can you describe any physical sensations you experienced at that time... the location of any areas of your body of, how we say, reduced muscle tone?.... What did you want to do? ... Now that you're sitting in the therapy room, can you feel the weakness from that time? Could you try to move your legs ... your arms.... They are so heavy.... So you couldn't move and keep her safe?... And you felt so desperate....

An accurate moment-by-moment reconstruction of what the person perceived, thought, felt, experienced in the body, and the resulting interpretations, including what they then did (or wanted to do), results in a much clearer picture of how the event unfolded.

Step Back and Look From an Allocentric Perspective – Visualize the Multiplicity of Factors

Often the detailed Narrative Exposure delving deep into the nature of our experiencing and behavior, reveals the multitude of factors that caused event histories. Looking at different people's responsibilities and circumstances that led to this outcome, can serve as a useful tool for analyzing the various agents that contributed to an incident (Figure 46). This leads to the allocation of the real percentage of one's own wrongdoing or failure, which is framed in proportion to other people and circumstances involved in the incident. Its key function is to visualize the distribution of "liability" among the different parties involved. The survivor only ever had a certain amount of responsibility for the incident, taking into account the influence of other people, factors, and forces.

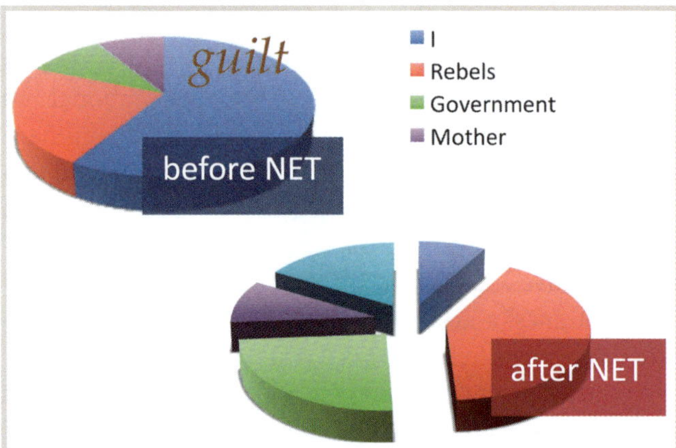

Figure 46. Before revisiting the event, the survivor has placed most of the blame and responsibility on themselves. After the detailed analysis of the past, the proportional allocation will have become more realistic and additional players may have been recognized (pastel blue).

Identify and Analyze Ethical Implications

Denn wir Überlebende wussten ganz genau, dass die (moralisch) Besten, die unter uns waren von dort (Ausschwitz) nicht herausgekommen sind – die Besten waren es, die nicht zurückgekehrt sind! [We survivors knew that the (morally) best of us died in Auschwitz. It was the (ones with the) best (behavior) who did not return!]

Victor Frankl, *Wer ein Warum zu leben hat [Man's Search for Meaning]*

Encourage discussion of the recovered trauma material and engage in an ethical debate regarding responsibility and guilt concepts. Address ethical dilemmas and potential conflicts between values or principles. The therapist creates a safe environment for participants to reflect on their ethical positions, socialization factors (childhood, environment), duties, omissions, and underlying motives. Consider the available options in this context and the reasons for choosing them, objectively analyzing the values and the reasoning underlying each option. The best plan of action should have been determined based on these values and reasons, and now is the chance to redress. It is crucial to maintain a logical and unbiased approach when considering these issues. Ethical beliefs guiding decision making may stem from religion, culture, or personal opinions. It is important to recognize that beliefs change over time, and that some individuals may hold different beliefs to one's own. Ethical issues may arise due to differences in beliefs. Disagreements over what is considered right or wrong, personal beliefs, and organizational values can all contribute to ethical issues. Survivors may act in ways they believe are ethical; however, others may disagree, resulting in conflict and tension. In addition, individuals may face ethical dilemmas when they have to choose between courses of action that have both positive and negative consequences. For reparation, it can be important to talk to people who are affected by the issue, researching the issue, and/or reading about the issue. This may involve taking a stand on the issue, trying to take action, or to raise awareness. In NET, however, there is no homework. The therapist might help the survivor to understand that these feelings are not pathological in a clinical sense, and the therapist can often help to find a way to become active. In this way the therapist may encourage the survivor to come up with a *giving back* plan themselves.

Create Opportunities for Giving Back to the Social Group

Discussing how much of the blame a person must assign to themselves is not intended to shift blame to others. Nor is a meticulous narrative intended to find apologetic motives in the story after the fact and to attribute all actions or omissions to other people and forces. This would not aid the survivor in reconciling themselves with the past. Feeling guilty for the part the survivor is responsible for is a healthy reaction. If there is guilt, it should be acknowledged and categorized precisely. The extent of the guilt must be clearly named and described. Responsibility is never 100% or 0%. It is crucial to acknowledge, nevertheless, that not all emotions are prosocial. The survivor may have felt anger, frustration, envy, or a desire for advantage, or they may have solely focused on their own survival that day. Although understandable, it can be difficult to acknowledge. This is where therapists can offer empathy and important insights by asking relevant questions that balance the perspective.

Feelings of guilt are not pathological per se. Guilt-prone individuals are good at taking other people's perspectives; they tend to be empathic, resilient, with no heightened risk for psychiatric symptoms, but also to have a desire to take reparative action. The regret over wrong behavior and about the loss of control over outcome, together with the fear of social punishment for violating the norms and values leads to extreme feelings of despair and helplessness and worry about how to repair things. Consequently, talking therapy and cognitive work alone may fall short in the treatment of guilt reactions after trauma. Trying to talk someone out of guilt feelings neglects the biological need for control over social threats and being socially integrated with a helpful role – contributing to the group's thriving. Again, psychoeducation on the matter can help achieve self-acceptance. Depending on the liability, a meaningful social activity, a plan for redress and giving back to the community may be the best cure for this reason. A salutary exercise is the allocation of the real percentage of one's own wrongdoing or failure framed in proportion to that of other people and circumstances involved in the incident. In some, posttraumatic growth can even be facilitated by trauma-related guilt, because of embarking in prosocial activity or charity work.

Receiving the Narrative of the Victim

Guilty individuals can find a way to show accountability for their actions and remain included in the community through a testimony framework (Zehr, 2015; Zehr et al., 2022; McCluskey et al., 2008; Lodi et al., 2021). Perpetrators acknowledge their wrongdoing through their willingness to listen to, receive the narration, and take responsibility for victims' stories. Restorative justice can be guided by questions such as: who has been harmed, who has been hurt, and what are the needs of those affected? Answering these questions enables the perpetrator to understand the consequences of their behaviors and to repair the harm caused. Responsible parties and perpetrators help the injured party complete their storytelling to fill in the blanks and help the victim feel less guilty. Kirkman and colleagues suggest this promising approach, which requires further research to tackle the perpetrators of sexual violence and those affected by it (Gang et al., 2021). In the Narrative Exposure framework, the survivor and the offender complete an individual NET procedure to address their traumas within their life story chronologically, resulting in a thorough exploration of their life story. From there, they commence a professionally assisted restorative approach in careful steps.

Shame

Addressing shame involves dealing with the threat of social devaluation and signaling willingness to question one's identity. Humans, more than any other species, depend on bonds, information, and resources from others of their own species. They establish complex social hierarchies and engage in competition for status, resources, and mates, resulting in potential threats to the individual such as social exclusion, ostracism, and loss of status (Boyer & Bergstrom, 2011). Favorable valuation by others was a critical resource for our ancestors (Fessler, 2007). However, people who demonstrate shameless behavior can jeopardize the group's social connections, health, and overall social harmony. Without mastering physicality, adherence to good conduct, and willingness to question one's value to the group, there is no human social life.

Shame, although extremely embarrassing, with a painful focus on the "me"/"us" serves the adaptive function of evaluating our "self," our core identity (not our behavior, as is the case with guilt) and shaping us socially to defend the individual (and their group) against social devaluation. Shame has everything to do with social status, which we assess through the internalized view that the other person might have of us. Shame closely tracks the threat of devaluation by others, even across cultures (Sznycer et al., 2016). Feelings of shame indicate a suffered degradation, being consigned or dismissed to an inferior rank or position. In contrast to guilt, shamed individuals feel defeated and subordinate in the social hierarchy. This can either lead to acceptance of the lower position, or the feelings of inferiority can instead lead to anger, hostility, mistrust, and finally to aggression to restore one's social dominance (Gilbert, 2000; Fessler, 2001; Tangney et al., 1992; Sell et al., 2009). Hostility is considered the desire to get even.

Shame develops naturally in childhood before there is a sense of responsibility and guilt, or a will to make amends. Abusive attachment figures are not only sources of distress, but are usually also emotionally unavailable and not capable of mirroring, soothing, and mentalizing the traumatic experiences that they cause (Sekowski et al., 2020). Our childhood developmental history plays a large role in this, as do the social experiences we have in peer groups (Neuner, 2023; Sansen et al., 2015; Iffland et al., 2014). Shame signals surrender and withdrawal and can eliminate cues for counter aggression, which is important for smaller, younger, weaker, and more vulnerable individuals. As a consequence, youths with rejecting parents are more shame prone and less guilt prone than other youths (Stuewig & McCloskey, 2005).

In What Situations Do We Feel Ashamed – And Why Does That Make Sense?

The social emotion of envy, and its corresponding facial expression, is shown as anger when a person competes for the same rank as another, and the other expresses pride and dominance with an upright posture, when their claim to social status is recognized. In contrast, a stooped posture of shame signals submission as a result of a denied status claim. The lack of shame as a conscious self-regulatory mechanism for such essential aspects as physical desire, sexual behavior, toilet training, emotionality, and social interaction, among others, can lead to marginalization and stigmatizing social consequences for adults. Freud harshly stated: "The lack of shame is the first sign of insanity..." (Freud, 1906–1909/2010).

However, the opposite extreme is also daunting – that is, people who experience extreme and persistent anxiety associated with social or performance situations in which they are likely to be scrutinized and observed by others. Individuals with social anxiety disorder may have persistent fears of being judged, criticized, ridiculed, or humiliated. They feel threatened in exactly the above-mentioned areas: socializing, talking, eating, using the bathroom, being looked at, dating, etc. Childhood experiences may influence how we perceive social cues and situations, leading to a heightened sense of anxiety regarding how others perceive our behaviors, including actions such as being seen, speaking, eating, or using the bathroom. This sensitivity is particularly prevalent in social phobia or, conversely, the insensitivity of ignoring social cues in other pathologies. Expressing poorly regulated anger, misperceiving others (including their emotional expression and situational cues), and lacking empathy for others' feelings demonstrate the importance of emotional literacy (Denham, 2003), all of which need to be rehabilitated in trauma therapy.

Important Areas of Shame

Important areas of shame include situations where we are unable to hide or control the following

1. **Inability to control bodily functions:** These involve involuntary bodily processes, toileting, and bowel movements, etc. ("Others are disgusted with me"). The regulation of status claims and the evaluation process show that shame is associated with the feared loss of control over bodily functions, leading to embarrassment. Situations in which we embarrass ourselves can lead to (feared) social devaluation by others and intense shame feelings.
2. **Inability to control drives and instincts:** This sort of lack of control equates us with "animality": unbridled eating and drinking, sexual drive, display of genitals, uncontrolled and even addictive lust for hunting and aggression, greed (intense and selfish desire for something, especially wealth, power, or food), etc.
3. **Inability to control emotions:** High status personalities can be identified by the expression of confidence, calmness, and control. They feel comfortable whenever "on stage" and being the center of attention, while subordinate persons bow. Lower status individuals show lowering of the head, increased pulse, sweating, avoidance, and ambivalence in eye contact when they are afraid of showing themselves and fear being devalued (Kaufman, 2004). Shame-prone individuals become irritable or fidgety when looked at, because they fear the other person's social judgment will be negative. ("I feel horrified, when people look at me." "I am always so emotional, I'm not taken seriously.")
4. **When adults are unable to achieve autonomy:** This happens with remaining submissive into adulthood, with a need for care and constant reassurance, and an inability to make everyday decisions without advice and backing from others, clinging, and lacking auton-

omy. Feeling shame when being dependent on others for some reason ("I am disabled and feel like a burden." "I am old and useless." "Others despise me because I need help."). Signaling shame can minimize risk in social interactions, in which individuals perceive that the ratio of their *social value to their social burden to others* is at a critically low level (Allen & Badcock, 2003).

5. **Display and motives of rivalry for rank and sexual partner:** This includes any unjustified aspiration to an increase in rank or status and unauthorized pursuits of reproductive benefit. Loss of social status for reasons such as rivalry and the nontolerated attempt to gain advantages or rank are also part of this. For example, a woman's violation of cultural dress codes may be subject to labeling, because it is understood to be an unjustified pursuit of reproductive advantage ("Shame on her!"; see Arnocky & Vaillancourt, 2017, Arnocky et al., 2012; Vaillancourt & Sharma, 2011). Darwin (1872/1998; Ekman, 2009) on the other hand, pointed out that decency (sexual shyness as a sign of partner loyalty) and blushing from shame are considered desirable because they are social signals for accepting compliance. As well as when exploring reproductive status (flirting), to involuntarily offer subordination by blushing to a (potential mating) partner suggests chastity, sexual fidelity, and paternity assurance in species with internal fertilization, such as humans.

Shame is a signal of the willingness to control physicality, master autonomy, resist rivalry, and comply with higher-ranking individuals to avoid social devaluation. The fear of social devaluation protects individuals from making illegitimate claims to higher status and dominance. Individuals experiencing shame are ready to question their identity and feel bad about themselves ("How could *I* be like that?"), which is a key social competence. Under traumatic and adverse social conditions, however, the important function of shame can take on threatening proportions, as shown in expressions such as "I am a 'bad person,' 'low-ranking,' 'defective,' 'worthless,' 'evaluated negatively by others,'" or "I want to escape and hide" (Tangney & Dearing, 2003; Boyer & Bergstrom, 2011). This heightened awareness of social devaluation was used historically to apply public humiliation: social threats to inflict harm in order to sanction someone through obvious status loss. Detaining people in a pillory, scold's bridle, or gag, or physically exposing people to public punishment, including public nudity and other forms of humiliation, was commonplace not only in the Middle Ages, but also in many modern war and captivity situations where the "enemy" is subjected to brutal shaming. Shame is deliberately inflicted by perpetrators to humiliate the victim, for example, during torture (Pérez-Sales & Petersen, 2023; Elbert et al., 2011; Hensel-Dittmann, 2011; El-Khoury et al., 2021) and also in the control of certain groups within society, such as any minorities, and including in racism, homophobia, and misogyny.

The questioning of one's own identity may be aggressively resisted, and reflected in emotional coldness and deliberate ignorance of social cues. This can happen when individuals see no chance of being accepted by a significant other or of being reintegrated into the group. The pain of early and repeated shaming and dishonoring is extremely dangerous for the development of this behavior (Heinze, 2017; da Silva et al., 2015; Nyström & Mikkelsen, 2013). A problematic calibration of social emotions, especially shame, is characteristic of personality disorders. Harsh, rejecting parenting in childhood is related to shame in adolescence. Repeated social defeat during childhood can result in (suppressed) anger, and reactive impulsivity, leading to a personality that is prone to blame, hurt, and to revictimize itself (Langer & Neuner, 2021). In some cases, appetitively violent individuals threaten, attack and kill other people as a violent way to gain dominance and (re-)establish status (Elbert et al., 2017a, 2017b; Tangney et al., 1992). Shame, being an emotion that affects one's entire being, does not in these cases motivate repair of perceived failure (unlike guilt; Sekowski et al., 2020). Shame has been connected to hiding, denying, and escaping, which interferes with an empathic connection to other persons. Shame and devaluation lead to low self-esteem (nothing to lose) that carries the risk of a desire to reinstate social status through acts full of hate and revenge, as described by several authors (Gilligan, 2003; Scheff, 2011; Leary et al., 2003; Websdale, 2010).

The importance of the basic ability to feel guilt is undisputed in research. However, the significance of shame in shaping socially emotionally appropriate behavior related to physical cleanliness, hygiene, sexual conduct, and recognition of one's place within the community is frequently underrated.

Treating Trauma-Related Shame With NET – In Victims and Offenders

Psychoeducation Regarding Understanding and Function of Shame Feelings and Expressions

When treating people who have experienced social devaluation, it is important to have a psychoeducational understanding of the effects of humiliation and degradation, as well as the biological functions of shame feelings and behavior.

Social emotions are universal, but their expressions and appropriateness vary across cultures. To provide effective trauma therapy, it is crucial for therapists to be knowledgeable about various cultural differences. They can seek advice from the survivor and interpreter. The cultures and subcultures in which an individual has grown, resides, and holds status play a significant role (relevant others!).

NET With Past Events That Evoked Shame and Anger at Rejection

The basic NET approach is to shower with praise and allow corrective relationship experiences. Therapists want to be emotionally available and possess the ability to mirror, soothe, and help mentalize the perceptions, thoughts, and emotions of the narrator during NET in order to deal with the unmentalized, pervasive, self-conscious emotions of shame-prone individuals (see above The Human Condition and How We Relate to Our Experiencing). The NET therapist's close "exposure conversation" style is supportive, empathic, and involved, and therefore the survivor feels accepted. Social appreciation in the therapeutic contact, as well as narrative and sensitive processing of hurtful moments of rejection, are also key. Rejection can unleash immense anger (Leary et al., 2006; Armenti & Babcock, 2021). The survivor is likely to be talking about the most shameful moments for the first time, and being met with empathy and care rather than rejection is an enormously reparative experience that can also inspire confidence in re-engaging in social relationships.

Note: Do not attempt to force the survivor to confront the traumatic situation aggressively where they were humiliated, and beware to ask them to repeat a shameful body position. Shame does not become emotionally and physiologically habituated (a decrease in response to a stimulus after repeated exposure) when confronted extensively, but instead becomes increasingly unbearable. However, the therapist wants to invite the shame-prone individual to look at them and check the eyes are friendly and not rejecting.

If a survivor becomes silent, provide helpful words and emotional support to overcome their speechlessness. Ensure to maintain the narrative for traumatized victims as well as perpetrators, and complete the storytelling.

Step Back and Look From an Allocentric Perspective

If we step back and look from an allocentric perspective, who should be ashamed?! Pointing out human rights violations can be an effective strategy for overcoming avoidance, along with taking an ethical stand. Redirecting shame toward the perpetrator can help balance the social power dynamic and prompt reflection ("Who should feel shame, the rapist or you?"). While reading the narrative, survivors often experience, for the first time, the previously suppressed anger at being humiliated. This is an important step in recovery. The therapist makes sure to support the process of exploring these sensations, putting these hurt feelings and perceived insults into words, and assigning their anger a time and place where it belongs, in the past.

Identify and Analyze the Ethical Implications

Since shame goes along with loss of social status and group exclusion it is important to discuss with offenders their tendency to reinstate dominance and a rank through aggression when they feel humiliated (see Müller-Bamouh et al., 2016). "... the destruction of shame causes a disinhibition in all other areas, a brutality and disregard for the personality of one's fellow human being." (Freud, 1906–1909/2010, p. 149). Showing remorse without claiming higher social status can only work if one is (re) connected to the social group in a meaningful way. Questioning one's own identity and violent self-image should be part of trauma therapy with perpetrators.

Create Opportunities to Feel One's Value to the Community, Group, or Society

The therapist reinforces self-confident behavior of the survivor during the therapy sessions. To gain an understanding of social recognition, it is essential to engage in therapeutic communication, relate personal experiences with specific details, and sensitively process previous experiences of social rejection, to enjoy a corrective relationship experience. Ultimately, obtaining social validation from external sources is crucial, as it is the only way to mitigate suffering. Learning to publicly show self-confidence alongside social support can counter the suffering of social pain and allow the individual to regain their dignity. The evidence supports the use of interventions that increase self-perceived status and minimize the impact of low status (Troop & Hiskey, 2013; Gilbert &

Procter, 2006; Harman & Lee, 2010; Lee, 2009). Validation should not solely come from professional therapists, but also from the social community and significant others. Publicly displaying self-confidence through real-life strategies for social support and improving social status can help counter the pain of social suffering and aid in regaining dignity.

Other Challenges During the Narration Process

Narrator Is Withholding Information

In general, if a narrator withholds information from the therapist or chooses not to disclose certain information, the storytelling obviously cannot proceed. The participant's internal attention is alternatively focused on what is not to be said. Storytellers may unintentionally withhold information. They may feel that the information is irrelevant or that the content is too confusing to articulate. Things may come to mind that they dismiss. They assume that it is not important to the work being done on the traumatic event or that it is unrelated. Whether this information is relevant can only be determined if the person dares to speak freely about all that they are experiencing.

Here are some examples of why a survivor might withhold information:

- The incident occurred in early childhood. The person had no cognitive framework or knowledge base to interpret the meaning of the physical sensations from that time. The adult still experiences the body sensations, but because they were not given meaning at the time, the origin of the sensations is unknown.
- The participant is afraid that the information shared will come back to someone else, such as the partner.
- It is assumed that the therapist will not understand or accept what they are trying to say.
- Shame, social pain, or guilt prevent the patient from talking about the experiences.
- The narrator feels too much unpleasant arousal, such as a rapid heartbeat, and wants to avoid this feeling.

The therapist may ask any of the following questions to elicit unspoken material:

"Did something come to mind that you did not mention?"
"Did you think of something that is hard to tell me about?"
"Is there anything else you're thinking about right now?"
"I just saw your eyes moving.... Did you see something in front of your eyes just now?"

The individual needs to feel safe enough in the relationship with the therapist to say whatever comes to mind. If the therapist refrains from judging and from interpreting, the person is more likely to feel safe enough to speak openly. It may be necessary for the therapist to work on safety issues, both exploring the survivor's fears and concerns, and providing the reassurance and confidentiality of a good therapeutic alliance.

There Seems to Be No Physiological and Emotional Relief

Sometimes it seems that the narrative has progressed well according to the therapist, but the narrator's arousal level and emotional tension remain high. In such cases, more often than not, it is highly likely that exposure was not done correctly. Usually this is a sign that not all key hot spots of an event have been explored in depth. Something important has not been put into words. Embarrassing or shameful events that have occurred may have remained hidden during the telling of the trauma-related story.

The following are other potentially important issues that a therapist might focus on to uncover a missing link. Here is a checklist for ways to support emotional processing:

- Review the sensory information contained in the incident. This may include visual images of the incident, somatosensory sensations, olfactory cues (smells), or physical pain experienced during the incident.
- Focus on what the survivor is paying attention to (sometimes a survivor will repeat things that the therapist did not pay much attention to).
- Review intentions during the incident, including conflicting or embarrassing ones.
- Review actions taken during the incident. Did the survivor regret taking certain actions? Were there actions the person would have liked to take but could not?
- Look for evidence of the individual's cognitions and interpretations *during* the event(s): thoughts, assumptions, decisions, religious beliefs, expectations, ideas, and conclusions made during the incident. What were they thinking at the time? On what basis were decisions made? What did they believe was happening? What did they think would happen next?
- Look for perceptions and interpretations since the event(s): Thoughts, assumptions, decisions, beliefs,

expectations, ideas, and conclusions made after the experiences. What does the participant believe about their condition? What do they think will happen to them if they are exposed to trauma material or have a flashback? What assumptions have they made about why this happened to them?
- Look for puzzles in the story. Is there information being given that could not have been available to them at the time or since then?
- Observe incongruities in the storyline. Look for examples of people or things that should have been present at the time, or vice versa, but were not. Look for events that should have taken place, but did not. Listen for events that took place, but should not have.
- Check on practical or existential questions that arise from the incident. What does the client feel about the larger meaning of their life? What does the incident mean in terms of their day-to-day life?
- Ask about anything the person wanted to communicate but did not or could not during or after the event.
- Ask about anything the person may have found out about themselves as a result of the incident.
- Notice strategies that the survivor uses to cope with the incident.

In these cases, the therapist carefully formulates their own questions to enable the narrator to evaluate material that has not been forthcoming. The idea is to recover a missing feature of the incident and incorporate it into the narrative. The following questions are examples. They only make sense in the context of an individual's narrative:

"Was there anything you wanted to say at the time of the incident but didn't?"

"Was there anything you wanted to do at the time of the incident and didn't?"

"Were you aware of anything else going on around you at the time of the incident while you were trying to ...?"

"Did this experience, at the time of the incident, raise questions for you?"

"You didn't mention any feelings when you talked about this situation.... Were you experiencing any emotions at the time of the incident?"

"Did you promise anything to yourself or others at the time of the incident?"

"How did you react when the man said that at the time of the incident?"

Take a closer look

Over session time, and at the latest when reviewing the story (i.e., reading it back), the narrative should improve in content and focus, and become more comprehensive, complete, detailed, and insightful. The person's level of arousal should become calmer toward the end of the storytelling. If this is true, there is no need for the therapist to intervene with questions. Sometimes, however, the therapist needs to help the person to go deeper and to allow more exploration and dwelling on the hot spot to enhance comprehension and integration ("Take me to your place of fear, (name)...." "Let us stay with that feeling and tell me about that...." "Help me understand...." "Help me make the connection to....")

After you have said something, let it sink in (effective pausing). Reassure the other person that you are listening (give subtle feedback indicating attention). Be sensitive moment for moment to the changing felt experiences which flow in this other person, move about delicately, and be a confident companion.

Therapist's Avoidance

Therapists will want to be aware of the behavior they might employ unwillingly to protect themselves from some horror they are listening to. The therapist might build up resistance as a defense mechanism, or might overly identify with and feel sorry for the survivor. The first is called joining the *fraternity of nonbelievers*. This happens when one does not want to shatter one's own deeply held beliefs that people are inherently good beings or that the world is a safe place. Listening to the survivor's narrative about the cruelty of perpetrators contradicts these beliefs. The second trap is called the *pitfall of sorrow*. This pitfall involves the therapist feeling more sympathy than empathy for the person's emotions. Other authors have noted that denial is a common way for mental health professionals and paraprofessionals to cope with the problems they face, reduce cognitive dissonance, and maintain self-esteem.

De Waal (1988) proposed two forms of denial. The first form of denial involves the therapist's rejection of responsibility. The therapist consciously chooses not to take responsibility for people's suffering or for the effectiveness and outcome of treatment interventions. As in major natural disasters, treating each of hundreds of thousands of people as an individual would paralyze even the most balanced helper (Harrell-Bond, 2002). As with the survivors themselves, some sort of coping mechanism is employed to blunt the truth of this realization. The second form of denial is when helpers rationalize away the truth erroneously – for instance, by convincing themselves that refugees or people of color from certain cultures, due to their accustomed suffering, would not experience pain or death equally. Harrell-Bond (1986) commented on this excuse, saying that there is perhaps no more dramatic way to express psychological distance or to deny a common humanity.

Survivors are likely to feel emotionally rejected by the therapist's defenses. Storytellers quickly recognize the listener's inability to cope with the emotionally shocking facts of the traumatic event. In order not to hurt, overwhelm, or horrify the therapist, people who have been victimized or offended by others tend to unconsciously minimize their version to a more socially acceptable story. The therapist must be professionally reflective about their mental capacity to handle the testimony they are about to hear. To take on the challenging task of guiding someone through trauma memory-focused work, therapists need to receive adequate supervision, intervision, and support, and feel physically and mentally healthy. When therapists realize that they cannot ultimately do this work and make decisions on the job, that is something courageous and decisive.

The same applies to the therapist's professional handling of brief episodes of emotional outbursts or flashbacks, or brief states of reactive psychosis in the participant. The therapist must not be afraid of such emotions. When the victim's painful feelings find an appropriate way to be expressed in a warm and understanding environment, they will naturally subside. As a rule of thumb, healthy, expressive crying lasts no longer than 10–15 minutes. The therapist will comfort a person who is crying and invite the person to allow the experience of whatever emotions are coming up. Expressions of anger should be even shorter, as they usually mask some underlying pain that will surface next. It is important, however, not only to feel the emotions, but to put them into words and to contextualize them in the story of the past.

Self-reflection for the therapist

Questions therapists might ask themselves before beginning trauma-focused work:

- Am I aware that the survivor is likely to find their story incommunicable?
- Am I ready to hear this person's story? Might the story relate to my own personal experiences? Will it activate parts of my own fear network?
- What kind of support do I need?
- Am I really convinced that the survivor will benefit from being exposed (again) to the traumatic memories?
- Do I need peer support or supervision?
- Am I aware of and know how I will deal with pitfalls: (1) maintaining a conspiracy of silence and (2) overidentifying with the survivor?

6 The Role of Interpreters in NET

Precise narration and empathic listening may require the assistance of an interpreter during treatment. Research has documented that effective, trauma-focused therapy can still be administered with the help of a language mediator. From our own research with adult refugees, asylum seekers, and refugee children, we have ample evidence that the inclusion of a trained interpreter does not necessarily hinder the efficacy of treatment for trauma memory-related disorders (Adenauer et al., 2011; Stenmark, et al., 2013; Hensel-Dittmann et al., 2011; Morath et al., 2014; Neuner et al., 2010; Ruf et al., 2010; Schauer et al., 2006).

However, the use of a language mediator inevitably alters the conventional therapist–narrator dynamic. When using interpreters in any talking therapy there are a number of things to bear in mind.

- Interpreter have a *clearly defined role* and task within the therapy. These should be explained to both the interpreter and the participant before the therapy begins. The therapist is responsible for the interpreter's role and well-being. Interpreters should not become "informal" social workers for everyday problems outside the therapy sessions.
- The interpreter is bound to all *contractual agreements* between the participant and the therapist, including confidentiality and ethical principles.
- We recommend that interpreters limit their tasks to the actual translation in a treatment setting. It is essential to *seek a word-for-word translation* and silence for what has not been said. The translator should interpret everything in the first person. This will allow therapists to evaluate mental processes such as coherence and to understand emotional reactions accurately. It would not be sufficient to merely translate the meaning. If a sentence is not understood by the translator, or cannot be translated for the therapist, the translator will consult the therapist immediately. The ideal interpreter for exposure work should act as a neutral voice, without their own opinions or interpretations. If the interpreter notices misunderstandings and barriers to understanding (e.g., due to mutual cultural ignorance) that hinder communication between therapist and survivor without either of them realizing it, we welcome the interpreter's explaining that in detail. The process of translation creates a temporal delay between observing the narrator's facial expressions and gestures, and receiving their verbal communication. Clinicians must train themselves to pay close attention to nonverbal cues and then connect them to the language used.
- Ideally, the survivor's preferred (native) language should be the same as the interpreter's. At minimum, the interpreter should possess familiarity with the living and cultural conditions in the survivor's country of origin to comprehend nonverbal communication forms, such as gestures, and culturally bound social emotions, such as pride, guilt, and shame, and be capable of relaying them to the therapist. Translators require practical and social skills, alongside theoretical knowledge of both cultures and languages.

Thoughts and perceptions that the translator may have on the therapeutic process can be discussed in a *separate meeting with the translator* alone. The concerns and helpful ideas of the interpreter should be given sufficient attention. Typically, they come from the same cultural background as the narrator, which can be helpful since they are familiar with the local conditions. However, the interpreter's opinions about the survivor's statements may be biased. In addition, they will need supervision and professional support from the therapist, since interpreters are often from the same ethnic group as the narrator and might have had similar (traumatic) experiences. Interpreters who *present with symptoms of traumatic stress* must not be employed for translation work and should be offered trauma memory-focused therapy themselves. The *mental health* of the interpreter should be monitored. This includes asking the language mediator how much they are stressed by hearing the narrator's stories. Learning about horror in their home country may not only reduce the concentration of the interpreter on the therapeutic process, but may also be absorbed by them or overwhelm their own feelings or re-experiences. We therefore consider it essential to clarify this before starting therapy.

- Interpreters must receive *comprehensive training* (Ruf-Leuschner et al., 2015).
  The language mediator should undergo training in essential concepts, including fear network, building block, adverse and traumatic events, imaginary exposure, and more, to be fully prepared for trauma-focused work prior to beginning translation services. The translation work necessitates trust in the therapist's process on the part of the mediator. To establish trust and facilitate accurate translation, the therapist explains the posttraumatic mental health concepts, including PTSD and depression, and the therapeutic approach, to the interpreter prior to beginning the therapy session. Any possible issues that might arise during therapy are discussed with the translator prior to the session in order to prepare them, such as if the individual experiences dissociative symptoms or avoidance. Appropriate consent is established between the therapist and the interpreter whenever possible.
- The language mediator often establishes a rapport with the narrator faster because the therapist cannot directly communicate with the survivor or use subtle cues. Such circumstances can disrupt the therapeutic relationship. Also, *a three-way constellation* may cause conflicts of loyalty and destabilize the translator's authority, making role allocation more crucial. The seating arrangement is crucial, with the therapist and narrator sitting facing each other, maintaining strong eye contact.
- The interpreter for therapeutic sessions must *not be related to, or have a personal acquaintance with,* the participant, in order to ensure objectivity and lack of bias. Many of the traumatic experiences encountered by survivors of all genders are emotionally charged and shame-ridden, making it unfeasible to discuss them in the presence of a familiar person. Furthermore, survivors commonly refrain from confiding details about traumatic events to their loved ones to avoid causing them emotional distress.
- This new situation of three people involved is a particular challenge for some therapists who are used to working alone. But it is not only an obstacle but also an opportunity. It slows down the density of information: The exchange takes more time and therefore allows for more precise reflection and tracing, as well as very precise verbalization, a desirable effect in psychotherapy. In addition, the therapist has the opportunity to observe the translator's reactions to the narrative. This can lead to interesting clues. Furthermore, a third person as an observer helps to keep the work on track along the timeline and not to avoid what is on the plate next.

A trained interpreter refrains from conveying personal opinions; however, they are present in the room as a third party who listens to what is being said. Many times, this is the survivor's first experience of having somebody from their culture who empathizes with and respectfully listens to their suffering. The interpreter's obligation to remain neutral and task oriented helps to reduce fear of disbelief, stigmatization, shame, and guilt.

Acknowledgments: Chapter 6 is based on a piece that we wrote together with Dr. Martina Ruf-Leischner (Ruf-Leuschner et al., 2015).

7 Teaching Narrative Exposure

Small Group Facilitation Guidance Note for Experienced Therapists Giving NET Training

This note has been drafted by the taskforce How to Facilitate Training at the NET Institute (https://www.net-institute.org). Members of the taskforce are Drs. Kathleen McBride (Australia & Ireland), Katy Robjant (UK), Elisabeth Kaiser (Germany), Vittoria Ardino (Italy), Maggie Schauer (Germany & Italy), and Thomas Elbert (Germany & Italy).

Training in NET ideally does not only include lectures and demonstrations but also asks participants to practice the Narrative Exposure cycle in small groups of 3–5 people, facilitated with by experienced trainers. This format has been successfully tested and used for 20 years in countless NET workshops around the globe and is now illustrated below to provide insight into our best practice model for running this small group facilitation at the NET Institute. Our small group work intends to give participants a safe and supportive learning environment that promotes active participation, learning by doing, with feedback, self-exploration, discussion, and critical reflection. Since we know that we are diving into people's private biographies, we want to ensure that our group facilitators are skilled, empathic, and well versed in managing the dynamics that a group can bring (Table 6).

Table 6. Small group facilitation structure

Time	Topics	Process
Beginning	Welcome & introductions "Break the ice"	Facilitator introduction – Your name, role during this session, experience using NET. Participants' introductions – Name, I am doing right now, preferred work role during this session. (Keep it brief!)
Within first 15 minutes	Purpose of small group work	• Frame task for this small group – for example, "We are here to practice processing a stone by applying Narrative Exposure in the next 90 minutes. We will explore a traumatic or otherwise arousing and/or meaningful life event (please adhere to outline in course schedule) by applying Narrative Exposure." • Distribute roles – for example, "One of you has the opportunity to take on the role of client, one of you the role of NET therapist, one of you will write the narrative and finally we will have a good observer, too. I will remain as a facilitator of the group and support the therapist." • **Important:** recognize the crossover of personal and professional levels and encourage participants to choose what they want to share in a confidential group space. • Recognize power dynamics. If there is a manager in the group, at an apt time in the training, emphasize that the purpose of the group is to try something new and learn, rather than assessing work performance.

Table 6. Small group facilitation structure

Time	Topics	Process
		• Express confidentiality – for example, "Whatever is shared in this group will stay in this group, please do not carry this information outside the group. Should you run into problems based on what was shared here, please only contact me or one of the other facilitators at NET Institute." • Explain – for example, "In addition, the purpose of narrating is to develop professional counseling skills rather than personal therapy; however, we definitely want to do justice to the narrator in terms of their own self-experience and see that they have an enriching experience." • Explain the type of frightening or highly arousing memory that is best utilized for practice and for the group participants as learners. Ideally, a memory that: – evokes some fear or other arousing emotion but is not too raw, highly personal, or recent. Give example of what has worked well in past groups – for example, transportation accident, rock climbing accident, attack by a dog, robbery by strangers, etc. – has a clear peak of arousal and an event arch with a clear beginning, middle, and end. Best for beginners is an event that has only one arousal peak; – happened only once and on a particular day and time; – is relatively well recalled. Try not to invite processing of interpersonal trauma, like early childhood abuse or neglect, domestic violence, rape by friend, etc., since these events usually happened more than once and have a large fear network.
Within first 15 minutes	Distribution of roles: Client, Therapist, Writer, & Observers	Recruit the client volunteer – FIRST Question: "Who has a frightening or highly emotional event that you are willing to share with the group?" Tell participants that this is also an important opportunity for experiential learning, as placing yourself in the client's shoes can give you a real understanding of the client's experience and often allows you to feel fears and/or avoidance you may have noticed your clients to experience similarly in the process. Allow some silence for participants to identify an event and consider whether or not they would like to share it in the small group. Talk again about the fact that this group will keep confidentiality. Also mention again that you will support the therapist at all times, so the client will have the full benefit of a NET session. Ask each participant for a brief and contained overview (Lifeline style) about the event: How old were you? Location? What happened? Actively check if there is a suitable type of emotional memory for practice. Remember to point out that you are looking for an experience that can yield most benefit in terms of learning how to apply the method of Narrative Exposure, as well as bringing most benefit for the client in terms of learning as well as processing. Please do not promise that a participant who was not selected to share an event will be able to do this in subsequent small groups within the training.

Table 6. Small group facilitation structure

Time	Topics	Process
		Caveat: Be very careful to not frustrate volunteers when you have to turn them down. Participants who are rejected when they are already engaged in their emotional memory may later become agitated or angry. Therefore, do not heat up several participants' hot memory unnecessarily. Do not inquire about emotions when deciding which event to take on. Decide quickly, transparently, and in a calm and allocentric manner. The decision rests entirely with you as a facilitator, do not involve the group in this process. For example: "Andrea, if it is ok with you, I would like us to get to know your experience of the bike accident when you were 10 years old. There is no personal preference intended here, but it sounds like an experience where Andrea can profit most and all of us will have a beneficial learning experience in terms of the application of NET as a method. Ok now, let's start…." Recruiting the therapist volunteer – SECOND Question for the "client": "Who in the group would you like to choose as your therapist?" Point out that this does not indicate any personal preference but is solely a choice based on this moment and small group practice. OR Question to the group: "Who would like to have a try at being the therapist? Who has not yet had the chance during the training to go into the therapist's role?" Be encouraging and validating of their existing skills and offer tandem work. Remind participants that you, the group facilitator, will continuously be there to support and coach the "therapist." Recruiting the narration writer – THIRD Instruct the testimony writer to write down the story chronologically (not the conversation!). Advising the observers – LAST The rest of the group participants take on the role of good observers. Tell the observers that you expect them: • To mute their audio but leave their cameras on. It is not safe in an online exposure setting to be unable to see what is going on behind the screen on the observers' side. We want everyone to always make themselves visible during attendance of our NET trainings. Participants have been informed about this requirement upon registration for the course. Bad Internet reception is no reason to go black. The "client" should have control over who is watching. Therefore, participants who switch off their camera during a personal narration of a client are asked to switch their camera back on. If this is ignored, please send the person to the waiting room; • To be prepared to give feedback to the therapist at the end; • To stay in tune with their own emotional experience and have the inner observer notice what happens; • To be ready to give feedback to the observed process and what else they have noticed about the application of the Narrative Exposure cycle; • To practice the write-up of the narration and be ready to read the narration back to the client at the end.

Table 6. Small group facilitation structure

Time	Topics	Process
		Now briefly explain the learning process & the facilitator's role • Facilitator says: "I will be here to always support you (the therapist). Should you get stuck or have a question, you can ask me for a 'time out' by turning to me, we will have a brief discussion, we can explore the best way forward, and you can resume your task and move on. If you get really stuck, you can also ask me to take over for a few moments, but I am sure you won't need this." • Offer encouragement and lower expectations of getting everything "right." Learning is about giving it a try and reflecting. Repeat that you are there at all times to support – for example, "If you are genuinely interested and curious, the arch of the event will unfold, and it will be clear what questions to ask – they come naturally. It's really about being curious and getting all the details of the event, it's like making a good old-style movie in chronological sequence of what has happened. In one sentence: Let's talk about this experience without omitting any part." • Remind the group that in a real-life NET process, the therapist will already have built a relationship with the client and completed psychoeducation, assessment, and a Lifeline, often even explored some minor events before attempting to process a big trauma stone. However, today the therapist is coming in cold, so this is not how we usually do it in NET therapy. The stone or stick is chosen out of the biography of the person for training purposes. • Probably the best way for the facilitator to support the therapist during the session is via the chat box function: "Please, would the therapist and all observers open their chat box. I will now repeat briefly how the Narrative Exposure cycle is applied, after you have started with a brief body scan: life time episode, year, month, day, time of the day the worst moment in the event happened (so we can start the exploration 1–2 hrs before), building the context, thoughts, emotions, body sensations, meaning back then, pendulum to the here and now, making a summary and next guiding question to build more context and drive the exploration forward until the end. Now that we remember the task, I would like to tell the therapist, that I will support you by offering key words in writing like 'body back then.' This means, e.g., that you are invited to phrase a question about the body sensation at that moment in the past. Should you want to explore another level, that is, of course, up to you. Please take my prompts as suggestions only. Please, dear client, unlike all the others, please keep your chat box closed. You only want to listen to the therapist and try to answer each next question as best you can. Please know that we will take very good care of you." • The facilitator can also interject with direct questions and give directions by voice. Remember that this causes quite a big disturbance to the therapist–client process. However, this might be necessary, especially if the therapist does not adhere to the Narrative Exposure cycle.

Table 6. Small group facilitation structure

Time	Topics	Process
		• Remember to praise the therapist again and again whenever there is a good prompt that causes meaningful and deep exploration of the event. • Remember to help guide the exploration to a safe point at the end. • Tell your observers not to interfere, since at the end of the session, there will be time for feedback and discussion. • Announce the timing: "we now have about 50 minutes for the narration." • The facilitator might remind the therapist in time (!) with a chat message when running over time. • Check that observers' audios are muted and cameras are on, and that client and therapist have pinned each other on screen. Remind observers to leave their camera on throughout. Observers can practice writing a narrative (optional), and the session can include a read back of the narrative if there is time (optional).
Next 40+ minutes	Practicing an exposure narration	The practice begins and the facilitator guides actively, listens well, and provides encouragement, feedback, and direction in relation to the key aspects of the Narrative Exposure method.
8–10 minutes	First Feedback	The facilitator expresses gratitude to the narrator and permits a degree of emotional sharing between the audience, narrator, therapist, and observer. It is essential that the storyteller receive social inclusion and compassion from the group.
10–15 minutes	Reading back	The writer of the narrative reads the story back to the narrator closely guided by the facilitator
15–20 minutes	Debriefing and reflection	Explain the feedback process • The facilitator thanks the client and therapist and suggests they can now relax. "Client and therapist, please lean back and relax now. You have worked really well. You can now listen to our good observers' comments. At the very end, we will come back to you one more time, first to the therapist and finally to our client, to hear how all of this has unfolded for you." • The facilitator now gives some validating and empathic feedback, normalizing and legitimizing what has happened during the Narrative Exposure session. They express praise to both client and therapist for having accepted their roles. • Now, one by one, the observers are invited to give their feedback in relation to what they have learned in the process, what they noticed the therapist doing well, etc. **Important:** do not allow the client's life to be further "analyzed" in any way. Finally, the therapist and then the client have their say. Next, invite the narrator to listen to the story being read back now *chronologically*. Teach the testimony writer to read slowly sentence by sentence and to check in with the client regularly.

Table 6. Small group facilitation structure

Time	Topics	Process
		Observer feedback Questions: "What did you notice? What worked well? Anything you are hesitant / uncertain about?" Actively name and encourage all observers to contribute. Recognize the positive skills demonstrated. Discuss any areas of uncertainty and any questions. Therapist feedback Questions: "What was the experience like for you? What did you think went well? Was there anything you found tricky? Did you have any concerns?" (do not allow them to talk about the personal side of the event. Focus on the technique). Client feedback Questions: "What was your experience like as the client? What helped you to share?" Gain feedback from the client's perspective about any therapist concerns – for example, "Theresa says she is worried that she has bombarded you with too many questions. How was that for you in reality?" Finally; your feedback comes last: Identify any key learnings that can be reflected on. If therapist made mistakes, talk about them in terms of "what we can do instead/or as an improvement." **Important:** Please refer any general questions regarding the method of NET to the Q&A in the plenary. Encourage the group to take any remaining questions and discussion points back to the main group as we aim for a commonly shared concept of learning!
	Closing the small group	Encourage participants to buddy with other staff at work and continue to practice Lifelines, and flower and stone narrations. Talk about the benefits of forming an intervision group – even online. End on a positive note, and thank the group for their participation.

The basic method of facilitating NET small groups has been developed over decades of learning and experience, together with numerous wonderful participants showing us how they benefited most. We draw on principles from trauma-informed practice, group dynamics, adult education and reflective experiential learning.

Small Group Practice Learning Objectives

The core objective of small group work is to practice and develop therapeutic skills for the Narrative Exposure of a traumatic, stressful, and fearful memory (stone); a traumatic, (appetitively) aggressive, and acting-out memory (stick), or a major positive memory (flower).

These NET skills include:

- Therapeutic relationship building through attuned listening, acceptance, and genuine curiosity.
- Giving brief psychoeducation so the client is supported and encouraged to narrate a stone, stick, candle, flower.
- Placing the traumatic event as embedded in the context of a life time episode.
- Identifying the point that marked the onset of the trauma, going in slow motion and spending enough time in the hot spot to enable integration.
- Connecting hot memories (implicit fragmented sensory-perceptual trauma memories) with cold memories (explicit memory anchored to a time and place).
- Exploring sensations (sight, sound, smell, taste, touch), cognitions, emotions, physiological responses, and meaning connected to a specific time and place.

- Assisting clients to pendulate and distinguish between the past and present.
- Strategies to counter avoidance and dissociative responses.
- Finding a *safe enough place* in the arch of the event line to end the narration.
- Meaning making – distinguishing the past from the present. What did the traumatic event mean back then? What does it mean now?
- Learning how to structure and time a Narrative Exposure session.
- Recording the narration for the client's testimony.
- Practicing the reading (retelling or reviewing) of the exposed event.

Small training groups consist of 3–5 participants in which one person volunteers as a narrator, another person takes the role of a therapist (or trauma counselor), and a third person writes the testimony. The others are observers. Small groups can be done by a video link (e.g., Zoom breakout room during a workshop) or in a face-to face setting. The phrase "small group work" refers to a single round of Narrative Exposure followed by feedback and discussion.

Retelling the Narrative

In retelling the narrative during small group work (10 minutes), if there was an observer designated to write down the narration, we invite them the read the essay out loud. Experience has shown that this step is very settling, comforting, and affirming for the volunteer-narrator, no only for patients in therapy, but also for the workshop participants. On the one hand, this process allows for mentalization and self-compassion; on the other hand, it is a good practice of this important NET part for real-life therapeutic situations.

The narrative of the event is carefully and slowly(!) read to the client. When reading what we have written down about the event, we want to check in again and again with the client whether we have captured and written down everything correctly. The therapist is interested in how the narrator (now listener) feels about hearing their own experience read back to them. This is a unique and new feeling. In this way, this reading back and sometimes reciprocal retelling of the event in first person and past tense ollows a structured, chronological event line.

Important: Tell your participants that this reading back the narrative is done at the beginning of the next NET session usually. But since we will not meet again in this small group formation, we are aiming to give the narrator a complete process and learn how to read back together.

Further Tips for Feedback and Reflection

Feedback and reflection offer an interactive process of exploring NET therapeutic benefits, issues, and challenges. By linking these with NET concepts, a greater understanding of the narration process can be gained. Facilitators explore with the group the details of practice learnings that have emerged.

It is very useful to encourage the therapist to raise any concerns they have had about the client's experience of the narration process and then ask the client what their experience was.

Therapists trained in less directive and structured modalities are often concerned that the client will experience the therapist as being rude and interrogative, whereas the person in the role of a client often reports that the process was felt to be affirming and containing. *So make sure you debrief the observers first, the therapist second, and the client last!*

This feedback structure also allows negative feedback to be provided in a more depersonalized way. After the observers, therapist, and client have given feedback, the facilitator can identify and highlight key issues that they have observed. Stay away from giving negative feedback. Rather say: "I noticed that the therapist was really good in ...; however, there were a couple of things we will want to add to the process, and these are..."

Overall, facilitators seek to enable participants to extract practice learnings from the small groups, so that therapists in training feel more confident and skilled in using NET in their own work.

It would be greatly beneficial to have consistent safeguarding procedures in place, and to carefully consider the implications of training practice in relation to participants' need for confidentiality and future work contexts. It is also important to remember that therapists in training are not using a technique, but rather sharing real stories from their lives.

References

Abbott, H. P. (2020). *The Cambridge introduction to narrative*. Cambridge University Press. https://doi.org/10.1017/9781108913928

Adenauer, H., Catani, C., Gola, H., Keil, J., Ruf, R., Schauer, M., & Neuner, F. (2011). Narrative exposure therapy for PTSD increases top-down processing of aversive stimuli: Evidence from a randomized controlled treatment trial. *BMC Neuroscience*, *12*, 127.

Agger, I. (1994). *Trauma and testimony among refugee women: A psycho-social exploration*. Zed Books.

Agger, I., & Jensen, S. B. (1990). Testimony as ritual and evidence in psychotherapy for political prisoners. *Journal of Traumatic Stress*, *3*, 115–130. https://doi.org/10.1002/jts.2490030109

Ainamani, H. E., Elbert, T., Olema, D. K., & Hecker, T. (2020). Gender differences in response to war-related trauma, PTSD, and the dose response effect – a study among the Congolese refugees in Uganda. *BMC Psychiatry*, *20*(1), 1–9. https://doi.org/10.1186/s12888-019-2420-0

Ainamani, H. E., Weierstall-Pust, R., Bahati, R., Otwine, A., Tumwesigire, S., & Rukundo, G. Z. (2022). Post-traumatic stress disorder, depression and the associated factors among children and adolescents with a history of maltreatment in Uganda. *European Journal of Psychotraumatology, 13*(1), Article 2007730. https://doi.org/10.1080/20008198.2021.2007730

Allen, N. B., & Badcock, P. B. (2003). The social risk hypothesis of depressed mood: evolutionary, psychosocial, and neurobiological perspectives. *Psychological Bulletin*, *129*(6), 887. https://doi.org/10.1037/0033-2909.129.6.887

American Psychiatric Association. (1994). *Diagnostic and statistical manual of mental disorders* (4th ed.).

American Psychiatric Association. (2013). *Diagnostic and statistical manual of mental disorders* (5th ed.).

Anda, R. F., Felitti, V. J., Bremner, J. D., Walker, J. D., Whitfield, Ch., Perry, B. D., Dube, Sh. R., & Giles, W. H. (2006) The enduring effects of abuse and related adverse experiences in childhood: A convergence of evidence from neurobiology and epidemiology. *European Archives of Psychiatry and Clinical Neuroscience*, *256*, 174–186. https://doi.org/10.1007/s00406-005-0624-4

Andersen, S. L., & Teicher, M. H. (2008). Stress, sensitive periods and maturational events in adolescent depression. *Trends in Neurosciences*, *31*, 183–191. https://doi.org/10.1016/j.tins.2008.01.004

Archibald, J. A. (2008). An indigenous storywork methodology. In J. G. Knowles, & A. L. Cole (Eds.), *Handbook of the arts in qualitative research: Perspectives, methodologies, examples, and issues* (pp. 371–393). Sage. https://doi.org/10.59962/9780774855440

Armenti, N. A., & Babcock, J. C. (2021). Borderline personality features, anger and intimate partner violence: an experimental manipulation of rejection. *Journal of Interpersonal Violence*, *36*, 5–6. https://doi.org/10.1177/0886260518771686

Arnocky, S., Sunderani, S., Miller, J. L., & Vaillancourt, T. (2012). Jealousy mediates the relationship between attractiveness comparison and females' indirect aggression. *Personal Relationships*, *19*(2), 290–303. https://doi.org/10.1111/j.1475-6811.2011.01362.x

Arnocky, S., & Vaillancourt, T. (2017). Sexual competition among women: A review of the theory and supporting evidence. In M. L. Fisher, *The Oxford handbook of women and competition* (pp. 25–39). Oxford University Press.

Assari, S. (2020). Family socioeconomic status and exposure to childhood trauma: Racial differences. *Children*, *7*(6), 57. https://doi.org/10.3390/children7060057

Augsburger, M., Dohrmann, K., Schauer, M., & Elbert, T. (2017). Relations between traumatic stress, dimensions of impulsivity, and reactive and appetitive aggression in individuals with refugee status. *Psychological Trauma: Theory, Research, Practice, and Policy*, *9*(S1), 137.

Augsburger, M., Meyer-Parlapanis, D., Bambonyé, M., Elbert, T., & Crombach, A. (2015). Appetitive aggression and adverse childhood experiences shape violent behavior in females formerly associated with combat. *Frontiers of Psychology*, *6*, 1756. https://doi.org/10.3389/fpsyg.2015.01756

Aysazci-Cakar, F., Schroder, T., & Hunt, N. (2023). Practical feasibility of Narrative Exposure Therapy in Syrian refugee population residing in Turkiye: A focus group study. *International Journal of Social Sciences (IJSS)/Uluslararasi Sosyal Bilimler Dergisi*, *7*(32), 1–25. https://doi.org/10.52096/usbd.7.32.01

Azoulay, R., Avigadol, L., & Gilboa-Schechtman, E. (2023). Social anxiety and accumulation of status loss events: The role of adulthood experiences. *British Journal of Clinical Psychology*, *62*(2), 518–524. https://doi.org/10.1111/bjc.12417

Babad, S., Zwilling, A., Carson, K. W., Fairchild, V., Razak, S., Robinson, G., & Nikulina, V. (2021). Risk-taking propensity and sensation seeking in survivors of adverse childhood experiences. *Journal of interpersonal violence*, *36*(19–20), NP10670–NP10687.

Baddely, A. L. (1990). *Human memory*. Allyn & Bacon. https://doi.org/10.1177/0886260519876035

Badour, C. L., Dutton, C. E., Wright, J. J., Jones, A. C., & Feldner, M. T. (2020). Shame proneness, negative cognitions, and posttraumatic stress among women with a history of sexual trauma. *Journal of Aggression, Maltreatment & Trauma*, *29*(6), 699–713. https://doi.org/10.1080/10926771.2020.1725211

Bateman, A., & Fonagy, P. (2013). Mentalization-based treatment. *Psychoanalytic Inquiry*, *33*(6), 595–613. https://doi.org/10.1080/07351690.2013.835170

Bates, D. (2022, June). *Storytelling in counseling is often the key to successful outcomes*. Psychotherapy.net. https://www.psychotherapy.net/blog/title/storytelling-in-counseling-is-often-the-key-to-successful-outcomes

Bauer, P. J. (1996). What do infants recall of their lives? Memory for specific events by one- to two-years-olds. *American Psychologist*, *51*, 29–41. https://doi.org/10.1037/0003-066X.51.1.29

Bailey, R., Dugard, J., Smith, S. F., & Porges, S. W. (2023). Appeasement: Replacing Stockholm syndrome as a definition of a survival strategy. *European Journal of Psychotraumatology*, *14*(1), 2161038. https://doi.org/10.1080/20008066.2022.2161038

Beck, A. T., & Clark, D. A. (2015). Anxiety and depression: An information processing perspective. In A. T. Beck & D. A. Clark (Eds.), *Anxiety and self-focused attention* (pp. 41–54). Routledge.

Bedard-Gilligan, M., Kaysen, D., Cordero, R. M., Huh, D., Walker, D., Kaiser-Schauer, E., Robjant, K., Saluskin, K., & Pearson, C. (2022). Adapting narrative exposure therapy with a tribal community: A community-based approach. *Journal of Clinical Psychology*, *78*(11), 2087–2108. https://doi.org/10.1002/jclp.23395

Behnke, A., Rojas, R., Karabatsiakis, A., & Kolassa, I.-T. (2020). Childhood maltreatment compromises resilience against occupational trauma exposure: A retrospective study among emergency medical service personnel. *Child Abuse & Neglect*, *99*, 104248. https://doi.org/10.1016/j.chiabu.2019.104248

Beltrán, R., & Begun, S. (2014). 'It is medicine' narratives of healing from the Aotearoa Digital Storytelling as Indigenous Media Project (ADSIMP). *Psychology and Developing Societies*, *26*(2), 155–179. https://doi.org/10.1177/0971333614549137

Ben Jelloun, T. (2001). *Cette aveuglante absence de lumière* [This blinding absence of light]. Éditions du Seuil.

Bettelheim, B. (1986). *Surviving the Holocaust.* Fontana.

Bichescu, D., Neuner, F., Schauer, M., & Elbert, T. (2007). Narrative Exposure Therapy of political imprisonment-related chronic trauma-spectrum disorders. *Behaviour Research and Therapy*, *45*, 2212–2220. https://doi.org/10.1016/j.brat.2006.12.006

Bichescu-Burian, D. M. (2012). A trauma-related dissociation model may explain psychopathology of the difficult-to-treat BPD patients. *Procedia-Social and Behavioral Sciences*, *33*, 95–99. https://doi.org/10.1016/j.sbspro.2012.01.090

Bisbey, S., & Bisbey, L. B. (1998). *Brief therapy for post-traumatic stress disorder: Traumatic incident reduction and related techniques.* Wiley.

Bisson, J. I., Roberts, N. P., Andrew, M., Cooper, R., & Lewis, C. (2013). Psychological therapies for chronic post-traumatic stress disorder (PTSD) in adults. *Cochrane Database of Systematic Reviews.* https://doi.org/10.1002/14651858.CD003388.pub4

Bjornestad, A., Brown, L., & Weidauer, L. (2019). The relationship between social support and depressive symptoms in Midwestern farmers. *Journal of Rural Mental Health*, *43*(4), 109. https://doi.org/10.1037/rmh0000121

Bjornsson, A. S., Hardarson, J. P., Valdimarsdottir, A. G., Gudmundsdottir, K., Tryggvadottir, A., Thorarinsdottir, K., Wessman, I., Sigurjonsdottir, Ó., Davidsdottir, S., & Thorisdottir, A. S. (2020). Social trauma and its association with posttraumatic stress disorder and social anxiety disorder. *Journal of Anxiety Disorders*, *72*, 102228. https://doi.org/10.1016/j.janxdis.2020.102228

Blanchard, E. B., Hickling, E. J., Forneris, C. A., Taylor, A. E., Buckley, T. C., Loos, W. R., & Jaccard, J. (1997). Prediction of remission of acute posttraumatic stress disorder in motor vehicle accident victims. *Journal of Traumatic Stress*, *10*, 215–234. https://doi.org/10.1002/jts.2490100205

Blazer, D. G., & Wallace, R. B. (2016). Cognitive aging: What every geriatric psychiatrist should know. *American Journal of Geriatric Psychiatry*, *24*, 776–81. https://doi.org/10.1016/j.jagp.2016.06.013

Blevins, C. A., Weathers, F. W., Davis, M. T., Witte, T. K., & Domino, J. L. (2015). The Posttraumatic Stress Disorder Checklist for DSM-5 (PCL-5): Development and initial psychometric evaluation. *Journal of Traumatic Stress*, *28*(6), 489–498. https://doi.org/10.1002/jts.22059

Bock, J., Helmeke, C., Ovtscharoff, W., Gruß, M., & Braun, K. (2003). Frühkindliche emotionale Erfahrungen beeinflussen die funktionelle Entwicklung des Gehirns. [Early childhood emotional experiences influence the functional development of the brain] *NeuroForum*, *2*, 51–57. https://doi.org/10.1515/nf-2003-0203

Boden, D., & Del Vento Bielby, D. (1983). The past as resource: A conversational analysis of elderly talk. *Human Development*, *26*(6), 308–319. https://doi.org/10.1159/000272892

Bonne, O., Brandes, D., Gilboa, A., Gomori, J. M., Shenton, M. E., Pitman, R. K., & Shalev, A. Y. (2001). Longitudinal MRI study of hippocampal volume in trauma survivors with PTSD. *American Journal of Psychiatry*, *158*, 8. https://doi.org/10.1176/appi.ajp.158.8.1248

Boyer, P., & Bergstrom, B. (2011). Threat-detection in child development: An evolutionary perspective. *Neuroscience & Biobehavioral Reviews*, *35*(4), 1034–1041. https://doi.org/10.1016/j.neubiorev.2010.08.010

Bracha, H. S. (2004). Freeze, flight, fight, fright, faint: adaptionist perspectives on the acute stress response spectrum. *CNS Spectrum*, *9*, 679–685. https://doi.org/10.1017/S1092852900001954

Breithaupt, F., Li, B., & Kruschke, J. K. (2022). Serial reproduction of narratives preserves emotional appraisals. *Cognition and Emotion*, *36*(4), 581–601, https://doi.org/10.1080/02699931.2022.2031906

Bremner, J. D. (2002). *Does stress damage the brain? Understanding trauma-related disorders from a mind-body perspective.* W. W. Norton.

Bremner, J. D., Krystal, J. H., Southwick, S. M., & Charney, D. S. (1995). Functional neuroanatomical correlates of the effects of stress on memory. *Journal of Traumatic Stress*, *8*, 527–545. https://doi.org/10.1002/jts.2490080403

Bremner, J. D., Randall, P., Vermetten, E., Staib, L., Bronen, R. A., Mazure, C., Capelli, S., McCarthy, G., Innis, R. B., & Charney, D. S. (1997). Magnetic resonance imaging-based measurement of hippocampal volume in posttraumatic stress disorder related to childhood physical and sexual abuse: A preliminary report. *Biological Psychiatry*, *41*, 23–32.

Bremner, J. D., Vythilingam, M., Vermetten, E., Southwick, S. M., McGlashan, T., Nazeer, A., Khan, S., Vaccarino, L. V., Soufer, R., Garg, P. K., Ng, C. K., Staib, L. H., Duncan, J. S., & Charney, D. S. (2003). MRI and PET study of deficits in hippocampal structure and function in women with childhood sexual abuse and posttraumatic stress disorder. *American Journal of Psychiatry*, *160*, 924–932.

Brewin, C. R. (2001). A cognitive neuroscience account of posttraumatic stress disorder and its treatment. *Behaviour Research and Therapy*, *39*, 373–393. https://doi.org/10.1016/S0005-7967(00)00087-5

Brewin, C. R. (2016). Coherence, disorganization, and fragmentation in traumatic memory reconsidered: A response to Rubin et al. (2016). *Journal of Abnormal Psychology*, *125*(7), 1011–1017. https://doi.org/10.1037/abn0000154

Brewin, C. R., Andrews, B., & Valentine, J. D. (2000). Meta-analysis of risk factors for posttraumatic stress disorder in trauma-exposed adults. *Journal of Consulting and Clinical Psychology*, *68*, 748–766. https://doi.org/10.1037/0022-006X.68.5.748

Brewin, C. R., Dalgleish, T., & Joseph, S. (1996). A dual representation theory of posttraumatic stress disorder. *Psychological Review*, *103*, 670–686. https://doi.org/10.1037/0033-295X.103.4.670

Brewin, C. R., Gregory, J. D., Lipton, M., & Burgess, N. (2010). Intrusive images in psychological disorders: Characteristics, neural mechanisms, and treatment implications. *Psychological Review*, *117*(1), 210. https://doi.org/10.1037/a0018113

Bryant-Davis, T. (2019). The cultural context of trauma recovery: Considering the posttraumatic stress disorder practice guideline and intersectionality. *Psychotherapy*, *56*(3), 400. https://doi.org/10.1037/pst0000241

Buchanan, T. W., & Lovallo, W. R. (2001). Enhanced memory for emotional material following stress-level cortisol treatment in humans. *Psychoneuroendocrinology*, *26*, 307–317. https://doi.org/10.1016/S0306-4530(00)00058-5

Burri, A., Maercker, A., Krammer, S., & Simmen-Janevska, K. (2013). Childhood trauma and PTSD symptoms increase the risk of cognitive impairment in a sample of former indentured child laborers in old age. *PLOS ONE*, *8*(2), e57826. https://doi.org/10.1371/journal.pone.0057826

Cahill, L., Babinsky, R., Markowitsch, H. J., & McGaugh, J. L. (1995). The amygdala and emotional memory. *Nature*, *377*, 295–296. https://doi.org/10.1038/377295a0

Cahill, L., Prins, B., Weber, M., & McGaugh, J. L. (1994). Beta-adrenergic activation and memory for emotional events. *Nature*, *371*, 702–704. https://doi.org/10.1038/371702a0

Campos, R. C., Besser, A., & Blatt, S. J. (2013). Recollections of parental rejection, self-criticism and depression in suicidality. *Archives of Suicide Research*, *17*(1), 58–74. https://doi.org/10.1080/13811118.2013.748416

Capaldi, D. M., Knoble, N. B., Shortt, J. W., & Kim, H. K. (2012). A systematic review of risk factors for intimate partner violence. *Partner Abuse*, *3*(2), 231–280. https://doi.org/10.1891/1946-6560.3.2.231

Cardinal, R. N., Parkinson, J. A., Hall, J., & Everitt, B. J. (2002). Emotion and motivation: The role of the amygdala, ventral striatum, and prefrontal cortex. *Neuroscience & Biobehavioral Reviews*, *26*, 321–352. https://doi.org/10.1016/S0149-7634(02)00007-6

Carlson, C. M. (1984). Reminiscing: Toward achieving ego integrity in old age. *Social Casework*, *65*(2), 81–89. https://doi.org/10.1177/104438948406500203

Caspi, A., Houts, R. M., Belsky, D. W., Harrington, H., Hogan, S., Ramrakha, S., Poulton, R., & Moffitt, T. E. (2016). Childhood forecasting of a small segment of the population with large economic burden. *Nature Human Behaviour*, *1*(1), 0005. https://doi.org/10.1038/s41562-016-0005

Castles, S., & Miller, M. J. (1993). *The age of migration: International population movements in the modern world*. Guilford Press.

Catani, C., Gerwirtz, A. H., Wieling, E., Schauer, E., Elbert, T., & Neuner, F. (2010). Tsunami, war, and cumulative risk in the life of Sri Lankan school children. *Child Development*, *81*, 1176–1191. https://doi.org/10.1111/j.1467-8624.2010.01461.x

Catani, C., Schauer, E., Elbert, T., Missmahl, I., Bette, J. P., & Neuner, F. (2009). War trauma, child labor, and family violence: Life adversities and PTSD in a sample of school children in Kabul. *Journal of Traumatic Stress*, *22*, 163–171. https://doi.org/10.1002/jts.20415

Centers for Disease Control and Prevention (CDC). (2024). *National intimate partner and sexual violence survey (NISVS)*. https://www.cdc.gov/nisvs/about/

Chessell, Z. J., Brady, F., Akbar, S., Stevens, A., & Young, K. (2019). A protocol for managing dissociative symptoms in refugee populations. *The Cognitive Behaviour Therapist*, 12.

Choi, K. R., Ford, J. D., Briggs, E. C., Munro-Kramer, M. L., Graham-Bermann, S. A., & Seng, J. S. (2019). Relationships between maltreatment, posttraumatic symptomatology, and the dissociative subtype of PTSD among adolescents. *Journal of Trauma & Dissociation*, *20*(2), 212–227. https://doi.org/10.1080/15299732.2019.1572043

Cienfuegos, J., & Monelli, C. (1983). The testimony of political repression as a therapeutic instrument. *American Journal of Orthopsychiatry*, *53*, 43–51.

Cloitre, M., Cohen, L. R., Ortigo, K. M., Jackson, C., & Koenen, K. C. (2020). *Treating survivors of childhood abuse and interpersonal trauma: STAIR narrative therapy*. Guilford Press.

Cloitre, M., Shevlin, M., Brewin, C. R., Bisson, J. I., Roberts, N. P., Maercker, A., Karatzias, T., & Hyland, P. (2018). The International Trauma Questionnaire: Development of a self-report measure of ICD-11 PTSD and complex PTSD. *Acta Psychiatrica Scandinavica*, *138*(6), 536–546. https://doi.org/10.1037/t73478-000

Coleman, P. G. (1989). Ageing and life history: The meaning of reminiscence in late life. *Sociological Review*, *37*(Suppl 1), 120–143. https://doi.org/10.1111/j.1467-954X.1989.tb03340.x

Conradt, E., Carter, S. E., & Crowell, S. E. (2020). Biological embedding of chronic stress across two generations within marginalized communities. *Child Development Perspectives*, *14*(4), 208–214. https://doi.org/10.1111/cdep.12382

Conway, M. A. (2001). Sensory-perceptual episodic memory and its context: autobiographical memory. *Philosophical Transactions of the Royal Society of London Series B: Biological Science*, *356*, 1375–1384.

Conway, M. A., & Pleydell-Pearce, C. W. (2000). The construction of autobiographical memories in the self-memory system. *Psychological Review*, *107*, 261–288. https://doi.org/10.1037/0033-295X.107.2.261

Cooper, D. K., Wieling, E., & Pfeiffer, A. (2019). Bioecological implications of narrative exposure therapy in low-resource settings: Individual, family, community, and socio-political contexts. *Australian and New Zealand Journal of Family Therapy*, *40*, 353–367. https://doi.org/10.1002/anzf.1392

Copeland, W. E., Gaydosh, L., Hill, S. N., Godwin, J., Harris, K. M., Costello, E. J., & Shanahan, L. (2020). Associations of despair with suicidality and substance misuse among young adults. *JAMA Network Open*, *3*(6), e208627–e208627. https://doi.org/10.1001/jamanetworkopen.2020.8627

Courtois, C. A., & Ford, J. D. (2009). *Treating complex traumatic stress disorders: An evidence-based guide*. Guilford Press.

Crombach, A., & Elbert, T. (2014). Controlling offensive behavior using narrative exposure therapy: A randomized controlled trial of former street children. *Clinical Psychological Science*, *3*(2), 270–282. https://doi.org/10.1177/2167702614534239

Cunningham, M., & Cunningham, J. D. (1997). Patterns of symptomatology and patterns of torture and trauma experiences in resettled refugees. *Australian and New Zealand Journal of Psychiatry*, *31*, 555–565. https://doi.org/10.3109/00048679709065078

Darwin, C. (1998). *The expression of the emotions in man and animals*. Oxford University Press. (Original work published 1872).

Da Silva, D. R., Rijo, D., & Salekin, R. T. (2015). The evolutionary roots of psychopathy. *Aggression and Violent Behavior*, *21*, 85–96. https://doi.org/10.1016/j.avb.2015.01.006

Davies, S., Pettersson, T., & Öberg, M. (2022). Organized violence 1989–2021 and drone warfare. *Journal of Peace Research*, *59*(4), 593–610. https://doi.org/10.1177/00223433221108428

Davis, L. L., Schein, J., Cloutier, M., Gagnon-Sanschagrin, P., Maitland, J., Urganus, A., Guerin, A., Lefebvre, P., & Houle, C. R. (2022). The economic burden of posttraumatic stress disorder in the United States from a societal perspective. *The Journal of Clinical Psychiatry*, *83*(3), 21m14116. https://doi.org/10.4088/JCP.21m14116

Deacon, B. J., & Farrell, N. R. (2013). Therapist barriers to the dissemination of exposure therapy. In E. A. Storch & D. McKay (Eds.), *Handbook of treating variants and complications in anxiety disorders* (pp. 363–373). Springer. https://doi.org/10.1007/978-1-4614-6458-7_23

De Bellis, M. (2002). Developmental traumatology: a contributory mechanism for alcohol and substance use disorders. *Psychoneuroendocrinology*, *27*, 155–170. https://doi.org/10.1016/S0306-4530(01)00042-7

De Bellis, M. D., Baum, A. S., Birmaher, B., Keshavan, M. S., Eccard, C. H., Boring, A. M., Jenkins, F. J., & Ryan, N. D. (1999). AE Bennett Research Award. Developmental traumatology Part I: Biological stress systems. *Biological Psychiatry*, *45*(10), 1259–1270.

Delsol, C., & Margolin, G. (2004). The role of family-of-origin violence in men's marital violence perpetration. *Clinical Psychology Review*, *24*(1), 99–122. https://doi.org/10.1016/j.cpr.2003.12.001

Denham, S. A. (2003). Social and emotional learning, early childhood. In T. P. Gullotta, M. Bloom, J. Kotch, C. Blakely, L. Bond, G. Adams, C. Browne, W. Klein, & J. Ramos (Eds.), *Encyclopedia of primary prevention and health promotion* (pp. 1009–1018). Springer. https://doi.org/10.1007/978-1-4615-0195-4_147

Dennis, M. K., & Minor, M. (2019). Healing through storytelling: Indigenising social work with stories. *British Journal of Social Work*, *49*(6), 1472–1490. https://doi.org/10.1093/bjsw/bcz044

Derriennic, J. P. (1971). Theory and ideologies of violence. *Journal of Peace Research*, *8*, 361–374.

De Jongh, A. D., Resick, P. A., Zoellner, L. A., Van Minnen, A., Lee, C. W., Monson, C. M., Foa, E., Wheeler, K.,Broeke, E., Feeny, N., Rauch, S., Chard, K., Mueser, K., Sloan, D., Gaag, M., Rothbaum, B., Neuner, F., Roos, C., Hehenkamp, L., & Bicanic, I. A. (2016). Critical analysis of the current treatment guidelines for complex PTSD in adults. *Depression and anxiety*, *33*(5), 359–369

de Quervain, D. J.-F., Roozendaal, B., & McGaugh, J. L. (1998). Stress and glucocorticoids impair retrieval of long-term spatial memory. *Nature*, *394*, 787–790. https://doi.org/10.1038/29542

de Quervain, D. J.-F., Roozendaal, B., Nitsch, R. M., McGaugh, J. L., & Hock, C. (2000). Acute cortisone administration impairs retrieval of long-term declarative memory in humans. *Nature Neuroscience*, *3*, 313–314. https://doi.org/10.1038/73873

De Waal, A. (1988). *The sanity factor: Expatriate behavior on African relief programs* (Network Paper 2b, 1 RSC/QEH). Refugee Participation Network.

De Young, A. C., & Landolt, M. A. (2018). PTSD in children below the age of 6 years. *Current Psychiatry Reports*, *20*, 1–11. https://doi.org/10.1007/s11920-018-0966-z

Dhossche, D. M., Ross, C. A., Stoppelbein, L. (2012). The role of deprivation, abuse, and trauma in pediatric catatonia without a clear medical cause. *Acta Psychiatrica Scandinavica*, *125*, 25–32. https://doi.org/10.1111/j.1600-0447.2011.01779.x

Dix, J., & Fornells-Ambrojo, M. (2023). Therapists' experience of the lifeline in narrative exposure therapy. *Journal of Traumatic Stress*, *36*(1), 106–116. https://doi.org/10.1002/jts.22886

Doná, G., & Berry, J. W. (1999). Refugee acculturation and re-acculturation. *Refugees: Perspectives on the experience of forced migration*, *68*(4), 211–222.

Dube, S. R., Felitti, V. J., Chapman, D. P., Giles, W. H., & Anda, R. F. (2003). Childhood abuse, neglect and household dysfunction and the risk of illicit drug use: The Adverse Childhood Experience Study. *Pediatrics*, *111*, 564–572. https://doi.org/10.1542/peds.111.3.564

Dunmore, E., Clark, D. M., & Ehlers, A. (2001). A prospective examination of the role of cognitive factors in persistent posttraumatic stress disorder (PTSD) after physical or sexual assault. *Behaviour Research and Therapy*, *39*, 1063–1084. https://doi.org/10.1016/S0005-7967(00)00088-7

Dutra, L., Bureau, J.-F., Holmes, B., Lyubchik, A., & Lyons-Ruth, K. (2009). Quality of early care and childhood trauma: A prospective study of developmental pathways to dissociation. *Journal of Nervous and Mental Disease*, *197*, 383–390. https://doi.org/10.1097/NMD.0b013e3181a653b7

Dyregrov, A., Gupta, L., Gjestad, R., & Mukanoheli, E. (2000). Trauma exposure and psychological reactions to genocide among Rwandan children. *Journal of Traumatic Stress*, *13*, 3–21. https://doi.org/10.1023/A:1007759112499

Eckart, C., Stoppel, C., Kaufmann, J., Tempelmann, C., Hinrichs, H., Elbert, T., Heinze, H. J., & Kolassa, I. T. (2010). Structural alterations in lateral prefrontal, parietal and posterior midline regions of men with chronic posttraumatic stress disorder. *Journal of Psychiatry and Neuroscience*, *35*, 10010–10020. https://doi.org/10.1503/jpn.100010

Edgar, N. E., Bennett, A., Dunn, N. S., MacLean, S. E., & Hatcher, S. (2022). Feasibility and acceptability of Narrative Exposure Therapy to treat individuals with PTSD who are homeless or vulnerably housed: A pilot randomized controlled trial. *Pilot and Feasibility Studies*, *8*(1), Article 83. https://doi.org/10.1186/s40814-022-01043-x

Egeland, B. (2009). Taking stock: Childhood emotional maltreatment and developmental psychopathology. *Child Abuse & Neglect*, *33*, 22–26. https://doi.org/10.1016/j.chiabu.2008.12.004

Ehlers, A., & Clark, D. M. (2000). A cognitive model of posttraumatic stress disorder. *Behaviour Research and Therapy*, *38*, 319–345. https://doi.org/10.1016/S0005-7967(99)00123-0

Ekman, P. (1999). Basic emotions. *Handbook of Cognition and Emotion, 98*(45–60), 16. https://doi.org/10.1002/0470013494.ch3

Ekman, P. (2009). Darwin's contributions to our understanding of emotional expressions. *Philosophical Transactions of the Royal Society B: Biological Sciences, 364*(1535), 3449–3451.

Ekwonye, A. U. (2022). Compassionate presence sessions: A qualitative exploration of experiences of older adults and college students. *Aging and Health Research, 2*(3), Article 100087. https://doi.org/10.1016/j.ahr.2022.100087

Elbert, T., Hermenau, K., Hecker, T., Weierstall, R., & Schauer, M. (2012). FORNET: Behandlung von traumatisierten und nicht-traumatisierten Gewalttätern mittels Narrativer Expositionstherapie [FORNET: Treatment of traumatized and non-traumatized violent offenders using narrative exposure therapy]. In J. Endrass, A. Rossegger, F. Urbaniok, & B. Borchard (Eds.), *Interventionen bei Gewalt- und Sexualstraftätern: Risk-Management, Methoden und Konzepte der forensischen Therapie* (pp. 255–276). Medizinisch Wissenschaftliche Verlagsgesellschaft.

Elbert, T., Moran, J. K., & Schauer, M. (2017a). Appetitive aggression. In B. J. Bushman (Ed.), *Aggression and violence* (pp. 119–136). Taylor & Francis; Routledge.

Elbert, T., Moran, J. K., & Schauer, M. (2017b). Lust an Gewalt: Appetitive Aggression als Teil der menschlichen Natur [Lust for violence: Appetitive aggression as a fundamental part of human nature]. *e-Neuroforum*, 23(2), 77–84. https://doi.org/10.1515/nf-2016-0056

Elbert, T., & Rockstroh, B. (2003). Stress factors: The science of our flexible responses to an unpredictable world. *Nature, 421*, 477–478. https://doi.org/10.1038/421477a

Elbert, T., & Schauer, M. (2002). Burnt into memory. *Nature, 412*, 883. https://doi.org/10.1038/419883a

Elbert, T., & Schauer, M. (2014). Epigenetic, neural and cognitive memories of traumatic stress and violence. In S. Cooper & K. Ratele (Eds.), *Psychology serving humanity: Proceedings of the 30th international congress of psychology: Volume 2: Western psychology* (pp. 215–227). Psychology Press.

Elbert, T. & Schauer, M. (2021). Menschliche Aggressions- und Tötungsbereitschaft. Entstehung, Folgen und Behandlung menschlicher Gewalt- und Tötungsbereitschaft [Human readiness for aggression and killing. Origin, consequences, and treatment of human readiness to use violence and kill]. *Psychotherapie Aktuell, 13*(2), 43–49.

Elbert, T., & Schauer, M. (2022). Epigenetisch gestützte Vererbung von Trauma- und Gewalterfahrungen. [Epigenetically supported inheritance of trauma and violence experiences.] In J. Müller, M. Ruf-Leuschner, B. Grimmer, C. Knaevelsrud, & B. Dammann (Eds.), *Traumafolgen: Forschung und therapeutische Praxis*. Kohlhammer.

Elbert, T., Schauer, M., & Moran, J. K. (2018). Two pedals drive the bi-cycle of violence: reactive and appetitive aggression. *Current Opinion in Psychology, 19*, 135–138. https://doi.org/10.1016/j.copsyc.2017.03.016

Elbert, T., Schauer, M., & Neuner, F. (2015). Narrative exposure therapy (NET) – Reorganizing memories of traumatic stress, fear and violence. In U. Schnyder & M. Cloitre (Eds.), *Evidence based treatments for trauma-related psychological disorders: A practical guide for clinicians* (pp 229–253). Springer. https://doi.org/10.1007/978-3-319-07109-1_12

Elbert, T., Schauer, M., & Neuner, F. (2022). Narrative exposure therapy (NET): Reorganizing memories of traumatic stress, fear, and violence. In U. Schnyder & M. Cloitre (Eds.), *Evidence based treatments for trauma-related psychological disorders: A practical guide for clinicians* (pp. 255–280). Springer International. https://doi.org/10.1007/978-3-030-97802-0_12

Elbert, T., Schauer, M., Ruf, M., Weierstall, R., Neuner, F., Rockstroh, B., & Junghöfer, M. (2011). The tortured brain: Imaging neural representations of traumatic stress experiences using RSVP with affective pictorial stimuli. *Zeitschrift für Psychologie, 219*, 167–174. https://doi.org/10.1027/2151-2604/a000064

Elbert, T., Schauer, M., Schauer, E., Huschka, B., Hirth, M., & Neuner, F. (2009). Trauma-related impairment in children: An epidemiological survey in Sri Lankan provinces affected by two decades of civil war and unrest. *Child Abuse & Neglect, 33*, 238–246. https://doi.org/10.1016/j.chiabu.2008.02.008

Elbert, T., Weierstall, R., & Schauer, M. (2010). Fascination violence – On mind and brain of man hunters. *European Archives of Psychiatry and Clinical Neuroscience, 260,* S100–S105. https://doi.org/10.1007/s00406-010-0144-8

Elbert, T., Wilker, S., Schauer, M., & Neuner, F. (2017). Dissemination psychotherapeutischer Module für traumatisierte Geflüchtete [Dissemination of psychotherapeutic modules for traumatized refugees]. *Nervenarzt, 88*, 26–33 https://doi.org/10.1007/s00115-016-0245-3

El-Khoury, J., Haidar, R., & Barkil-Oteo, A. (2021). Psychological torture: Characteristics and impact on mental health. *International Journal of Social Psychiatry, 67*(5), 500–506. https://doi.org/10.1177/0020764020961800

Emmelkamp, P. M. G. (2023). *Mental health of refugees: Etiology and treatment*. Springer. https://doi.org/10.1007/978-3-031-34078-9

Ertl, V., Pfeiffer, A., Saile, R., Schauer, E., Elbert, T., & Neuner, F. (2010). Validation of a mental health assessment in an African conflict population. *Psychological Assessment, 22*, 318–324. https://doi.org/10.1037/a0018810

Ertl, V., Pfeiffer, A., Schauer, E., Elbert, T., & Neuner, F. (2011). Community-implemented trauma therapy for former child soldiers in Northern Uganda: A randomized controlled trial. *JAMA, 206*, 503–512. https://doi.org/10.1001/jama.2011.1060

Fang, X., Brown, D. S., Florence, C. S., & Mercy, J. A. (2012). The economic burden of child maltreatment in the United States and implications for prevention. *Child Abuse & Neglect, 36*(2), 156–165. https://doi.org/10.1016/j.chiabu.2011.10.006

Farley, M., & Keaney, J. C. (1997). Physical symptoms, somatization, and dissociation in women survivors of childhood sexual assault. *Women Health, 25*, 33–45. https://doi.org/10.1300/J013v25n03_03

Fazel, M., Stratford, H. J., Rowsell, E., Chan, C., Griffiths, H., & Robjant, K. (2020). Five applications of narrative exposure therapy for children and adolescents presenting with post-traumatic stress disorders. *Frontiers in Psychiatry*, 11. https://doi.org/10.3389/fpsyt.2020.00019

Felitti, V. J., Anda, R. F., Nordenberg, D., Williamson, D. F., Spitz, A. M., Edwards, V., Koss, M. P., & Marks, J. S. (1998). Relationship of childhood abuse and household dysfunction to many of the leading causes of death in adults. The Adverse Childhood Experiences (ACE) Study.*American Journal of Preventive Medicine*, *14*(4), 245–258. https://doi.org/10.1016/s0749-3797(98)00017-8.

Felitti, V. J., Anda, R. F., Nordenberg, D., Williamson, D. F., Spitz, A. M., Edwards, V., Koss, M. P., & Marks, J. S. (2019). Reprint of: Relationship of childhood abuse and household dysfunction to many of the leading causes of death in adults: The adverse childhood experiences (ACE) study. *American Journal of Preventive Medicine*, *56*(6), 774–786. https://doi.org/10.1016/j.amepre.2019.04.001

Fernández, S., Saguy, T., & Halperin, E. (2015). The paradox of humiliation. *Personality and Social Psychology Bulletin*, *41*(7), 976–988. https://doi.org/10.1177/0146167215586195

Fessler, D. M. T. (2001). Emotions and cost/benefit assessment: The role of shame and self esteem in risk taking. In R. Selten & G. Gigerenzer (Eds.), *Bounded rationality: The adaptive toolbox* (pp. 191–214). MIT University Press.

Fessler, D. M. T. (2007). From appeasement to conformity: Evolutionary and cultural perspectives on shame, competition, and cooperation. In J. L. Tracy, R. W. Robins, & J. P. Tangney (Eds.), *The self-conscious emotions: Theory and research*. Guilford Press.

Finch, J., Ford, C., Grainger, L., & Meiser-Stedman, R. (2020). A systematic review of the clinician-related barriers and facilitators to the use of evidence-informed interventions for post-traumatic stress. *Journal of Affective Disorders*, *263*, 175–186. https://doi.org/10.1016/j.jad.2019.11.143

Foa, E. B., & Kozak, M. J. (1986). Emotional processing of fear: Exposure to corrective information. *Psychological Bulletin*, *99*, 20–35. https://doi.org/10.1037/0033-2909.99.1.20

Foa, E. B., Molnar, C., & Cashman, L. (1995). Change in rape narratives during exposure therapy for posttraumatic stress disorder. *Journal of Traumatic Stress*, *4*, 675–690. https://doi.org/10.1002/jts.2490080409

Foa, E. B., & Rothbaum, B. O. (1998). *Treating the trauma of rape: Cognitive-behavioral therapy for PTSD*. Guilford Press.

Foa, E. B., Zoellner, L. A., Feeny, N. C., Hembree, E. A., & Alvarez-Conrad, J. (2002). Does imaginal exposure exacerbate PTSD symptoms? *Journal of Consulting and Clinical Psychology*, *70*(4), 1022. https://doi.org/10.1037/0022-006X.70.4.1022

Fosse, R., Skjelstad, D. V., Schalinski, I., Thekkumthala, D., Elbert, T., Aanondsen, C. M., Greger, H. K., & Joszefiak, T. (2020). Measuring childhood maltreatment: Psychometric properties of the Norwegian version of the Maltreatment and Abuse Chronology of Exposure (MACE) scale. *PLOS ONE*, *15*(2), e0229661. https://doi.org/10.1371/journal.pone.0229661

Franck, L., Molyneux, N., & Parkinson, L. (2016). Systematic review of interventions addressing social isolation and depression in aged care clients. *Quality of Life Research*, *25*, 1395–1407. https://doi.org/10.1007/s11136-015-1197-y

Frank, A. W. (2013). *The wounded storyteller: Body, illness and ethics*. University of Chicago Press.

Frankl, E. V. (1959). *Man's search for meaning: An introduction to logotherapy*. Beacon Press Boston. (Original work published 1946 in German)

Freud, S. (1906–1909/2010). *Gesammelte Werke* [Collected Works] (Vol. 7). Fischer Verlag.

Friedman, M. J., Resick, P. A., Bryant, R. A., & Brewin, C. R. (2011). Considering PTSD for DSM-5. *Depression and Anxiety*, *28*(9), 750–769. https://doi.org/10.1002/da.20767

Friskie, S. M. (2020). The healing power of storytelling: Finding identity through narrative. *Arbutus Review*, *11*(1), 19–27. https://doi.org/10.18357/tar111202019324

Frost, R., Hyland, P., McCarthy, A., Halpin, R., Shevlin, M., & Murphy, J. (2019). The complexity of trauma exposure and response: Profiling PTSD and CPTSD among a refugee sample. *Psychological Trauma: Theory, Research, Practice, and Policy*, *11*(2), 165–175. https://doi.org/10.1037/tra0000408

Furukawa, E., Tangney, J., & Higashibara, F. (2012). Cross-cultural continuities and discontinuities in shame, guilt, and pride: A study of children residing in Japan, Korea and the USA. *Self and Identity*, *11*(1), 90–113. https://doi.org/10.1080/15298868.2010.512748

Gambetta, D. (1999, June 1). Primo Levi's last moments: On that tragic Saturday, only his body was smashed. *Boston Review*., https://www.bostonreview.net/articles/diego-gambetta-primo-levi-last-moments/

Gang, D., Loff, B., Naylor, B., & Kirkman, M. (2021). A call for evaluation of restorative justice programs. *Trauma, Violence, & Abuse*, *22*(1), 186–190. https://doi.org/10.1177/1524838019833003

Gensichen, J., Schmidt, K., Schauer, M., & Elbert, T. (2023). Posttraumatische Belastungsströrung (PTBS) [Posttraumatic stress disorder (PTSD)]. In J. Gensichen, M. Härter, & M. Berger (Eds.), *Psychologische Kurzinterventionen für die Hausarztpraxis und die Psychosomatische Grundversorgung* (Chapter 8, pp. 91–100). Elsevier Health Sciences.

Gensichen, J., Schultz, S., Adrion, C. Schmidt, K., Schauer, M., Lindemann, D., Unruh, N., Kosilek, R. P., Schneider, A., Scherer, M., Bergmann, A., Heintze, C., Joos, S., Briegel, J., Scherag, A., König, H. H., Brettschneider, C., Schulze, T. G., Mansmann, U., Linde, K., ...& Elbert, T. (2018). Effect of a combined brief narrative exposure therapy with case management versus treatment as usual in primary care for patients with traumatic stress sequelae following intensive care medicine: study protocol for a multicenter randomized controlled trial (PICTURE). *Trials*, *19*, 480. https://doi.org/10.1186/s13063-018-2853-7

Gergely, G., Fonagy, P., Jurist, E., & Target M. (2002). Affect regulation, mentalization, and the development of the self. *International Journal of Psychoanalysis*, *77*, 217–234.

Gilbert, P. (2000). The relationship of shame, social anxiety and depression: The role of the evaluation of social rank. *Clinical Psychology & Psychotherapy*, *7*(3), 174–189. https://doi.org/10.1002/1099-0879(200007)7:3<174::AID-CPP236>3.0.CO;2-U

Gilbert, P., & Procter, S. (2006). Compassionate mind training for people with high shame and self-criticism: Overview and pilot study of a group therapy approach. *Clinical Psychology & Psychotherapy*, *13*, 353–379. https://doi.org/10.1002/cpp.507

Gilligan, J. (2003). Shame, guilt, and violence. *Social Research: An International Quarterly*, *70*(4), 1149–1180. https://doi.org/10.1353/sor.2003.0053

Gilligan, J. (2020). Shame: The emotions and morality of violence. In M. Vogel (Ed.), *Crime, inequality and the State* (pp. 245–250). Routledge. https://doi.org/10.4324/9781003060581-18

Goessmann, K., Ibrahim, H., Saupe, L. B., & Neuner, F. (2021). Toward a contextually valid assessment of partner violence: development and psycho-sociometric evaluation of the gendered violence in partnerships scale (GVPS). *Frontiers in Psychology, 11*, Article 607671. https://doi.org/10.3389/fpsyg.2020.607671

Gottvall, M., Vaez, M., & Saboonchi, F. (2019). Social support attenuates the link between torture exposure and post-traumatic stress disorder among male and female Syrian refugees in Sweden. *BMC International Health and Human Rights, 19*, 1–11. https://doi.org/10.1186/s12914-019-0214-6

Gratz, K. L., Latzman, R. D., Tull, M. T., Reynolds, E. K., & Lejuez, C. W. (2011). Exploring the association between emotional abuse and childhood borderline personality features: the moderating role of personality traits. *Behavior Therapy, 42*(3), 493–508. https://doi.org/10.1016/j.beth.2010.11.003

Greene, N. R., & Naveh-Benjamin, M. (2023). Adult age-related changes in the specificity of episodic memory representations: A review and theoretical framework. *Psychology and Aging, 38*(2), 67. https://doi.org/10.1037/pag0000724

Haag, A. C., Celi, S., & Landolt, M. A. (2019). Trauma and PTSD in preschool-aged children. *Anxiety in preschool children: Assessment, Treatment, and Prevention*, 143.

Haferkamp, L., Bebermeier, A., Möllering, A., & Neuner, F. (2015). Dissociation is associated with emotional maltreatment in a sample of traumatized women with a history of child abuse. *Journal of Trauma Dissociation, 16*(1), 86–99. https://doi.org/10.1080/15299732.2014.959149

Hailes, H. P., Yu, R., Danese, A., & Fazel, S. (2019). Long-term outcomes of childhood sexual abuse: An umbrella review. *The Lancet Psychiatry, 6*(10), 830–839.

Hamby, S., Elm, J. H., Howell, K. H., & Merrick, M. T. (2021). Recognizing the cumulative burden of childhood adversities transforms science and practice for trauma and resilience. *American Psychologist, 76*(2), 230. https://doi.org/10.1037/amp0000763

Harandi, T. F., Taghinasab, M. M., & Nayeri, T. D. (2017). The correlation of social support with mental health: A meta-analysis. *Electronic Physician, 9*(9), 5212. https://doi.org/10.19082/5212

Hariri, A. R., Bookheimer, S. Y., & Mazziotta, J. C. (2000). Modulating emotional response: Effects of a neocortical network on the limbic system. *Neuroreport, 11*, 43–48. https://doi.org/10.1097/00001756-200001170-00009

Harman, R., & Lee, D. (2010). The role of shame and self-critical thinking in the development and maintenance of current threat in post-traumatic stress disorder. *Clinical Psychology and Psychotherapy, 17*, 13–24. https://doi.org/10.1002/cpp.636

Harrell-Bond, B. (2002). Can humanitarian work with refugees be humane? *Human Rights Quarterly, 24*, 51–85. https://doi.org/10.1353/hrq.2002.0011

Harrell-Bond, B. E. (1986). *Imposing aid: Emergency assistance to refugees.* Oxford University Press.

Harvey, A. G., & Bryant, R. A. (1999). A qualitative investigation of the organization of traumatic memories. *British Journal of Clinical Psychology, 38*, 401–405. https://doi.org/10.1348/014466599162999

Harvey, J. H., Carlson, H. R., Huff, T. M., & Green, M. A. (2001). Embracing their memory: The construction of accounts of loss and hope. In R. A. Neimeyer (Ed.), *Meaning reconstruction & the experience of loss* (pp. 231–243). American Psychological Association. https://doi.org/10.1037/10397-012

Hawkins, J. D., Herrenkohl, T. I., Farrington, D. P., Brewer, D., Catalano, R. F., Harachi, T. W., & Cothern, L. (2000). Predictors of youth violence. *Juvenile Justice Bulletin, 4*, 1–10.

Hecker, T., Fetz, S., Ainamani, H., & Elbert, T. (2015). The cycle of violence: Associations between exposure to violence, trauma-related symptoms and aggression – findings from Congolese refugees in Uganda. *Journal of Traumatic Stress, 28*(5), 448–455.

Hecker, T., Hermenau, K., Crombach, A., & Elbert, T. (2015). Treating traumatized offenders and veterans by means of narrative exposure therapy. *Frontiers in Psychiatry, 6*, 80. https://doi.org/10.3389/fpsyt.2015.00080

Heinze, P. (2017). Psychopathy, unconscious shame and attachment: Considering the psychodynamics of psychopathy. *Psychodynamic Practice, 23*(1), 7–32. https://doi.org/10.1080/14753634.2016.1269663

Hensel-Dittman, D., Schauer, M., Ruf, M., Catani, C., Odenwald, M., Elbert, T., & Neuner, F. (2011). The treatment of traumatized victims of war and torture: A randomized controlled comparison of narrative exposure therapy and stress inoculation training. *Psychotherapy and Psychosomatics, 80*(6), 345–352. https://doi.org/10.1159/000327253

Herman, J. L. (1992). *Trauma and recovery: From domestic abuse to political terror.* Basic Books.

Hermenau, K., Hecker, T., Maedl, A., Schauer, M., & Elbert, T. (2013). Growing up in armed groups: trauma and aggression among child soldiers in DR Congo. *European Journal of Psychotraumatology, 4*(1), Article 21408. https://doi.org/10.3402/ejpt.v4i0.21408

Hermenau, K., Hecker, T., Ruf, M., Schauer, E., Elbert, T., & Schauer, M. (2011). Childhood adversity, mental ill-health and aggressive behavior in an African orphanage: Changes in response to trauma-focused therapy and the implementation of a new instructional system. *Child and Adolescent Psychiatry and Mental Health, 5*, 29. https://doi.org/10.1186/1753-2000-5-29

Hermenau, K., Hecker, T., Schaal, S., Maedl, A., & Elbert, T. (2013). Addressing post-traumatic stress and aggression by means of narrative exposure: A randomized controlled trial with ex-combatants in the Eastern DRC. *Journal of Aggression, Maltreatment & Trauma, 22*(8), 916–934. https://doi.org/10.1080/10926771.2013.

Heron, R. L., & Eisma, M. C. (2021). Barriers and facilitators of disclosing domestic violence to the healthcare service: a systematic review of qualitative research. *Health & Social Care in the Community, 29*(3), 612–630. https://doi.org/10.1111/hsc.13282

Herron, J. L., & Venner, K. L. (2023). A systematic review of trauma and substance use in American Indian and Alaska Native individuals: Incorporating cultural considerations. *Journal of Racial and Ethnic Health Disparities, 10*(2), 603–632. https://doi.org/10.1007/s40615-022-01250-5

Hijazi, A. M., Lumley, M. A., Ziadni, M. S., Haddad, L., Rapport, L. J., & Arnetz, B. B. (2014). Brief narrative exposure therapy for posttraumatic stress in Iraqi refugees: A preliminary randomized clinical trial. *Journal of Traumatic Stress, 27*, 314–322. https://doi.org/10.1002/jts.21922

Hinsberger, M., Holtzhausen, L., Sommer, J., Kaminer, D., Elbert, T., Seedat, S., Augsburger, M., Schauer, M., & Weierstall, R. (2020). Long-term effects of psychotherapy in a context of continuous community and gang violence: Changes in aggressive attitude in high-risk South African adolescents. *Behavioural and Cognitive Psychotherapy*, 1–13. https://doi.org/10.1017/S1352465819000365

Hinsberger, M., Holtzhausen, L., Sommer, J., Kaminer, D., Elbert, T., Seedat, S., Wilker, S., Crombach, A., & Weierstall, R. (2017). Feasibility and effectiveness of narrative exposure therapy and cognitive behavioral therapy in a context of ongoing violence in South Africa. *Psychological Trauma: Theory, Research, Practice, and Policy*, *9*(3), 282–291. https://doi.org/10.1037/tra0000197

Hinsberger, M., Sommer, J., Kaminer, D., Holtzhausen, L., Weierstall, R., Seedat, S., Madikane, S., & Elbert, T. (2016). Perpetuating the cycle of violence in South African low-income communities: Attraction to violence in young men exposed to continuous threat. *European Journal of Psychotraumatology*, *7*(1), Article 29099.

Hollifield, M., Verbillis-Kolp, S., Farmer, B., Toolson, E. C., Woldehaimanot, T., Yamazaki, J., Holland, A., St. Clair, J., & SooHoo, J. (2013). The Refugee Health Screener-15 (RHS-15): Development and validation of an instrument for anxiety, depression, and PTSD in refugees. *General Hospital Psychiatry*, *35*(2), 202–209. https://doi.org/10.1037/t66025-000

Holmes, J. (2018). Suicide and deliberate self-harm: When attachments fail. In M. Pompili, (Ed.), *Phenomenology of suicide: Unlocking the suicidal mind*. (pp. 113–129). Springer.

Howe, M. L., Courage, M. L., & Peterson, C. (1994). How can I remember when “I” wasn't there: Long-term retention of traumatic experiences and emerge of the cognitive self. *Consciousness and Cognition*, *3*, 327–355. https://doi.org/10.1006/ccog.1994.1019

Hughes, K., Bellis, M. A., Hardcastle, K. A., Sethi, D., Butchart, A., Mikton, C., Jones, L., Dunne, M. P. (2017). The effect of multiple adverse childhood experiences on health: A systematic review and meta-analysis. *Lancet Public Health*, *2*(8), e356–e366. https://doi.org/0.1016/S2468-2667(17)30118-4.

Ibrahim, H., Catani, C., & Neuner, F. (2021). The posttraumatic stress interview for children (KID-PIN): Development and validation of a semi-structured interview of PTSD symptoms among displaced children in the Middle East. *PeerJ*, *9*, e12403. https://doi.org/10.7717/peerj.12403

Ibrahim, H., Ertl, V., Catani, C., Ismail, A. A., & Neuner, F. (2018). Trauma and perceived social rejection among Yazidi women and girls who survived enslavement and genocide. *BMC Medicine*, *16*(1), 154. https://doi.org/10.1186/s12916-018-1140-5

Iffland, B., Sansen, L. M., Catani, C., & Neuner, F. (2012). Emotional but not physical maltreatment is independently related to psychopathology in subjects with various degrees of social anxiety: A web-based internet survey. *BMC Psychiatry*, *12*, 49. https://doi.org/10.1186/1471-244X-12-49

Iffland, B., Sansen, L. M., Catani, C., & Neuner, F. (2014). The trauma of peer abuse: Effects of relational peer victimization and social anxiety disorder on physiological and affective reactions to social exclusion. *Frontiers in Psychiatry*, *5*, 26. https://doi.org/10.3389/fpsyt.2014.00026

Imel, Z. E., Laska, K., Jakupcak, M., & Simpson, T. L. (2013). Meta-analysis of dropout in treatments for posttraumatic stress disorder. *Journal of Consulting and Clinical Psychology*, *81*(3), 394. https://doi.org/10.1037/a0031474

Inter-Agency Standing Committee. (2007). *IASC guidelines on mental health and psychosocial support in emergency settings*. ISAC. https://interagencystandingcommittee.org/sites/default/files/migrated/2020-11/IASC%20Guidelines%20on%20Mental%20Health%20and%20Psychosocial%20Support%20in%20Emergency%20Settings%20%28English%29.pdf

Isele, D., Teicher, M. H., Ruf-Leuschner, M., Elbert, T., Kolassa, I. T., Schury, K., & Schauer, M. (2014). KERF: An instrument for measuring adverse childhood experiences: Construction and psychometric evaluation of the German MACE (Maltreatment and Abuse Chronology of Exposure) scale. *Zeitschrift für Klinische Psychologie und Psychotherapie*, *43*(2), 121–130. https://www.testarchiv.eu/en/test/9008437

Jacob, N., Neuner, F., Maedl, A., Schaal, S., & Elbert, T. (2014). Dissemination of psychotherapy for trauma spectrum disorders in postconflict Settings: A randomized controlled trial in Rwanda. *Psychotherapy and Psychosomatics*, *83*(6), 354.

Jacob, N., Wilker, S., & Isele, D. (2017). Narrative Expositionstherapie zur Behandlung von Traumafolgestörungen. [Narrative exposure therapy for the treatment of trauma-related disorders]. *Swiss Archives of Neurololgy, Psychiatry and Psychotherapy*, *168*(4), 99–106. https://doi.org/10.1159/000365114

Jaffee, S. R. (2005). Family violence and parent psychopathology: Implications for children's socioemotional development and resilience. In S. Goldstein & R. B. Brooks (Eds.), *Handbook of Resilience in Children* (pp. 149–163). Springer. https://doi.org/10.1007/0-306-48572-9_10

Jaycox, L. H., Foa, E. B., & Morral, A. R. (1998). Influence of emotional engagement and habituation on exposure therapy for PTSD. *Journal of Consulting and Clinical Psychology*, *66*, 185–192. https://doi.org/10.1037/0022-006X.66.1.185

Jeste, D. V., Di Somma, S., Lee, E. E., Nguyen, T. T., Scalcione, M., Biaggi, A., Daly, R., Liu, J., Tu, X., Ziedonis, D., Glorioso, D., Antonini, P., & Brenner, D. (2021). Study of loneliness and wisdom in 482 middle-aged and oldest-old adults: A comparison between people in Cilento, Italy and San Diego. USA. *Aging & Mental Health*, *25*(11), 2149–2159. https://doi.org/10.1080/13607863.2020.

Jeste, D. V., Lee, E. E., Palmer, B. W., & Treichler, E. B. H. (2020). Moving from humanities to sciences: A new model of wisdom fortified by sciences of neurobiology, medicine, and evolution. *Psychological Inquiry*, *31*(2), 134–143. https://doi.org/10.1080/1047840X.2020.1757984

Johnson, J. G., Smailes, E. M., Cohen, P., Brown, J., & Bernstein, D. P. (2000). Associations between four types of childhood neglect and personality disorder symptoms during adolescence and early adulthood: Findings of a community-based longitudinal study. *Journal of Personality Disorders*, *14*(2), 171–187. https://doi.org/10.1521/pedi.2000.14.2.171

Jones, D. P. H., & Krugman, R. D. (1986). Can a three-year-old child bear witness to her sexual assault and attempted murder? *Child Abuse & Neglect*, *10*, 253–258. https://doi.org/10.1016/0145-2134(86)90086-4

Jongedijk, R. A., Schauer, M., & Elbert, T. (2014). Dissociatie en NET [Dissociation in NET]. In R. A. Jongedijk (Ed.), *Levensverhalen en psychotrauma. Narratieve Exposure Therapie in theorie en praktijk* (pp. 265–277). Uitgeverij Boom.

Julian, J. M., Held, J. I., Hixson, K., & Conn, B. M. (2023). The implementation of narrative exposure therapy (NET) for transgender and gender diverse adolescents and young adults. *Journal of Child & Adolescent Trauma, 16*, 795–804. https://doi.org/10.1007/s40653-023-00530-4

Kaiser, E., Dohrmann, K., Rockstroh, B., Elbert, T., & Schauer, M. (2025). *NAT Narrative Trauma Work – Praxishandbuch* [Practical guide to NAT Narrative Trauma Work]. Beltz Verlag.

Kaltenbach, E., Chisholm, M., Xiong, T., Thomson, D., Crombach, A., & McGrath, P. J. (2021). Online narrative exposure therapy for parents of children with neurodevelopmental disabilities suffering from posttraumatic stress symptoms: Study protocol of a randomized controlled trial. *European Journal of Psychotraumatology, 12*(1), 1991650. https://doi.org/10.1080/20008198.2021.1991650

Kaltenbach, E., Härdtner, E., Hermenau, K., Schauer, M., Elbert, T. (2017). Efficient identification of mental health problems in refugees in Germany: the Refugee Health Screener. *European Journal of Psychotraumatology, 8*(Suppl 2), 1–12. http://doi.org/10.1080/20008198.2017.1389205 https://doi.org/10.1080/20008198.2017.1389205

Kaltenbach, E., Hermenau, K., Schauer, M., Dohrmann, K., Elbert, T., & Schalinski, I. (2020). Trajectories of posttraumatic stress symptoms during and after Narrative Exposure Therapy (NET) in refugees. *BMC Psychiatry, 20*, 1–14. https://doi.org/10.1186/s12888-020-02720-y

Kaltenbach, E., Patrick, J., McGrath, P., Schauer, M., Kaiser, E., Crombach, A., & Robjant, K. (2021). Practical guidelines for online Narrative Exposure Therapy (e-NET) – A short-term treatment for posttraumatic stress disorder adapted for remote delivery. *European Journal of Psychotraumatology, 12*(1). https://doi.org/10.1080/20008198.2021.1881728

Kaltenbach, E., Schauer, M., Hermenau, K., Elbert, T., & Schalinski, I. (2018). Course of mental health in refugees: A one year panel survey. *Frontiers in Psychiatry, 9*, 352. https://doi.org/10.3389/fpsyt.2018.00352

Kaminer, D. (2006). Healing processes in trauma narratives: a review. *South African Journal of Psychology, 36*(3), 481–499. https://doi.org/10.1177/008124630603600304

Karunakara, U., Neuner, F., Schauer, M., Singh, K., Hill, K., Elbert, T., & Burnham, G. (2004). Traumatic events and symptoms of post-traumatic stress disorder amongst Sudanese nationals, refugees and Ugandan nationals in the West Nile. *African Health Sciences, 4*, 83–93.

Kaufman, G. (2004). *The psychology of shame: Theory and treatment of shame-based syndromes*. Springer.

Kealy, D., Rice, S. M., Ogrodniczuk, J. S., & Spidel, A. (2018). Childhood trauma and somatic symptoms among psychiatric outpatients: Investigating the role of shame and guilt. *Psychiatry Research, 268*, 169–174. https://doi.org/10.1016/j.psychres.2018.06.072

Keane, T. M., Zimering, R. T., & Caddell, J. M. (1985). A behavioural formulation of posttraumatic stress disorder in combat veterans. *Behaviour Therapist, 8*, 9–12.

Kecala, N. M., Goodman, B. F., & Griffin, M. G. (2022). Dissociation as a distinct peritraumatic coping response: A preliminary analysis. *Journal of Trauma & Dissociation, 24*(1), 79–94. https://doi.org/10.1080/15299732.2022.2117262.

Kelly, A. E. (2002). *The psychology of secrets*. Springer. https://doi.org/10.1007/978-1-4615-0683-6

Kessler, R. C., Sonnega, A., Bromet, E., Hughes, M., & Nelson, C. B. (1995). Posttraumatic stress disorder in the National Comorbidity Survey. *Archives of General Psychiatry, 52*, 1048–1060. https://doi.org/10.1001/archpsyc.1995.03950240066012

Kiburi, S. K., Molebatsi, K., Obondo, A., & Kuria, M. W. (2018). Adverse childhood experiences among patients with substance use disorders at a referral psychiatric hospital in Kenya. *BMC Psychiatry, 18*(1), 1–12. https://doi.org/10.1186/s12888-018-1780-1

Kiecolt-Glaser, J. K., Preacher, K. J., MacCallum, R. C., Atkinson, C., Malarkey, W. B., & Glaser, R. (2003). Chronic stress and age-related increases in the proinflammatory cytokine IL-6. *Proceedings of the National Academy of Sciences USA, 100*, 9090–9095. https://doi.org/10.1073/pnas.1531903100

Kilpatrick, D. G., Resnick, H. S., Milanak, M. E., Miller, M. W., Keyes, K. M., & Friedman, M. J. (2013). National estimates of exposure to traumatic events and PTSD prevalence using DSM-IV and DSM-5 criteria. *Journal of Traumatic Stress, 26*(5), 537–547. https://doi.org/10.1002/jts.21848

Kinzie, J. D., Sack, W. H., Angell, R. H., & Clarke, G. (1989). A three-year follow-up of Cambodian young people traumatized as children. *Journal of the American Academy of Child and Adolescent Psychiatry, 28*, 501–504. https://doi.org/10.1097/00004583-198907000-00006

Kinzl, J. F., Traweger, C., & Biebl, W. (1995). Family background and sexual abuse associated with somatization. *Psychotherapy and Psychosomatics, 64*, 82–87. https://doi.org/10.1159/000288995

Kleim, B., Ehlers, A., & Glucksman, E. (2007). Early predictors of chronic post-traumatic stress disorder in assault survivors. *Psychological Medicine, 37*, 1457–1467. https://doi.org/S003329170 7001006

Köbach, A., Carleial, S., Elbert, T., Schmitt, S., & Robjant, K. (2021). Treating trauma and aggression with Narrative Exposure Therapy in former child and adult soldiers: a randomised controlled trial in Eastern DR Congo. *Journal of Consulting and Clinical Psychology, 89*(3), 143–155. https://doi.org/10.1037/ccp0000632

Köbach, A., Schaal, S., Hecker, T., & Elbert, T. (2017). Psychotherapeutic intervention in the demobilization process: addressing combat-related mental injuries with narrative exposure in a first and second dissemination stage. *Clinical Psychology and Psychotherapy, 24*(4), 807–825. https://doi.org/10.1002/cpp.1986

Köbach, A., Schauer, M., & Elbert, T. (2016). *Checklist for Threats to Human Life* (THL). University of Konstanz.

Koenig, A., Schury, K., Reister, F., Köhler-Dauner, F., Schauer, M., Ruf-Leuschner, M., Ziegenhain, U., Fegert, J., & Kolassa, I. T. (2016). Psychosoziale Risiken für das Kindeswohl bei werdenden Müttern mit Missbrauchs- und Vernachlässigungserfahrungen in der eigenen Kindheit [Psychosocial risk factors for child welfare among postpartum mothers with a history of childhood maltreatment and neglect]. *Geburtshilfe und Frauenheilkunde, 76*(03), 261–267.

Kolassa, I. T., & Elbert, T. (2007). Structural and functional neuroplasticity in relation to traumatic stress. *Current Directions in Psychological Science*, *16*, 326–329. https://doi.org/10.1111/j.1467-8721.2007.00529.x

Kolassa, I. T., Ertl, V., Kolassa, S., Onyut, L. P., & Elbert, T. (2010). Spontaneous remission from PTSD depends on the number of traumatic event types experienced. *Psychological Trauma: Theory, Research, Practice, and Policy*, *2*, 169–174. https://doi.org/10.1037/a0019362

Kolassa, I. T., Wienbruch, C., Neuner, F., Schauer, M., Ruf, M., Odenwald, M., & Elbert, T. (2007). Altered oscillatory brain dynamics after repeated traumatic stress. *BMC Psychiatry*, *7*, 56. https://doi.org/10.1186/1471-244X-7-56

Koss, M. P., Tromp, S., & Tharan, M. (1995). Traumatic memories: Empirical foundations, forensic and clinical implications. *Clinical Psychology: Science and Practice*, *2*(2), 111–132. https://doi.org/10.1111/j.1468-2850.1995.tb00034.x

Kozlowska, K., Walker, P., McLean, L., & Carrive, P. (2015). Fear and the defense cascade: clinical implications and management. *Harvard Review of Psychiatry*, *23*, 263–287. https://doi.org/10.1097/HRP.0000000000000065

Krusemark, E. A., & Li, W. (2011). Do all threats work the same way? Divergent effects of fear and disgust on sensory perception and attention. *Journal of Neuroscience*, *31*, 3429–3434. https://doi.org/10.1523/JNEUROSCI.4394-10.2011

Kubany, E. S., Haynes, S. N., Abueg, F. R., Manke, F. P., Brennan, J. M., & Stahura, C. (1996). Development and validation of the Trauma-Related Guilt Inventory (TRGI). *Psychological Assessment*, *8*(4), 428. https://doi.org/10.1037/1040-3590.8.4.428

Kubany, E. S., & Ralston, T. (2008). *Treating PTSD in battered women: A step-by-step manual for therapists and counselors*. New Harbinger.

Landmann, H., Gaschler, R., & Rohmann, A. (2019). What is threatening about refugees? Identifying different types of threat and their association with emotional responses and attitudes towards refugee migration. *European Journal of Social Psychology*, *49*(7), 1401–1420. https://doi.org/10.1002/ejsp.2593

Lang, P. J. (1977). Imagery in therapy: An information processing analysis of fear. *Behavior Therapy*, *8*, 862–866. https://doi.org/10.1016/S0005-7894(77)80157-3

Lang, P. J. (1979). A bio-informational theory of emotional imagery. *Psychophysiology*, *16*(6), 495–512. https://doi.org/10.1111/j.1469-8986.1979.tb01511.x

Lang, P. J. (1984). Dead Souls: Or why the neurobehavioral science of emotion should pay attention to cognitive science. In Th. Elbert, B. Rockstroh, W. Lutzenberger, & N. Birbaumer (Eds.), *Self-regulation of the brain and behaviour* (pp. 255–272). Springer. https://doi.org/10.1007/978-3-642-69379-3_18

Lang, P. J. (1993). The network model of emotion: Motivational connections. In R. Wyer & T. Scrull (Eds.), *Advances in social cognition, VI*. Lawrence Erlbaum Associates.

Lange, T. M. (2020). Trans-affirmative narrative exposure therapy (TA-NET): A therapeutic approach for targeting minority stress, internalized stigma, and trauma reactions among gender diverse adults. *Practice Innovations*, *5*(3), 230. https://doi.org/10.1037/pri0000126

Langer, L., & Neuner, F. (2021). The mediating processes of revictimization after child abuse in a sample of adult women. *Journal of Family Trauma, Child Custody & Child Development*, *18*(2), 162–183. https://doi.org/10.1080/26904586.2021.1886221

Lanius, R. A., Boyd, J. E., McKinnon, M. C., Nicholson, A. A., Frewen, P., Vermetten, E., ... & Spiegel, D. (2018). A review of the neurobiological basis of trauma-related dissociation and its relation to cannabinoid-and opioid-mediated stress response: A transdiagnostic, translational approach. *Current Psychiatry Reports*, *20*(12), 1–14. https://doi.org/10.1007/s11920-018-0983-y

Laplanche, J., & Pontalis, J. B. (2018). *The language of psychoanalysis*. Routledge.

Laub, D. (1991). Truth and testimony the process and the struggle. *American Imago*, *48*(1), 75–91.

Leach, C. W. (2017). Understanding shame and guilt. In L. Woodyatt, E. Worthington, Jr., M. Wenzel, & B. Griffin (Eds), *Handbook of the psychology of self-forgiveness* (pp. 17–28). Springer. https://doi.org/10.1007/978-3-319-60573-9_2

Leary, M. R., Kowalski, R. M., Smith, L., & Phillips, S. (2003). Teasing, rejection, and violence: Case studies of the school shootings. *Aggressive Behavior*, *29*(3), 202–214. https://doi.org/10.1002/ab.10061

Leary, M. R., Tambor, E. S., Terdal, S. K., & Downs, D. L. (1995). Self-esteem as an interpersonal monitor: The sociometer hypothesis. *Journal of Personality and Social Psychology*, *68*, 518–530. https://doi.org/10.1037/0022-3514.68.3.518

Leary, M. R., Twenge, J. M., & Quinlivan, E. (2006). Interpersonal rejection as a determinant of anger and aggression. *Personality and Social Psychology Review*, *10*(2), 111–132. https://doi.org/10.1207/s15327957pspr1002_2

LeDoux, J. E. (2000). Emotion circuits in the brain. *Annual Review of Neuroscience*, *23*, 155–184. https://doi.org/10.1146/annurev.neuro.23.1.155

Lee, D. A. (2009). Compassion-focussed cognitive therapy for shame-based trauma memories and flashbacks in post-traumatic stress disorder. In N. Grey (Ed.), *A casebook of cognitive therapy for traumatic stress reactions* (pp. 230–246). Routledge.

Lee, E. E., Govind, T., Ramsey, M., Wu, T. C., Daly, R., Liu, J., Tu, X. M., Paulus, M. P., Thomas, M. L., & Jeste, D. V. (2021). Compassion toward others and self-compassion predict mental and physical well-being: A 5-year longitudinal study of 1090 community-dwelling adults across the lifespan. *Translational Psychiatry*, *11*(1), Article 397. https://doi.org/10.1038/s41398-021-01491-8

Leeners, B., Rath, W., Block, E., Görres, G., & Tschudin, S. (2014). Risk factors for unfavorable pregnancy outcome in women with adverse childhood experiences. *Journal of Perinatal Medicine*, *42*(2), 171–178. https://doi.org/10.1515/jpm-2013-0003

Lely, J., Van den Bout, J., Ter Heide, J. J., Van der Aa, N., Knipscheer, J. W., & Kleber, R. J. (2017). Narrative exposure therapy vs. present-centered therapy with older adults: Results from an RCT. *Innovation in Aging*, *1*(Suppl 1), 58.

Lely, J. C. G., De la Rie, S. M., Knipscheer, J. W., & Kleber, R. J. (2019). Stronger than my ghosts: A qualitative study on cognitive recovery in later life. *Journal of Loss and Trauma*, *24*(4), 369–382. https://doi.org/10.1080/15325024.2019.1603008

Lely, J. C. G., Knipscheer, J. W., Moerbeek, M., Ter Heide, F. J. J., Van den Bout, J., & Kleber, R. J. (2019). Randomised controlled trial comparing narrative exposure therapy with present-centered therapy for older patients with post-traumatic stress disorder. *British Journal of Psychiatry, 214*(6), 369–377. https://doi.org/10.1192/bjp.2019.59

Lely, J. C. G., Ter Heide, F. J. J., Moerbeek, M., Knipscheer, J. W., & Kleber, R. J. (2022). *Psychopathology and resilience in older adults with posttraumatic stress disorder: A randomized controlled trial comparing narrative exposure therapy and present-centered therapy, European Journal of Psychotraumatology, 13*(1). https://doi.org/10.1080/20008198.2021.2022277

Leskela, J., Dieperink, M., & Thuras, P. (2002). Shame and posttraumatic stress disorder. *Journal of Traumatic Stress, 15*(3), 223–226. https://doi.org/10.1023/A:1015255311837

Letourneau, E. J., Brown, D. S., Fang, X., Hassan, A., & Mercy, J. A. (2018). The economic burden of child sexual abuse in the United States. *Child Abuse & Neglect, 79*, 413–422. https://doi.org/10.1016/j.chiabu.2018.02.020

Levi, P. (1963). *La tregua* [The reawakening]. Einaudi.

Lewis, C., Roberts, N. P., Gibson, S., & Bisson, J. I. (2020). Dropout from psychological therapies for post-traumatic stress disorder (PTSD) in adults: Systematic review and meta-analysis. *European Journal of Psychotraumatology, 11*(1), 1709709. https://doi.org/10.1080/20008198.2019.1709709

Lieb, K., Zanarini, M., Linehan, M. M., & Bohus, M. (2004). Borderline personality disorder. *The Lancet, 364*, 453–461. https://doi.org/10.1016/S0140-6736(04)16770-6

Lieberman, M. D., Eisenberger, N. I., Crockett, M. J., Tom, S. M., Pfeifer, J. H., & Way, B. M. (2007). Putting feelings into words: Affect labeling disrupts amygdala activity to affective stimuli. *Psychological Science, 18*, 421–428. https://doi.org/10.1111/j.1467-9280.2007.01916.x

Lieberman, M. D., Hariri, A., Jarcho, J. M., Eisenberger, N. I., & Bookheimer, S. Y. (2005). An fMRI investigation of race-related amygdala activity in African-American and Caucasian-American individuals. *Nature Neuroscience, 8*, 720–722. https://doi.org/10.1038/nn1465

Lodi, E., Perrella, L., Lepri, G. L., Scarpa, M. L., & Patrizi, P. (2021). Use of restorative justice and restorative practices at school: A systematic literature review. *International Journal of Environmental Research and Public Health, 19*(1), 96. https://doi.org/10.3390/ijerph19010096

Macfie, J., Cicchetti, D., & Toth, S. L. (2001). The development of dissociation in maltreated preschool-aged children. *Development and Psychopathology, 13*(2), 233–254. https://doi.org/10.1017/S0954579401002036

Madigan, S., Bakermans-Kranenburg, M., van IJzendoorn, M., Moran, G., Pederson, D., & Benoit, D. (2006). Unresolved states of mind, anomalous parental behavior, and disorganized attachment: A review and metaanalysis of a transmission gap. *Attachment and Human Development, 8*, 89–111. https://doi.org/10.1080/14616730600774458

Maercker, A., & Bachem, R. (2013). Life-review interventions as psychotherapeutic techniques in psychotraumatology. *European Journal of Psychotraumatology, 4*(1), 19720. https://doi.org/10.3402/ejpt.v4i0.19720

Maercker, A., Cloitre, M., Bachem, R., Schlumpf, Y. R., Khoury, B., Hitchcock, C., & Bohus, M. (2022). Complex post-traumatic stress disorder. *The Lancet, 400*(10345), 60–72. https://doi.org/10.1016/S0140-6736(22)00821-2

Maercker, A., & Zöllner, T. (2002). Life-Review-Therapie als spezifische Form der Behandlung posttraumatischer Belastungsstörungen im Alter [Life review therapy as a specific form of treatment for post-traumatic stress disorder in old age]. *Verhaltenstherapie und Verhaltensmedizin, 23*(2), 213–225.

Malaktaris, A. L., & Lynn, S. J. (2019). The phenomenology and correlates of flashbacks in individuals with posttraumatic stress symptoms. *Clinical Psychological Science, 7*(2), 249–264. https://doi.org/10.1177/2167702618805081

Malkki, L. H. (1995). *Purity and exile: Violence memory, and national cosmology among Hutu refugees in Tanzania.* University of Chicago Press. https://doi.org/10.7208/chicago/9780226190969.001.0001

Margolin, G., & Gordis, E. B. (2000). *The effects of family and community violence on children, Annual Review of Psychology, 51*, 445–479. https://doi.org/10.1146/annurev.psych.51.1.445

Marlow, K., Schröder, T., Tickle, A., & Renton, J. (2022). Adapting the protocol for narrative exposure therapy for adults with mild intellectual disabilities. *British Journal of Learning Disabilities, 51*(3), 334–343 https://doi.org/10.1111/bld.12479

Marshall, G. N., Jaycox, L. H., Engel, C. C., Richardson, A. S., Dutra, S. J., Keane, T. M., Rosen, R. C., & Marx, B. P. (2019). PTSD symptoms are differentially associated with general distress and physiological arousal: Implications for the conceptualization and measurement of PTSD. *Journal of Anxiety Disorders, 62*, 26–34. https://doi.org/10.1016/j.janxdis.2018.10.003.

Maslow, A. H. (1954). *Motivation and personality.* Harper and Row.

Matz, K., Junghöfer, M., Elbert, T., Weber, K., Wienbruch, C., & Rockstroh, B. (2010). Adverse experiences in childhood influence brain responses to emotional stimuli in adult psychiatric patients. *International Journal of Psychophysiology, 75*, 277–286. https://doi.org/10.1016/j.ijpsycho.2009.12.010

Mauritz, M. W., Goossens, P. J., Jongedijk, R., Vermeulen, H., & van Gaal, B. (2022). Investigating the efficacy and experiences with narrative exposure therapy in severe mentally ill patients with comorbid post-traumatic stress disorder receiving flexible assertive community treatment: A mixed methods study. *Frontiers in Psychiatry*, 13. https://doi.org/10.3389/fpsyt.2022.804491

Mauritz, M. W., van Gaal, B. G., Goossens, P. J., Jongedijk, R. A., & Vermeulen, H. (2021). Treating patients with severe mental illness with narrative exposure therapy for comorbid post-traumatic stress disorder. *BJPsych Open, 7*(1). https://doi.org/10.1192/bjo.2020.124

Mauritz, M. W., Van Gaal, B. G., Jongedijk, R. A., Schoonhoven, L., Nijhuis-van der Sanden, M. W., & Goossens, P. J. (2016). Narrative exposure therapy for posttraumatic stress disorder associated with repeated interpersonal trauma in patients with severe mental illness: a mixed methods design. *European Journal of Psychotraumatology, 7*(1), 32473. https://doi.org/10.3402/ejpt.v7.32473

Mayer, B. (2020). *Trauma und geistige Beeinträchtigung: eine Studie zur Anwendung der NET (Narrativen Expositionstherapie) bei Menschen mit geistiger oder psychischer Beeinträchtigung* [Trauma and mental impairment: a study on the use of NET (Narrative Exposure Therapy) with people with intellectual or mental impairment.] Universität Konstanz.

Mayer, B., Elbing, U., & Ostermann, T. (2023). Trauma treatment using Narrative Exposure Therapy adapted to persons with intellectual disabilities or severe chronic mental disorders – A randomised controlled pilot study with an embedded observational study. *Journal of Intellectual Disability Research*, *67*(11), 1096–1112. https://doi.org/10.1111/jir.13076

Mayer, B., & Needham, I. (2011). "Discovering the real story within": A case study of the diagnostic correction of alleged intellectual disability to post traumatic stress disorder. In I. Needham, H. Nijman, T. Palmstierna, & R. Almvik (Eds.), *Proceedings of the 7th European Congress on Violence in Clinical Psychiatry* (pp. 333–337). Kavanah.

McClelland, J. L., McNaughton, B. L., & O'Reilly, R. C. (1995). Why there are complementary learning systems in the hippocampus and neocortex: Insights from the successes and failures of connectionist models of learning and memory. *Psychological Review*, *102*, 419–457. https://doi.org/10.1037/0033-295X.102.3.419

McCluskey, G., Lloyd, G., Kane, J., Riddell, S., Stead, J., & Weedon, E. (2008). Can restorative practices in schools make a difference? *Educational Review*, *60*(4), 405–417. https://doi.org/10.1080/00131910802393456

McEwen, B. S. (2002). *The end of stress as we know it*. Joseph Henry Press; Dana Press.

McGaugh, J. L. (2002). Memory consolidation and the amygdala: A systems perspective. *Trends in Neuroscience*, *25*, 456. https://doi.org/10.1016/S0166-2236(02)02211-7

McGrath, P. J., Lingley-Pottie, P., Thurston, C., MacLean, C., Cunningham, C., Waschbusch, D. A., Watters, C., Stewart, S., Bagnell, A., Santor, D., & Chaplin, W. (2011). Telephone-based mental health interventions for child disruptive behavior or anxiety disorders: randomized trials and overall analysis. *Journal of the American Academy of Child and Adolescent Psychiatry*, *50*(11), 1162–1172. https://doi.org/10.1016/j.jaac.2011.07.013.

McGuire, A. P., Gauthier, J. M., Anderson, L. M., Hollingsworth, D. W., Tracy, M., Galea, S., & Coffey, S. F. (2018). Social support moderates effects of natural disaster exposure on depression and posttraumatic stress disorder symptoms: Effects for displaced and nondisplaced residents. *Journal of Traumatic Stress*, *31*(2), 223–233. https://doi.org/10.1002/jts.22270

McKinnon, M. C., Boyd, J. E., Frewen, P. A., Lanius, U. F., Jetly, R., Richardson, J. D., & Lanius, R. A. (2016). A review of the relation between dissociation, memory, executive functioning and social cognition in military members and civilians with neuropsychiatric conditions. *Neuropsychologia*, *90*, 210–234. https://doi.org/10.1016/j.neuropsychologia.2016.07.017

McLaughlin, K. A., & Lambert, H. K. (2017). Child trauma exposure and psychopathology: Mechanisms of risk and resilience. *Current Opinion in Psychology*, *14*, 29–34. https://doi.org/10.1016/j.copsyc.2016.10.004

McLean, L. M., & Gallop, R. (2003). Implications of childhood sexual abuse for adult borderline personality disorder and complex posttraumatic stress disorder. *American Journal of Psychiatry*, *160*, 2, 369–371. https://doi.org/10.1176/appi.ajp.160.2.369

McLeer, S. V., Callaghan, M., Henry, D., & Wallen, J. (1994). Psychiatric disorders in sexually abused children. *Journal of the American Academy of Child & Adolescent Psychiatry*, *33*, 313–319. https://doi.org/10.1097/00004583-199403000-00003

McLeer, S. V., Dixon, J. F., Henry, D., Ruggiero, K., Escovitz, K., Niedda, T., & Scholle, R. (1998). Psychopathology in non-clinically referred sexually abused children. *Journal of the American Academy of Child & Adolescent Psychiatry*, *37*, 1326–1333. https://doi.org/10.1097/00004583-199812000-00017

Meaney, M. (2008). Maternal care and hippocampal plasticity: Evidence for experience-dependent structural plasticity, altered synaptic functioning, and differential responsiveness to glucocorticoids and stress. *Journal of Neuroscience*, *28*(23), 6037–6045. https://doi.org/10.1523/JNEUROSCI.0526-08.2008

Meaney, M., Aitken, D., van Berkel, C., Bhatnagar, C., & Sapolsky, R. (1988). Effects of neonatal handling on age-related impairments associated with the hippocampus. *Science*, *239*, 766–770. https://doi.org/10.1126/science.3340858

Merrick, M. T., Ports, K. A., Ford, D. C., Afifi, T. O., Gershoff, E. T., & Grogan-Kaylor, A. (2017). Unpacking the impact of adverse childhood experiences on adult mental health. *Child Abuse & Neglect*, *69*, 10–19. https://doi.org/10.1016/j.chiabu.2017.03.016

Metcalfe, J., & Jacobs, W. (1996). A hot-system/cool-system view of memory under stress. *PTSD Research Quarterly*, *7*, 1–3.

Misch, P., Phillips, M., Evans, P., & Berelowitz, M. (1993). Trauma in pre-school children: A clinical account. In G. Forrest (Ed.), *Trauma and crisis management*. ACPP Publications.

Morath, J., Gola, H., Sommershof, A., Hamuni, G., Kolassa, S., Catani, C., Adenauer, H., Ruf-Leuschner, M., Schauer, M., Elbert, T., Groettrup, M., & Kolassa, I. T. (2014). The effect of trauma-focused therapy on the altered T cell distribution in individuals with PTSD. Evidence from a randomized controlled trial. *Journal of Psychiatric Research*, *54*, 1–10.

Morath, J., Moreno-Villanueva, M., Hamuni, G., Kolassa, S., Ruf, M., Schauer, M., Elbert, T., Bürkle, A., & Kolassa, I. T. (2014). Effects of psychotherapy on DNA strand break accumulation originating from traumatic stress. *Psychotherapy & Psychosomatics*, *83*, 289–297. https://doi.org/10.1159/000362739

Mørkved, N., & Thorp, S. R. (2018). The treatment of PTSD in an older adult Norwegian woman using narrative exposure therapy: A case report. *European Journal of Psychotraumatology*, *9*(1), 1414561. https://doi.org/10.1080/20008198.2017.1414561

Morrison, J. (1989). Childhood sexual histories of women with somatization disorder. *American Journal of Psychiatry*, *146*, 239–241. https://doi.org/10.1176/ajp.146.2.239

Müller-Bamouh, V., Ruf-Leuschner, M., Dohrmann, K., Schauer, M., & Elbert, T. (2016). Are experiences of family and of organized violence predictors of aggression and violent behavior? A study with unaccompanied refugee minors. *European Journal of Psychotraumatology*, *7*(1), 27856. https://doi.org/10.3402/ejpt.v7.27856

Muris, P., & Meesters, C. (2014). Small or big in the eyes of the other: On the developmental psychopathology of self-conscious emotions as shame, guilt, and pride. *Clinical Child and Family Psychology Review*, *17*, 19–40. https://doi.org/10.1007/s10567-013-0137-z

Nader, K., Schafe, G. E., & LeDoux, J. E. (2000). Fear memories require protein synthesis in the amygdala for consolidation after retrieval. *Nature*, *406*, 722. https://doi.org/10.1038/35021052

Nandi, C., Crombach, A., Bambonyé, M., Elbert, T., Weierstall, R. (2015). Predictors of post-traumatic stress and appetitive aggression in active soldiers and former combatants. *European Journal of Psychotraumatology 2015*, *6*, 26553. https://doi.org/10.3402/ejpt.v6.26553

Nandi, C., Elbert, T., Bambonye, M., Weierstall, R., Reichert, M., Zeller, A., & Crombach, A. (2017). Predicting domestic and community violence by soldiers living in a conflict region. *Psychological Trauma: Theory, Research, Practice, and Policy*, *9*(6), 663–671. https://doi.org/10.1037/tra0000262

Narvaez, J. C. M., Remy, L., Bermudez, M. B., Scherer, J. N., Ornell, F., Surratt, H., Kurtz, S. P., & Pechanski, F. (2019). Re-traumatization cycle: Sexual abuse, post-traumatic stress disorder and sexual risk behaviors among club drug Users. *Substance Use & Misuse*, *54*(9), 1499–1508. https://doi.org/10.1080/10826084.2019.1589521

Neuner, F. (2012). Safety first? Trauma exposure in PTSD. In *Exposure therapy: Rethinking the model: Refining the method* (pp. 299–312). Springer.

Neuner, F. (2016). *Clinican's corner: I want to hear your story: The identity of narrative exposure therapy*. Interational Society for Traumatic Stress Studies: Blogs: StressPoints. https://istss.org/clinicians-corner-i-want-to-hear-your-story-the-identity-of-narrative-exposure-therapy-professor-dr-frank-neuner/

Neuner, F. (2023). Physical and social trauma: Towards an integrative transdiagnostic perspective on psychological trauma that involves threats to status and belonging. *Clinical Psychology Review*, *99*, 102219. https://doi.org/10.1016/j.cpr.2022.102219

Neuner, F., & Elbert, T. (2007). The mental health disaster in conflict settings: Can scientific research help? *BMC Public Health*, *7*, 275. https://doi.org/10.1186/1471-2458-7-275

Neuner, F., Kurreck, S., Ruf, M., Odenwald, M., Elbert, T., & Schauer, M. (2010). Can asylum-seekers with post-traumatic stress disorder be successfully treated? A randomized controlled pilot study. *Cognitive Behavior Therapy*, *39*, 81–91. https://doi.org/10.1080/16506070903121042

Neuner, F., Onyut, P. L., Ertl, V., Odenwald, M., Schauer, E., & Elbert, T. (2008). Treatment of posttraumatic stress disorder by trained lay counselors in an African refugee settlement: A randomized controlled trial. *Journal of Consulting and Clinical Psychology*, *76*, 686–694. https://doi.org/10.1037/0022-006X.76.4.686

Neuner, F., Schauer, E., Catani, C., Ruf, M., & Elbert, T. (2006). Post-Tsunami stress: A study of posttraumatic stress disorder in children living in three severely affected regions in Sri Lanka. *Journal of Traumatic Stress*, *19*, 339–347. https://doi.org/10.1002/jts.20121

Neuner, F., Schauer, M., & Elbert, T. (2011). Psychotherapy in war and crisis regions: Narrative exposure therapy and beyond. *ISTSS StressPoints*, *25*(1), 8–9.

Neuner, F., Schauer, M., & Elbert, T. (2018). Narrative Exposure Therapy (NET) as treatment for traumtized refugees and post-conflict populations. In N. Morina & A. Nickerson (Eds.), *Mental health of refugee and conflict-affected populations: Theory, research and clinical practice* (pp. 183–200). Springer Nature Switzerland. https://doi.org/10.1007/978-3-319-97046-2_9

Neuner, F., Schauer, M., Elbert, T., & Roth, W. T. (2002). A narrative exposure treatment as intervention in a Macedonia's refugee camp: A case report. *Journal of Behavioural and Cognitive Psychotherapy*, *30*, 205–209. https://doi.org/10.1017/S1352465802002072

Neuner, F., Schauer, M., Karunakara, U., Klaschik, C., Robert, C., & Elbert, T. (2004). Psychological trauma and evidence for enhanced vulnerability for PTSD through previous trauma in West Nile refugees. *BMC Psychiatry*, *4*, 34. https://doi.org/10.1186/1471-244X-4-34

Neuner, F., Schauer, M., Klaschik, C., Karunakara, U., & Elbert, T. (2004). A comparison of narrative exposure therapy, supportive counseling, and psychoeducation for treating posttraumatic stress disorder in an African refugee settlement. *Journal of Consulting and Clinical Psychology*, *72*, 579–587. https://doi.org/10.1037/0022-006X.72.4.579

Ni, T., Zhang, Y., Xue, S., Xu, W., & Tang, W. (2022). PTSD and depressive symptoms in Chinese adolescents exposed to multiple stressors from natural disasters, stressful life events, and maltreatment: A dose-response effect. *Frontiers in Psychology*, *13*, 1050260. https://doi.org/10.3389/fpsyg.2022.1050260

Nikdel, F., Arabzadeh, M., & Ghazanfari, N. (2016). The survey of relationship between memory self-efficacy and hope with quality of life in older adults of Kohgiluyeh and Boyer-Ahmad in 2016. *Journal of Gerontology*, *1*(2), 19–26. https://doi.org/10.18869/acadpub.joge.1.2.19

Nutt, D. J., & Malizia, A. L. (2004). Structural and functional brain changes in posttraumatic stress disorder. *Journal of Clinical Psychiatry*, *65*(Suppl 1), 11–17.

Nyström, M. B. T., & Mikkelsen, F. (2013). Psychopathy-related personality traits and shame management strategies in adolescents. *Journal of Interpersonal Violence*, *28*(3), 519–537 https://doi.org/10.1177/0886260512455512

O'Connor, L. E., Berry, J. W., Weiss, J., Schweitzer, D., & Sevier, M. (2000). Survivor guilt, submissive behaviour and evolutionary theory: The down-side of winning in social comparison. *Psychology and Psychotherapy: Theory, Research and Practice*, *73*(4), 519–530. https://doi.org/10.1348/000711200160705

Olavarrieta, G. A., & Benuto, L. (2022). Narrative exposure therapy: A case for use with refugees via telehealth with the use of an interpreter. *Clinical Case Studies*, 15346501221077703. https://doi.org/10.1177/15346501221077703

Olthuis, J. V., Kaltenbach, E., Giberson, E., Saryeddine, T., Asmundson, G. J. G., Carleton, R. N., Cramm, H., Crombach, A., Devlin, J., Mack, J., Lingley-Pottie, P., Rao, S., Sullivan, M., Wozney, L., & McGrath, P. J. (2023). Paraprofessional delivery of online narrative exposure therapy for firefighters. *Journal of Traumatic Stress*, *36*, 772–784.

Olthuis, J. V., Wozney, L., Asmundson, G. J., Cramm, H., Lingley-Pottie, P., & McGrath, P. J. (2016). Distance-delivered interventions for PTSD: A systematic review and meta-analysis. *Journal of Anxiety Disorders*, *44*, 9–26. https://doi.org/10.1016/j.janxdis.2016.09.010

Onyut, P. L., Neuner, F., Ertl, V., Schauer, E., Odenwald, M., & Elbert, T. (2009). Trauma, poverty and mental health among

Somali and Rwandese refugees living in an African refugee settlement – An epidemiological study. *Conflict and Health*, *3*, 6. https://doi.org/10.1186/1752-1505-3-6

Onyut, P. L., Neuner, F., Schauer, E., Ertl, V., Odenwald, M., Schauer, M., & Elbert, T. (2005). Narrative Exposure Therapy as a treatment for child war survivors with posttraumatic stress disorder: Two case reports and a pilot study in an African refugee settlement. *BMC Psychiatry*, *5*, 7. https://doi.org/10.1186/1471-244X-5-7

Orang, T., Ayoughi, S., Moran, J. K., Ghaffari, H., Mostafavi, S., Rasoulian, M., & Elbert, T. (2018). The efficacy of narrative exposure therapy in a sample of Iranian women exposed to ongoing intimate partner violence – A randomized controlled trial. *Clinical Psychology & Psychotherapy*, *25*(6), 827–841. https://doi.org/10.1002/cpp.2318

O'Rourke, N., Canham, S., Wertman, A., Chaudhury, H., Carmel, S., Bachner, Y. G., & Peres, H. (2016). Holocaust survivors' memories of past trauma and the functions of reminiscence. *The Gerontologist*, *56*(4), 743–752. https://doi.org/10.1093/geront/gnu168

Öst, L. G. (2002). Applied tension. In *Encyclopedia of psychotherapy* (pp. 103–108). Elsevier. https://doi.org/10.1016/B0-12-343010-0/00012-X

Ozer, E. J., Best, S. R., Lipsey, T. L., & Weiss, D. S. (2003). Predictors of posttraumatic stress disorder and symptoms in adults: A meta-analysis. *Psychological Bulletin*, *129*, 52–73. https://doi.org/10.1037/0033-2909.129.1.52

Papageorgiou, V., Frangou-Garunovic, A., Iordanidou, R., Yule, W., Smith, P., & Vostanis, P. (2000). War trauma and psycho-pathology in Bosnian refugee children. *European Child and Adolescent Psychiatry*, *9*, 84–90. https://doi.org/10.1007/s007870050002

Park, J. K., Park, J., Elbert, T., & Kim, S. J. (2020). Effects of narrative exposure therapy on posttraumatic stress disorder, depression, and insomnia in traumatized North Korean refugee youth. *Journal of Traumatic Stress*, *33*(3), 353–359. https://doi.org/10.1002/'jts.22492.

Pavlov, I. P. (1927). *Conditioned reflexes: An investigation of the physiological activity of the cerebral cortex* (G. V. Anrep, Trans. & Ed.). Oxford University Press.

Pearlman, L. A., & Mac Ian, P. S. (1995). Vicarious traumatization: An empirical study of the effects of trauma work on trauma therapists. *Professional Psychology: Research and Practice*, *26*(6), 558–565. https://doi.org/10.1037/0735-7028.26.6.558

Pech-Cárdenas, F. (2023). Indigenous wisdom: Re-story-ation to resist, resurge, and inspire. *Open Rivers: Rethinking Water, Place, & Community*, 23. https://openrivers.lib.umn.edu/article/indigenous-wisdom-re-story-ation/

Peltonen, K., & Kangaslampi, S. (2019). Treating children and adolescents with multiple traumas: a randomized clinical trial of narrative exposure therapy. *European Journal of Psychotraumatology*, *10*(1), 1558708. https://doi.org/10.1080/20008198.2018.1558708

Pennebaker, J. W., & Seagal, J. D. (1999). Forming a story: The health benefits of narrative. *Journal of Clinical Psychology*, *55*, 1243–1254. https://doi.org/10.1002/(SICI)1097-4679(199910)55:10<1243::AID-JCLP6>3.0.CO;2-N

Pennebaker, J. W., & Stone, L. D. (2004). Translating traumatic experiences into language: Implications for child abuse and long-term health. In L. J. Koenig, L. S. Doll, A. O'Leary, & W. Pequegnat (Eds.), *From child sexual abuse to adult sexual risk: Trauma, revictimization, and intervention* (pp. 201–216). American Psychological Association. https://doi.org/10.1037/10785-010

Pérez-Sales, P. (2017). Psychological torture: Definition, evaluation and measurement. Routledge Books. https://doi.org/10.4324/9781315616940

Pérez-Sales, P., & Petersen, H. D. (2023). Forensic assessment of psychological torture. *Encyclopedia of Forensic Sciences*, *2*, 493–502. https://doi.org/10.1016/B978-0-12-823677-2.00177-X

Peterson, C. (1996). The preschool child witness: Errors in account of traumatic injury. *Canadian Journal of Behavioural Science*, *28*, 36–42. https://doi.org/10.1037/0008-400X.28.1.36

Pittig, A., Kotter, R., & Hoyer, J. (2019). The struggle of behavioral therapists with exposure: Self-reported practicability, negative beliefs, and therapist distress about exposure-based interventions. *Behavior Therapy*, *50*(2), 353–366. https://doi.org/10.1016/j.beth.2018.07.003

Plessner, H. (1975). *Die Stufen des Organischen und der Mensch* [The stages of the organic and the human being]. de Gruyter.

Plessner, H. (2003). *Conditio humana* [The human condition]. Suhrkamp Verlag.

Porter, C., Palmier-Claus, J., Branitsky, A., Mansell, W., Warwick, H., & Varese, F. (2020). Childhood adversity and borderline personality disorder: A meta-analysis. *Acta Psychiatrica Scandinavica*, *141*(1), 6–20. https://doi.org/10.1111/acps.13118

Potter, F., Zehb, M., Dohrmann, K., Müller-Bamouh, V., Rockstroh, B., & Crombach, A. (2023). "It is worth hanging in there" – psychotherapeutic experiences shaping future motivation for outpatient psychotherapy with refugee clients in Germany. *BMC Psychiatry*, *23*(1), 503. https://doi.org/10.1186/s12888-023-05004-3

Potthast, N., Neuner, F., & Catani, C. (2014). The contribution of emotional maltreatment to alcohol dependence in a treatment-seeking sample. *Addictive Behaviors*, *39*(5), 949–958. https://doi.org/10.1016/j.addbeh.2014.01.015

Provençal, N., & Binder, E. B. (2015). The effects of early life stress on the epigenome: From the womb to adulthood and even before. *Experimental Neurology*, *268*, 10–20. https://doi.org/10.1016/j.expneurol.2014.09.001

Pugh, J. M. (2022). *Why do communities matter? A study looking at the role of communities in the lives of people with experience of torture and trafficking* [Doctoral dissertation, University of Leeds].

Pynoos, R. S., & Nader, K. (1989). Children's memory and proximity to violence. *Journal of the American Academy of Child & Adolescent Psychiatry*, *28*, 236–241. https://doi.org/10.1097/00004583-198903000-00015

Radtke, K. M., Schauer, M., Gunter, H. M., Ruf-Leuschner, M., Sill, J., Meyer, A., & Elbert, T. (2015). Epigenetic modifications of the glucocorticoid receptor gene are associated with the vulnerability to psychopathology in childhood maltreatment. *Translational Psychiatry*, *5*(5), e571. https://doi.org/10.1038/tp.2015.63

Reich, J. (2017). *Exploring movie construction & production: What's so exciting about movies?* Open SUNY Textbooks.

Reid, A. M., Bolshakova, M. I., Guzick, A. G., Fernandez, A. G., Striley, C. W., Geffken, G. R., & McNamara, J. P. (2017). Common barriers to the dissemination of exposure therapy for youth with anxiety disorders. *Community Mental Health Journal*, *53*, 432–437. https://doi.org/10.1007/s10597-017-0108-9

Reviere, S. L. (1996). *Memory of childhood trauma: A clinician's guide to the literature.* Guilford Press.

Robjant, K., & Fazel, M. (2010). The emerging evidence for Narrative Exposure Therapy: A review. *Clinical Psychology Reviews*, *30*, 1030–1039. https://doi.org/10.1016/j.cpr.2010.07.004

Robjant, K., Köbach, A., Schmitt, S., Chibashimba, A., Carleial, S., & Elbert, T. (2019). The treatment of posttraumatic stress symptoms and aggression in female former child soldiers using adapted Narrative Exposure therapy – a RCT in eastern Democratic Republic of CONGO. *Behaviour Research and Therapy*, *123*, 103482. https://doi.org/10.1016/j.brat.2019.103482

Robjant, K., Meyer, D., Kaiser, E., Kaltenbach, E., & Schauer, M. (2021). e-NET: Narrative Exposure Therapy online – The challenges and opportunities of delivering trauma therapy remotely. *Maltrattamento e Abuso all'Infanzia*, *22*(3), 69–85. https://doi.org/10.3280/MAL2020-003002

Robjant, K., Schmitt, S., Carleial, S., Elbert, T., Abreu, L., Chibashimba, A., Hinkel, H., Hoeffler, A., Rukundo Zeller, A., Rockstroh, B., & Köbach, A. (2022). NETfacts – An integrated intervention at the individual and collective level to treat communities affected by organized violence. *Proceedings of the National Academy of Sciences USA*, *119*(44), e2204698119. https://doi.org/10.1073/pnas.2204698119

Robjant, K., Schmitt, S., Elbert, T., Chibashimba, A., & Köbach, A. (2020). The NETfacts health system: An integrative approach to counter the mental sequelae of trauma and violence at the individual and community level. *Maltrattamento e Abuso all'Infanzia*, *3*, 63–72. https://doi.org/10.3280/MAL2020-003006

Roozendaal, B., de Quervain, D. J.-F., Ferry, B., Setlow, B., & McGaugh, J. L. (2001). Basolateral amygdala-nucleus accumbens interactions in mediating glucocorticoid enhancement of memory consolidation. *Journal of Neuroscience*, *21*, 2518–2525. https://doi.org/10.1523/JNEUROSCI.21-07-02518.2001

Roozendaal, B., Griffith, Q. K., Buranday, J., de Quervain, D. J.-F., & McGaugh, J. L. (2003). The hippocampus mediates glucocorticoid-induced retrieval impairments of spatial memory: Dependence on the basolateral amygdala. *Proceedings of the National Academy of Science USA*, *100*, 1328–1333. https://doi.org/10.1073/pnas.0337480100

Rosenthal, G. (1997). Traumatische Familienvergangenheiten [Traumatic family backgrounds]. In G. Rosenthal (Ed.), Der Holocaust im Leben von drei Generationen [The Holocaust in the lives of three generations]. Psycho-sozial-Verlag.

Ruf, M., & Schauer, M. (2012). Facing childhood trauma: Narrative exposure therapy within a cascade model of care. In J. Murray (Ed.), *Exposure therapy: New developments* (pp. 229–261). Nova Science.

Ruf, M., Schauer, M., Neuner, F., Catani, C., Schauer, E., & Elbert, T. (2010). Narrative exposure therapy for 7- to 16-year-olds – A randomized controlled trial with traumatized refugee children. *Journal of Traumatic Stress*, *23*, 437–445. https://doi.org/10.1002/jts.20548

Ruf-Leuschner, M., Brunnemann, N., Schauer, M., Pryss, R., Barnewitz, E., Liebrecht, M., Kratzer, W., Reichert, M., & Elbert, T. (2016). The KINDEX App – An instrument for assessment and immediate evaluation of psychosocial stressors in pregnant women in the daily practice of gynecologists, midwives, and in women's hospitals. *Verhaltenstherapie*, *26*, 171–181.

Ruf-Leuschner, M., Schauer, M., & Elbert, T. (2015). Raum für den Dritten: DolmetscherInnen in der Therapie von Flüchtlingen [Space for the third party: Interpreters in the therapy of refugees; special issue]. *Psychotherapie zu Dritt – über die Arbeit mit Dolmetschern in therapeutischen Gesprächen.*https://www.vivo.org/wp-content/uploads/2015/05/NTFN-Broschu%CC%88re_S22-28.pdf

Ruzek, J. I., Eftekhari, A., Rosen, C. S., Crowley, J. J., Kuhn, E., Foa, E. B., Hembree, E. A., & Karlin, B. E. (2014). Factors related to clinician attitudes toward prolonged exposure therapy for PTSD. *Journal of Traumatic Stress*, *27*(4), 423–429. https://doi.org/10.1002/jts.21945

Sachser, C., Berliner, L., Risch, E., Rosner, R., Birkeland, M. S., Eilers, R., Hafstad, G. S., Pfeiffer, E., Plener, P. L., & Jensen, T. K. (2022). The Child and Adolescent Trauma Screen 2 (CATS-2) – validation of an instrument to measure DSM-5 and ICD-11 PTSD and complex PTSD in children and adolescents. *European Journal of Psychotraumatology*, *13*(2), Article 2105580. https://doi.org/10.1080/20008066.2022.2105580

Sachser, C., Berliner, L., Holt, T., Jensen, T. K., Jungbluth, N., Risch, E., Rosner, R., & Goldbeck, L. (2017). International development and psychometric properties of the Child and Adolescent Trauma Screen (CATS). *Journal of Affective Disorders*, *210*, 189–195. https://doi.org/10.1016/j.jad.2016.12.040

Saigh, P. A. (1991). The development of post-traumatic stress disorder following four different types of traumatizations. *Behaviour Research & Therapy*, *29*, 213–216. https://doi.org/10.1016/0005-7967(91)90110-O

Saigh, P. A. (1992). The behavioural treatment of child and adolescent post-traumatic stress disorder. *Advances in Behaviour Research & Therapy*, *14*, 247–275. https://doi.org/10.1016/0146-6402(92)90004-8

Saigh, P. A., Yule, W., & Inamdar, S. C. (1996). Imaginal flooding of traumatized children and adolescents. *Journal of School Psychology*, *34*, 163–183. https://doi.org/10.1016/0022-4405(96)00005-2

Sanftenberg, L., Beutel, A., Friemel, C. M., Kosilek, R. P., Schauer, M., Elbert, T., ... & Gensichen, J. (2023). Barriers and opportunities for implementation of a brief psychological intervention for post-ICU mental distress in the primary care setting – Results from a qualitative sub-study of the PICTURE trial. *BMC Primary Care*, *24*(1), 113.

Sansen, L. M., Iffland, B., & Neuner, F. (2015). The trauma of peer victimization: Psychophysiological and emotional characteristics of memory imagery in subjects with social anxiety disorder. *Psychophysiology*, *52*(1), 107–116. https://doi.org/10.1111/psyp.12291

Sapolsky, R. M. (1999). Glucocorticoids, stress, and their adverse neurological effects: Relevance to aging. *Experimental Gerontology*, *34*(6), 721–732. https://doi.org/10.1016/S0531-5565(99)00047-9

Sayed, S., Iacoviello, B. M., & Charney, D. S. (2015). Risk factors for the development of psychopathology following trauma. *Current psychiatry reports*, *17*, 1–7.

Schaaf, K. K., & McCanne, T. R. (1994). Childhood abuse, body image disturbance, and eating disorders. *Child Abuse & Neglect*, *18*, 607–615. https://doi.org/10.1016/0145-2134(94)90011-6

Schaal, S., & Elbert, T. (2006). Ten years after the genocide: Trauma confrontation and posttraumatic stress in Rwandan adolescents. *Journal of Traumatic Stress*, *19*, 95–105. https://doi.org/10.1002/jts.20104

Schaal, S., Elbert, T., & Neuner, F. (2009). Narrative exposure therapy versus interpersonal psychotherapy: A pilot randomized controlled trial with Rwandan genocide orphans. *Psychotherapy and Psychosomatics*, *78*, 298–306. https://doi.org/10.1159/000229768

Schacter, D. L. (1996). *Searching for memory: The brain, the mind and the past.* Basic Books.

Schalinski, I., & Ardino, V. (2020). Recent developments of narrative exposure therapy. *Maltrattamento e abuso all'infanzia*, *2020* (3), 7–9.

Schalinski, I., Elbert, T., & Schauer, M. (2011). Female dissociative responding to extreme sexual violence in a chronic crisis setting: The case of Eastern Congo. *Journal of Traumatic Stress*, *24*, 235–238. https://doi.org/10.1002/jts.20631

Schalinski, I., Schauer, M., & Elbert, T. (2015). The Shutdown Dissociation Scale (Shut-D). *European Journal of Psychotraumatology*, *6*, 25652. https://doi.org/10.3402/ejpt.v6.25652

Schalinski, I., Schauer, M., & Elbert, T. (2016). *Shut-D – Shutdown Dissociation Scale* [Test description, questionnaire in German, English, Norwegian, and implementation instructions]. https://doi.org/10.23668/psycharchives.4596

Schalinski, I., Teicher, M. H., Nischk, D., Hinderer, E., Müller, O., & Rockstroh, B. (2016). Type and timing of adverse childhood experiences differentially affect severity of PTSD, dissociative and depressive symptoms in adult inpatients. *BMC Psychiatry*, *16*, 295. https://doi.org/10.1186/s12888-016-1004-5

Schalinski, I., Teicher, M. H., & Rockstroh, B. (2019). Early neglect is a key determinant of adult hair cortisol concentration and is associated with increased vulnerability to trauma in a transdiagnostic sample. *Psychoneuroendocrinology*, *108*, 35–42. https://doi.org/10.1016/j.psyneuen.2019.06.007

Schauer, E., Neuner, F., Elbert, T., Ertl, V., Onyut, L., Odenwald, M., & Schauer, M. (2004). Narrative exposure therapy in children – A case study. *Intervention*, *2*(1), 18–32.

Schauer, M. (2016, March). The mass refugee movement: Better reframed as mental health crisis? Global Perspectives of the International Society for Traumatic Stress Studies. *ISTSS StressPoints*. http://sherwood-istss.informz.net/admin31/content/template.asp?sid=48039&brandid=4463&uid=1019025605&mi=5471628&mfqid=26491997&ptid=0&ps=48039 https://doi.org/10.13140/RG.2.1.4113.1926

Schauer, M. (2018). Ik in de ogen van de ander: functies van schuld en schaamte na psychotrauma [Me in the eyes of the other: Functions of guilt and shame after psychotrauma] [Keynote Lecture at NtVP Annual Meeting 2018, Lunteren, NL]. *Impact Magazine*, *2*(2), 32–34.

Schauer, M. (2024). *Die einfachste Psychotherapie der Welt* [The simplest psychotherapy in the world]. Rowohlt Polaris.

Schauer, M., & Elbert, T. (2010). Dissociation following traumatic stress: Etiology and treatment. *Journal of Psychology*, *218*(2), 109–127. https://doi.org/10.1027/0044-3409/a000018

Schauer, M., Elbert, T., Gotthardt, S., Rockstroh, B., Odenwald, M., & Neuner, F. (2006). Wiedererfahrung durch Psychotherapie modifiziert Geist und Gehirn. [Re-experience through psychotherapy modifies mind and brain]. *Verhaltenstherapie*, *16*, 96–103. https://doi.org/10.1159/000093195

Schauer, M., Elbert, T., & Neuner, F. (2007). Interaktion von Neurowissenschaftlichen Erkenntnissen und Psychotherapeutischen Einsichten am Beispiel von Angst und traumatischem Stress [How neuroscientific findings and psychotherapeutic insights interact using the example of anxiety and traumatic stress]. In R. Becker & H.-P. Wunderlich (Eds.), *Wie wirkt Psychotherapie: Forschungsgrundlagen für die Praxis* (pp. 87–108). Thieme-Verlag.

Schauer, M., Neuner, F., & Elbert, T. (2005). *Narrative exposure therapy: A short-term intervention for traumatic stress disorders after war, terror, and torture.* Hogrefe & Huber Publishers.

Schauer, M., Neuner, F., & Elbert, T. (2011). *Narrative exposure therapy: A short-term treatment for traumatic stress disorders.* Hogrefe Publishing.

Schauer, M., Neuner, F., & Elbert, T. (2017). Narrative exposure therapy for children and adolescents (KIDNET). In M. Landolt, M. Cloitre, & U. Schnyder (Eds.), *Evidence-based treatments for trauma related disorders in children and adolescents* (pp. 227–250). Springer. https://doi.org/10.1007/978-3-319-46138-0_11

Schauer, M., Neuner, F., Karunakara, U., Klaschik, C., Robert, C., & Elbert, T. (2003). PTSD and the "building block" effect of psychological trauma among West Nile Africans. *ESTSS (European Society for Traumatic Stress Studies) Bulletin*, *10*(2), 5–6.

Schauer, M., & Robjant, K. (2018). Commentary on Scheidell et al. (2018): En-counting adversities; the 'building blocks' of psychopathology. *Addiction*, *113*(1), 57–58. https://doi.org/10.1111/add.14067

Schauer, M., Robjant, K., Elbert, T., & Neuner, F. (2020). Narrative exposure therapy (NET). In J. D. Ford & C. A. Courtois, (Eds.), *Treating complex traumatic stress disorders: An evidence-based guide* (pp. 309–331). Guilford Press.

Schauer, M., & Ruf-Leuschner, M. (2014). Die Lifeline in der Narrativen Expositionstherapie (NET) [Lifeline in Narrative Exposure Therapy]. *Psychotherapeut*, *59*, 226–238. https://doi.org/10.1007/s00278-014-1041-9

Schauer, M., Ruf-Leuschner, M., & Landolt, M. (2014). Dem Leben Gestalt geben: Die *Lifeline* in der Traumatherapie von Kindern und Jugendlichen. [Giving Gestalt to life: The Lifeline in trauma therapy for children and adolescents] In K. Priebe & A. Dyer (Eds.), *Metaphern, Geschichten und Symbole in der Traumatherapie* (pp. 177–186). Hogrefe.

Schauer, M., & Schalinski, I. (2022). Die Biologie des Überlebens – Ätiologie und Behandlung trauma-induzierter Dissoziation [The biology of survival: Etiology and treatment of trauma-induced dissociation]. In J. Müller, M. Ruf-Leuschner, B. Grimmer, C. Knaevelsrud, & B. Dammann (Eds), *Traumafolgen: Forschung und therapeutische Praxis* (pp. 58-81). Kohlhammer.

Schauer, M., & Schauer, E. (2010). Trauma-focused public mental-health interventions: A paradigm shift in humanitarian assistance and aid work. In E. Martz (Ed.), *Trauma rehabilitation after war and conflict* (pp. 361–430). Springer. https://doi.org/10.1007/978-1-4419-5722-1_16

Scheff, T. J. (2011). Social-emotional origins of violence: A theory of multiple killing. *Aggression and Violent Behavior, 16*(6), 453–460. https://doi.org/10.1016/j.avb.2011.03.007

Scheidell, J. D., Quinn, K., McGorray, S. P., Frueh, B. C., Beharie, N. N., Cottler, L. B., & Khan, M. R. (2018). Childhood traumatic experiences and the association with marijuana and cocaine use in adolescence through adulthood. *Addiction, 113*(1), 44–56. https://doi.org/10.1111/add.13921

Schmitt, S., Robjant, K., Elbert, T., Carleial, S., Hoeffler, A., Chibashimba, A., Hinkel, H., & Köbach, A. (2022). Breaking the cycles of violence with narrative exposure: development and feasibility of NETfacts, a community-based intervention for populations living under continuous threat. *PLOS, 17*(12), e0275421. https://doi.org/10.1371/journal.pone.0275421

Schnyder, U., Bryant, R. A., Ehlers, A., Foa, E. B., Hasan, A., Mwiti, G., Kristensen, C. H., Neuner, F., Oe, M., & Yule, W. (2016). Culture-sensitive psychotraumatology. *European Journal of Psychotraumatology, 7*(1), Article 31179.

Scoglio, A. A., Reilly, E. D., Girouard, C., Quigley, K. S., Carnes, S., & Kelly, M. M. (2022). Social functioning in individuals with post-traumatic stress disorder: A systematic review. *Trauma, Violence, & Abuse, 23*(2), 356–371. https://doi.org/10.1177/1524838020946800

Segerstrom, S. C., & Miller, G. E. (2004). Psychological stress and the human immune system: A meta-analytic study of 30 years of inquiry. *Psychological Bulletin, 130*, 601–630. https://doi.org/10.1037/0033-2909.130.4.601

Sekowski, M., Gambin, M., Cudo, A., Wozniak-Prus, M., Penner, F., Fonagy, P., & Sharp, C. (2020). The relations between childhood maltreatment, shame, guilt, depression and suicidal ideation in inpatient adolescents. *Journal of Affective Disorders, 276*, 667-677. https://doi.org/10.1016/j.jad.2020.07.056

Sell, A., Tooby, J., & Cosmides, L. (2009). Formidability and the logic of human anger. *Proceedings of the National Academy of Sciences USA, 106*(35), 15073–15078.

Serpeloni, F., Narrog, J. A., Pickler, B., Avanci, J. Q., Assis, S. G. D., & Köbach, A. (2023). Treating post-traumatic stress disorder in survivors of community and domestic violence using narrative exposure therapy: A case series in two public health centers in Rio de Janeiro/Brazil. *Ciência & Saúde Coletiva, 28*, 1619–1630.

Serpeloni, F., Radtke, K., de Assis, S. G., Henning, F., Nätt, D., & Elbert, T. (2017). Grandmaternal stress during pregnancy and DNA methylation of the third generation: an epigenome-wide association study. *Translational psychiatry, 7*(8), e1202–e1202. https://doi.org/10.1038/tp.2017.153

Serpeloni, F., Radtke, K. M., Hecker, T., Sill, J., Vukojevic, V., Assis, S., Schauer, M., Elbert, T., & Nätt, D. (2019). Does prenatal stress shape postnatal resilience? – An epigenome-wide study on violence and mental health in humans. *Frontiers in Genetics, Section Epigenomics and Epigenetics, 10*, 269. https://doi.org/10.3389/fgene.2019.00269

Shanahan, L., Hill, S. N., Gaydosh, L. M., Steinhoff, A., Costello, E. J., Dodge, K. A., Harris, K. M., & Copeland, W. E. (2019). Does despair really kill? A roadmap for an evidence-based answer. *American Journal of Public Health, 109*(6), 854–858. https://doi.org/10.2105/AJPH.2019.305016

Sharif, F., Jahanbin, I., Amirsadat, A., & Moghadam, M. H. (2018). Effectiveness of life review therapy on quality of life in the late life at day care centers of Shiraz, Iran: A randomized controlled trial. *International Journal of Community Based Nursing & Midwifery, 6*, 136–145.

Shin, S. H., McDonald, S. E., & Conley, D. (2018). Patterns of adverse childhood experiences and substance use among young adults: A latent class analysis. *Addictive Behaviors, 78*, 187–192. https://doi.org/10.1016/j.addbeh.2017.11.020

Shultz, J. M., Rechkemmer, A., Rai, A., & McManus, K. T. (2019). Public health and mental health implications of environmentally induced forced migration. *Disaster Medicine and Public Health Preparedness, 13*(2), 116–122. https://doi.org/10.1017/dmp.2018.27

Siehl, S., Robjant, K., & Crombach, A. (2021). Systematic review and meta-analyses of the long-term efficacy of narrative exposure therapy for adults, children and perpetrators. *Psychotherapy Research, 31*(6), 695–710. https://doi.org/10.1080/10503307.2020.1847345

Sloman, L., & Gilbert, P. (2000). *Subordination and defeat: An evolutionary approach to mood disorders and their therapy*. Routledge. https://doi.org/10.4324/9781410605207

Smaik, N. M., Simmons, L. A., Abdulhag, B., & Dardas, L. A. (2023). The feasibility and preliminary efficacy of narrative exposure therapy on post-traumatic stress disorder among Syrian refugees in Jordan. *International Journal of Nursing Sciences, 10*(4), 518–526. https://doi.org/10.1016/j.ijnss.2023.09.007

Smith, D., Schlaepfer, P., Major, K., Dyble, M., Page, A. E., Thompson, J., Chaudhary, N., Salali, G. D., Mace, R., Astete, L., Ngales, M., Vinicius, L., & Migliano, A. B. (2017). Cooperation and the evolution of hunter-gatherer storytelling. *Nature Communications, 8*(1), 1853. https://doi.org/10.1038/s41467-017-02036-8

Smolak, L., & Murnen, S. K. (2002). A meta-analytic examination of the relationship between child sexual abuse and eating disorders. *International Journal of Eating Disorders, 31*, 136–150. https://doi.org/10.1002/eat.10008

Somasundaram, D. J. (1993). *Child trauma*. University of Jaffna.

Sommer, J., Hinsberger, M., Elbert, T., Holtzhausen, L., Kaminer, D., Seedat, S., Mandikane, S., Weierstall, R. (2017). The interplay between trauma, substance abuse and appetitive aggression and its relation to criminal activity among high-risk males in South Africa. *Addictive Behaviors, 64*, 29–34. https://doi.org/10.1016/j.addbeh.2016.08.008

Sommer, J., Hinsberger, M., Weierstall, R., Holtzhausen, L., Kaminer, D., Seedat, S., Maercker, A., Madikane, S., & Elbert, T. (2016). Social acknowledgment of violent experiences and its role in PTSD and appetitive aggression among high-risk males in South Africa. *Clinical Psychological Science, 5*, 166–172. https://doi.org/10.1177/2167702616658634

Sommershof, A., Aichinger, H., Engler, E., Adenauer, H., Catani, C., Boneberg, E. M., Elbert, T., Groettrup, M., & Kolassa, I.-T. (2009). Substantial reduction of naïve and regulatory T cells following traumatic stress. . *Brain, Behavior, and Immunity, 23*, 1117–1124. https://doi.org/10.1016/j.bbi.2009.07.003

Sourander, A., McGrath, P. J., Ristkari, T., Cunningham, C., Huttunen, J., Lingley-Pottie, P., Hinkka-Yli-Salomäki, S., Kinnunen, M., Vuorio, J., Sinokki, A., Fossum, S., & Unruh, A. (2016). Internet-assisted parent training intervention for disruptive behavior in 4-year-old children: A randomized clinical trial. *JAMA Psychiatry, 73*(4), 378–387. https://doi.org/10.1001/jamapsychiatry.2015.3411

Spoont, M. R., Sayer, N. A., Kehle-Forbes, S. M., Meis, L. A., & Nelson, D. B. (2017). A prospective study of racial and ethnic variation in VA psychotherapy services for PTSD. *Psychiatric Services, 68*(3), 231–237. https://doi.org/10.1176/appi.ps.201600086

Spyridou, A., Schauer, M., & Ruf-Leuschner, M. (2014). Obstetric care providers assessing psychosocial risk factors during pregnancy: Validation of a short screening tool – the KINDEX Spanish Version. *Child and Adolescent Psychiatry and Mental Health, 8*, 30, https://doi.org/10.1186/s13034-014-0030-7

Spyridou, A., Schauer, M., & Ruf-Leuschner, M. (2015). Obstetric care providers are able to assess psychosocial risks, identify and refer high-risk pregnant women: Validation of a short assessment tool – the KINDEX Greek version. *BMC Pregnancy and Childbirth, 15*(1), 41. https://doi.org/10.1186/s12884-015-0462-y

Spyridou, A., Schauer, M., & Ruf-Leuschner, M. (2016). Prenatal screening for psychosocial risks in a high risk-population in Peru using the KINDEX interview. *BMC Pregnancy and Childbirth, 16*(1), 1. https://doi.org/10.1186/s12884-016-0799-x

Squire, L. R. (1994). Declarative and nondeclarative memory: Multiple brain systems supporting learning and memory. In D. L. Schacter & E. Tulving (Eds.), *Memory systems* (pp. 207–228). MIT Press.

Staub, E. (1998). Breaking the cycle of genocidal violence: Healing and reconciliation. In J. H. Harvey (Ed.), *Perspectives on loss: A source book: Death, dying, and bereavement* (pp. 231–238). Brunner/Mazel.

Steele, K. (2021). Beyond attachment. In D. J. Siegel, A. N. Schore, & L. Cozolino (Eds.), *Interpersonal neurobiology and clinical practice*. W. W. Norton.

Steensma, D. P. (2013). Stories we tell one another: Narrative reflection and the art of oncology. *American Society of Clinical Oncology Educational Book, 33*(1), e331–e335. https://doi.org/10.14694/EdBook_AM.2013.33.e331

Stenmark, H., Catani, C., Neuner, F., Elbert, T., & Holen, A. (2013). Treating PTSD in refugees and asylum seekers within the general health care system: A randomized controlled multicenter study. *Behaviour Research and Therapy, 51*(10), 641–647.

Stenmark, H., Guzey, I. C., Elbert, T., & Holen, A. (2014). Gender and offender status predicting treatment success in refugees and asylum seekers with PTSD. *European Journal of Psychotraumatology, 5*(1), 20803. https://doi.org/10.1016/j.brat.2013.07.002

Stevens, N. R., Miller, M. L., Soibatian, C., Otwell, C., Rufa, A. K., Meyer, D. J., & Shalowitz, M. U. (2020). Exposure therapy for PTSD during pregnancy: A feasibility, acceptability, and case series study of Narrative Exposure Therapy (NET). *BMC Psychology, 8*, 1–18. https://doi.org/10.1186/s40359-020-00503-4

Stotz, S. J., Elbert, T., Müller, V., & Schauer, M. (2015). The relationship between trauma, shame, and guilt: findings from a community-based study of refugee minors in Germany. *European Journal of Psychotraumatology, 6*(1), 25863. https://doi.org/10.3402/ejpt.v6.25863

Strijk, P., Jongedijk, R. A., & Bedawi, V. (2020). A new treatment approach for PTSD: High-intensive narrative exposure therapy (HI-NET). *Maltrattamento e abuso all'infanzia, 22*, (3), 51–62.

Stuewig, J., & McCloskey, L. A. (2005). The relation of child maltreatment to shame and guilt among adolescents: Psychological routes to depression and delinquency. *Child Maltreatment, 10*(4), 324–336. https://doi.org/10.1177/1077559505279308

Stuewig, J., Tangney, J. P., Kendall, S., Folk, J. B., Meyer, C. R., & Dearing, R. L. (2015). Children's proneness to shame and guilt predict risky and illegal behaviors in young adulthood. *Child Psychiatry & Human Development, 46*, 217–227. https://doi.org/10.1007/s10578-014-0467-1

Sullivan, M. A., Saylor, C. F., & Foster, K. Y. (1991). Post-hurricane adjustment of preschoolers and their families. *Advances in Behaviour Research and Therapy, 13*, 163–171. https://doi.org/10.1016/0146-6402(91)90004-T

Sznycer, D., Tooby, J., Cosmides, L., Porat, R., Shalvi, S., & Halperin, E. (2016). Shame closely tracks the threat of devaluation by others, even across cultures. *Proceedings of the National Academy of Sciences USA, 113*(10), 2625–2630. https://doi.org/10.1073/pnas.1514699113

Tandon, Y. (1984). Ugandan refugees in Kenya: A community of enforced self-reliance. *Disasters, 8*, 267–271. https://doi.org/10.1111/j.1467-7717.1984.tb00889.x

Tangney, J. P., & Dearing, R. L. (2003). *Shame and guilt: Emotions and social behavior*. Guilford Press.

Tangney, J. P., Stuewig, J., & Hafez, L. (2011). Shame, guilt, and remorse: Implications for offender populations. *Journal of Forensic Psychiatry & Psychology, 22*(5), 706–723. https://doi.org/10.1080/14789949.2011.617541

Tangney, J. P., Stuewig, J., & Mashek, D. J. (2007). Moral emotions and moral behavior. *Annual Review of Psychology, 58*, 345–372. https://doi.org/10.1146/annurev.psych.56.091103.070145

Tangney, J. P., Stuewig, J., Mashek, D., & Hastings, M. (2011). Assessing jail inmates' proneness to shame and guilt: Feeling bad about the behavior or the self? *Criminal Justice and Behavior, 38*(7), 710–734. https://doi.org/10.1177/0093854811405762

Tangney, J. P., Wagner, P., Fletcher, C., & Gramzow, R. (1992). Shamed into anger? The relation of shame and guilt to anger and self-reported aggression. *Journal of Personality and Social Psychology, 62*(4), 669–675. https://doi.org/10.1037/0022-3514.62.4.669

Teicher, M. H., Andersen, S. L., Polcari, A., Anderson, C. M., & Navalta, C. P. (2002). Developmental neurobiology of childhood stress and trauma. *Psychiatric Clinics of North America, 25*, 397–326. https://doi.org/10.1016/S0193-953X(01)00003-X

Teicher, M. H., Gordon, J. B., & Nemeroff, C. B. (2022). Recognizing the importance of childhood maltreatment as a critical factor in psychiatric diagnoses, treatment, research, prevention, and education. *Molecular Psychiatry, 27*(3), 1331–1338. https://doi.org/10.1038/s41380-021-01367-9

Teicher, M. H., & Parigger, A. (2015). The 'Maltreatment and Abuse Chronology of Exposure' (MACE) scale for the retrospective assessment of abuse and neglect during development. *PLOS ONE, 10*(2), e0117423. https://doi.org/10.1371/journal.pone.0117423

Terpou, B. A., Harricharan, S., McKinnon, M. C., Frewen, P., Jetly, R., & Lanius, R. A. (2019). The effects of trauma on brain and body: A unifying role for the midbrain periaqueductal gray. *Journal of Neuroscience Research*, *97*(9), 1110–1140. https://doi.org/10.1002/jnr.24447

Terr, L. C. (1988). What happens to early memories of trauma? A study of twenty children under age five at the time of documented traumatic events. *Journal of the American Academy of Child and Adolescent Psychiatry*, *27*, 96–104. https://doi.org/10.1097/00004583-198801000-00015

Terr, L. (1993). *Unchained memories*. Basic Books.

Tessler, M., & Nelson, K. (1994). Making memories: The influence of joint encoding on later recall by young children. *Consciousness and Cognition*, *3*, 307–326. https://doi.org/10.1006/ccog.1994.1018

Thabet, A. M., Thabet, S., & Vostanis, P. (2018). The relationship between trauma due to war, post-traumatic stress disorder and fears among Palestinian children. *EC Paediatrics, 7*(3), 171–178.

Thabet, A. A., & Vostanis, P. (1999). Post-traumatic stress reactions in children of war. *Journal of Child Psychology and Psychiatry*, *40*, 385–391. https://doi.org/10.1111/1469-7610.00456

Thekkumthala, D., Schalinski, I., Parigger, A., Ruf-Leuschner, M., Elbert, T. & Schauer, M. (2023). *KERF-I. Belastende Kindheitserfahrungen* [KERF-I. Adverse Childhood Experiences]. https://www.testarchiv.eu/en/test/9008437 (KERF-40-I)

Thekkumthala, D., Schauer, M., Ruf-Leuschner, M., Kraus, B., Gruber, M., & Elbert, T. (2019). Borderline personality disorder symptoms in relation to adverse childhood experiences and balance performance. *Mental Health & Prevention*, *14*, 200167. https://doi.org/10.1016/j.mhp.2019.200167

Thomson, I. (2019). *Primo Levi: The elements of a life*. Penguin Random House.

Torre, J. B., & Lieberman, M. D. (2018). Putting feelings into words: Affect labeling as implicit emotion regulation. *Emotion Review*, *10*(2), 116–124. https://doi.org/10.1177/1754073917742706

Tremblay, R. E., Japel, C., Perusse, D., Mcduff, P., Boivin, M., Zoccolillo, M., & Montplaisir, J. (1999). The search for the age of 'onset' of physical aggression: Rousseau and Bandura revisited. *Criminal Behaviour and Mental Health*, *9*, 8–23. https://doi.org/10.1002/cbm.28

Troop, N. A., & Hiskey, S. (2013). Social defeat and PTSD symptoms following trauma. *British Journal of Clinical Psychology*, *52*(4), 365–379. https://doi.org/10.1111/bjc.12022

Tseng, Y. T., Schaefke, B., Wei, P., & Wang, L. (2023). Defensive responses: Behaviour, the brain and the body. *Nature Reviews Neuroscience*, *24*(11), 655–671. https://doi.org/10.1038/s41583-023-00736-3

Tulving, E. (2001). Episodic memory and common sense: how far apart? *Philosophical Transactions of the Royal Society of London Series B: Biological Science*, *356*, 1505–1515. https://doi.org/10.1098/rstb.2001.0937

Turner, S. (1999). *Angry young men in camps: Gender, age and class relations among Burundian refugees in Tanzania* (Working Paper No. 9). Roskilde University, Institute of Development Studies.

Ullmann, E., Licinio, N., Bornstein, S. R., Lanzman, R. S., Kirschbaum, C., Sierau, S., Doehnert, C., Zimmermann, P., Kindler, H., Schauer, M., Ruf-Leuschner, M., Fegert, J. M., von Klitzing, K., & Ziegenhain, U. (2017). Counteracting posttraumatic LHPA activation in refugee mothers and their infants. *Molecular Psychiatry*, *23*, 2–5. https://doi.org/10.1038/mp.2017.235

UN General Assembly. (1984). *Convention against torture and other cruel, inhuman or degrading treatment or punishment*. https://www.ohchr.org/en/instruments-mechanisms/instruments/convention-against-torture-and-other-cruel-inhuman-or-degrading

UNICEF. (2001). *The state of the world's children 2001*.

UNICEF. (2022). *UNICEF global annual results report 2022*. https://www.unicef.org/media/143226/file/Global%20Annual%20Results%20Report%202022%20:%20Goal%20area%203.pdf

United Nations High Commissioner For Refugees. (2023). *Mid-year trends 2023*. https://www.unhcr.org/mid-year-trends-report-2023; https://www.unhcr.org/refugee-statistics

United Nations High Commissioner For Refugees. (2002). *Extensive abuse of West African refugee children reported*. https://www.unhcr.org/news/news-releases/extensive-abuse-west-african-refugee-children-reported

Vagi, K. J., Rothman, E. F., Latzman, N. E., Tharp, A. T., Hall, D. M., & Breiding, M. J. (2013). Beyond correlates: A review of risk and protective factors for adolescent dating violence perpetration. *Journal Of Youth And Adolescence*, *42*(4), 633–649. https://doi.org/10.1007/s10964-013-9907-7

Vaidya, N., Marquand, A. F., Nees, F., Siehl, S., & Schumann, G. (2024). The impact of psychosocial adversity on brain and behaviour: an overview of existing knowledge and directions for future research. *Molecular Psychiatry*. Advance online publication. https://doi.org/10.1038/s41380-024-02556-y

Vaillancourt, T., & Sharma, A. (2011). Intolerance of sexy peers: Intrasexual competition among women. *Aggressive behavior*, *37*(6), 569–577. https://doi.org/10.1002/ab.20413

van Boetzelaer, E., Browne, J. L., Vaid, S., Pellecchia, U., van de Kamp, J., Franco, O. H., & Baidjoe, A. Y. (2023). Elderly people in humanitarian crises, a forgotten population: A call for action. *PLOS Global Public Health*, *3*(7), e0002142. https://doi.org/10.1371/journal.pgph.0002142

Van der Kolk, B. A. (1989). The compulsion to repeat the trauma: Re-enactment, revictimization, and masochism. *Psychiatric Clinics of North America*, *12*(2), 389–411. https://doi.org/10.1016/S0193-953X(18)30439-8

van der Kolk, B. (1995). Dissociation and the fragmentary nature of traumatic memories: overview and exploratory study. *Journal of Traumatic Stress*, *8*, 4. https://doi.org/10.1002/jts.2490080402

van der Kolk, B. A. (1996). Trauma and memory. In B. A. van der Kolk, A. C. McFarlane, & L. Weisaeth (Eds.), *Traumatic stress*. Guilford Press.

Van Es, C. M., Velu, M. E., Sleijpen, M., van der Aa, N., Boelen, P. A., & Mooren, T. (2023). Trauma-focused treatment for traumatic stress symptoms in unaccompanied refugee minors: a multiple baseline case series. *Frontiers in Psychology*, *14*, 1125740.

Velu, M. E., Martens, I., Shahab, M., de Roos, C., Jongedijk, R. A., Schok, M., & Mooren, T. (2022). Trauma-focused treatments for refugee children: Study protocol for a randomized controlled trial of the effectiveness of KIDNET versus EMDR therapy versus a waitlist control group (KIEM). *Trials*, *23*(1), 1–11. https://doi.org/10.1186/s13063-022-06178-z

Volpe, E. M., Quinn, C. R., Resch, K., Douglas, V., & Cerulli, C. (2016). Assessing the feasibility and acceptability of narrative exposure therapy to address IPV-related mental health in parenting and pregnant adolescents. *Journal of Family Violence*, *32*, 439–452. https://doi.org/10.1007/s10896-016-9818-y

Volpe, E. M., Quinn, C. R., Resch, K., Sommers, M. S., Wieling, E., & Cerulli, C. (2017). Narrative exposure therapy: A proposed model to address IPV-related PTSD in parenting and pregnant adolescents. *Family & Community Health*, *40*(3), 258. https://doi.org/10.1097/FCH.0000000000000072

Wagenaar, W. A., & Groeneweg, J. (1990). The memory of concentration camp survivors. *Applied Cognitive Psychology*, *4*, 77–87. https://doi.org/10.1002/acp.2350040202

Walker, E. A., Katon, W. J., Hansom, J., Harrop-Griffiths, J., Holm, L., Jones, M. L., Hickok, L., & Jemelka, R. P. (1992). Medical and psychiatric symptoms in women with childhood sexual abuse. *Psychosomatic Medicine*, *54*, 658–664. https://doi.org/10.1097/00006842-199211000-00005

Watkins, J. G. (1971). The affect bridge. *The International Journal of Clinical and Experimental Hypnosis*, *19*(1), 21–27.

Weathers, F. W., Blake, D. D., Schnurr, P. P., Kaloupek, D. G., Marx, B. P., & Keane, T. M. (2013). *The Life Events Checklist for DSM-5 (LEC-5) – Standard* [Measurement instrument]. National Center for PTSD. https://www.ptsd.va.gov/professional/assessment/te-measures/life_events_checklist.asp

Weathers, F. W., Litz, B. T., Keane, T. M., Palmieri, P. A., Marx, B. P., & Schnurr, P. P. (2013). *The PTSD checklist for DSM-5 (PCL-5)*. https://www.ptsd.va.gov/professional/assessment/adult-sr/ptsd-checklist.asp

Webb, R. T., Antonsen, S., Carr, M. J., Appleby, L., Pedersen, C. B., & Mok, P. L. H. (2017). Self-harm and violent criminality among young people who experienced trauma-related hospital admission during childhood: A Danish national cohort study. *Lancet Public Health*, *2*(7), e314–e322. https://doi.org/10.1016/S2468-2667(17)30094-4

Webb, M., Heisler, D., Call, S., Chickering, S. A., & Colburn, T. A. (2007). Shame, guilt, symptoms of depression, and reported history of psychological maltreatment. *Child Abuse & Neglect*, *31*(11-12), 1143–1153. https://doi.org/10.1016/j.chiabu.2007.09.003

Websdale, N. (2010). *Familicidal hearts: The emotional styles of 211 killers*. Oxford University Press.

Weierstall, R., & Elbert, T. (2011). The Appetitive Aggression Scale. *European Journal of Psychotraumatology*, *2*, 8430. https://doi.org/10.3402/ejpt.v2i0.8430

Weierstall, R., Huth, S., Knecht, J., Nandi, C., & Elbert, T. (2012). Appetitive aggression as a resilience factor against trauma disorders: Appetitive aggression and PTSD in German World War II Veterans. *PLOS ONE*, *7*(12): e50891. https://doi.org/10.1371/journal.pone.0050891

Weine, S. M., Becker, D. F., McGlashan, T. H., Laub, D., Lazrove, S., & Vojvoda, D. (1995). Psychiatric consequences of "ethnic cleansing": Clinical assessments and trauma testimonies of newly resettled Bosnian refugees. *American Journal of Psychiatry*, *152*, 536–542.

Weine, S. M., Kulenovic, A. D., Pavkovic, I., & Gibbons, R. (1998). Testimony psychotherapy in Bosnian refugees: A pilot study. *American Journal of Psychiatry*, *155*, 1720–1726. https://doi.org/10.1176/ajp.155.12.1720

Weine, S., & Laub, D. (1995). Narrative constructions of historical realities in testimony with Bosnian survivors of "ethnic cleansing." *Psychiatry*, *58*, 246–260. https://doi.org/10.1080/00332747.1995.11024729

Weinhold, S. L., Göder, R., Pabst, A., Scharff, A. L., Schauer, M., Baier, P. C., Aldenhoff, J., Elbert, T., & Seeck-Hirschner, M. (2017). Sleep recordings in individuals with borderline personality disorder before and after trauma therapy. *Journal of Neural Transmission*, *124*, 99–107. https://doi.org/10.1007/s00702-016-1536-3

Weisman, O., Aderka, I. M., Marom, S., Hermesh, H., & Gilboa-Schechtman, E. (2011). Social rank and affiliation in social anxiety disorder. *Behaviour Research and Therapy*, *49*(6-7), 399–405. https://doi.org/10.1016/j.brat.2011.03.010

Westerhof, G. J., Alea, N., & Bluck, S. (2020). Narrative and identity: The importance of our personal past in later life. In A. K. Thomas & A. Gutchess (Eds.), *The Cambridge handbook of cognitive aging: A life course perspective* (pp. 383–399). Cambridge University Press. https://doi.org/10.1017/9781108552684.024

Widom, C. S. (1999). Posttraumatic stress disorder in abused and neglected children grown up. *American Journal of Psychiatry*, *156*, 1223–1229. https://doi.org/10.1176/ajp.156.8.1223

Widom, C. S., Czaja, S. J., & Paris, J. (2009). A prospective investigation of borderline personality disorder in abused and neglected children followed up into adulthood. *Journal of Personality Disorders*, *5*, 433–446 https://doi.org/10.1521/pedi.2009.23.5.433

Widom, C. S., & Morris, S. (1997). Accuracy of adult recollections of childhood victimization: Part II: Childhood sexual abuse. *Psychological Assessment*, *9*, 34–46. https://doi.org/10.1037/1040-3590.9.1.34

Widom, C. S., & Shepard, R. L. (1996). Accuracy of adult recollections of childhood victimization: Part I: Childhood physical abuse. *Psychological Assessment*, *8*, 412–421. https://doi.org/10.1037/1040-3590.8.4.412

Wiesel, E. (1996). *Interview: Holocaust survivor's storyteller.* Academy of Achievement, Museum of Living History. https://achievement.org/video/elie-wiesel-6/

Wilker, S., Catani, C., Wittmann, J., Preusse, M., Schmidt, T., May, T., Ertl, V., Doering, B., Rosner, R., Zindler, A., &Neuner, F. (2020). The efficacy of Narrative Exposure Therapy for Children (KIDNET) as a treatment for traumatized young refugees versus treatment as usual: Study protocol for a multi-center randomized controlled trial (YOURTREAT). *Trials*, *21*(1), 1–16.

Wilker, S., Kleim, B., Geiling, A., Pfeiffer, A., Elbert, T., & Kolassa, I. T. (2017). Mental defeat and cumulative trauma experiences predict trauma-related psychopathology: Evidence from a post-conflict population in Northern Uganda. *Clinical Psychological Science*, *5*, 974–984. https://doi.org/10.1177/2167702617719946

Wilker, S., Pfeiffer, A., Elbert, T., Ovuga, E., Karabatsiakis, A., Krumbholz, A., Thieme, D., Schelling, G., & Kollassa, I. T. (2016). Endocannabinoid concentrations in hair are associated with PTSD symptom severity. *Psychoneuroendocrinology*, *67*, 198–206. https://doi.org/10.1016/j.psyneuen.2016.02.010

Wilker, S., Pfeiffer, A., Kolassa, S., Koslowski, D., Elbert, T., & Kolassa, I. T. (2015). How to quantify exposure to traumatic stressors? Reliability and validity of measures for cumulative trauma exposure in a post-conflict population. *European Journal of Psychotraumatology*, *6*, 28306. https://doi.org/10.3402/ejpt.v6.28306

Williams, L. M., & Banyard, V. L. (1999). *Trauma and memory*. Sage.

Wittmann, J., Groß, M., Catani, C., Schmidt, T., Neldner, S., Wilker, S., May, T., Ertl, V., Rosner, R., Zindler, A., Odenwald, M., & Neuner, F. (2022). The efficacy of Narrative Exposure Therapy for Children (KIDNET) as a treatment for traumatized young refugees versus treatment as usual: Update to the study protocol for the multi-center randomized controlled trial YOURTREAT. *Trials*, *23*(1), 1–5

Wolitzky-Taylor, K., Fenwick, K., Lengnick-Hall, R., Grossman, J., Bearman, S. K., Arch, J., Miranda, J., & Chung, B. (2018). A preliminary exploration of the barriers to delivering (and receiving) exposure-based cognitive behavioral therapy for anxiety disorders in adult community mental health settings. *Community Mental Health Journal*, *54*, 899–911. https://doi.org/10.1007/s10597-018-0252-x

World Health Organization. (2017). *International classification of diseases – 11th revision.*

World Health Organization. (2021). *WHO's 7 policy recommendations on building resilient health systems*. https://www.who.int/news/item/19-10-2021-who-s-7-policy-recommendations-on-building-resilient-health-systems

Wyles, P., O'Leary, P., & Tsantefski, M. (2023). Bearing witness as a process for responding to trauma survivors: A review. *Trauma, Violence, & Abuse*, *24*(5), 3078–3093. https://doi.org/10.1177/15248380221124262

Zang, Y., Hunt, N., & Cox, T. (2013). A randomized controlled pilot study: The effectiveness of narrative exposure therapy with adult survivors of the Sichuan earthquake. *BMC Psychiatry*, *13*, 41. https://doi.org/10.1186/1471-244X-13-41

Zehr, H. (2015). *The little book of restorative justice: Revised and updated*. Simon & Schuster.

Zehr, H., MacRae, A., Pranis, K., & Amstutz, L. S. (2022). *The big book of restorative justice: Four classic justice & peacebuilding books in one volume*. Simon and Schuster.

Zlotnick, C., Rodriguez, B. F., Weisberg, R. E., Bruce, S. E., Spencer, M. A., Culpeper, L., & Keller, M. B. (2004). Chronicity in posttraumatic stress disorder and predictors over the course of posttraumatic stress disorder among primary care patients. *Journal of Nervous and Mental Disease*, *192*, 153–159. https://doi.org/10.1097/01.nmd.0000110287.16635.8e

Appendix and Online Supplementary Materials

The following materials for your book can be downloaded free of charge once you register on the Hogrefe website:

Appendix 1: Checklist for Threats to Human Life (THL)

Appendix 2: Examples of Narrations of Life Experiences Resulting From NET

In addition to the appendices, the following handouts that are printed as figures in the book are also part of the online supplementary materials.

Handout 1: Illustration of the Narrative Exposure Therapy (NET) process step-by-step (Figure 11)

Handout 2: The Narrative Exposure cycle (Figure 17)

Handout 3: Exposure conversation style – contrasting past with present, moving back and forth in time (Figure 20)

Handout 4: Readback is a mandatory step in NET (Figure 26)

Handout 5: Structure of Narrative Exposure sessions (Figures 28, 30, 31)

Handout 6: Steps of KIDNET (Figure 35 and Figure 37)

Handout 7: The procedure of the NETfacts health system (Figure 41)

Handout 8: Counteracting dissociation (Figure 45)

DOWNLOAD

How to proceed:

1. Go to www.hgf.io/media and create a user account. If you already have one, please log in.
2. Go to **My supplementary materials** in your account dashboard and enter the code below. You will automatically be redirected to the download area, where you can access and download the supplementary materials.

   Code: B-LC8ZAD

To make sure you have permanent direct access to all the materials, we recommend that you download them and save them on your computer.

Checklist for Threats to Human Life - THL

THL English
May 2016

Authors:
Anke Köbach
Thomas Elbert
Maggie Schauer

For the interviewer only: *The present questionnaire is a comprehensive instrument for the assessment of adverse life experiences with potential long-term effects on mental health. In the first part, the THL details sociodemographic data and details of familial crisis. The second part assesses life events that threatened the social or physical integrity of the interviewee as well as acts in which the interviewee intentionally threatened the integrity of him/herself or another person. The manual outlines the theoretical principles of the questionnaire and provides a detailed guide for the application and analysis of the questionnaire.*

Introduction: "Every person encounters challenging or stressful situations in the course of his or her life. Some of these life events are hard to forget and can even influence future feelings, thoughts and actions. Experiences associated with personal loss, fear, or disgust, as well as violence perpetrated against other human beings can be particularly difficult to deal with. I am now going to ask you some questions about your current life situation and then I will describe some experiences and ask if they apply to you. Of course, all information will remain strictly confidential."

Date:	
Code:	
Name of the interviewer:	
Interview with translation?	Yes ◯ No ◯
Language:	
Name of the translator:	

SOCIODEMOGRAPHIC DATA

PERSONAL INFORMATION

Date of birth:	
Sex:	male ◯ female ◯
Country and town of birth:	
Nationality:	
Native language:	
Religious affiliation:	Yes ◯ No ◯
If yes:	Islam ◯ Christianity ◯ Hinduism ◯ Buddhism ◯ Judaism ◯ other ◯ n.a. ◯
Did you ever have to leave your home and seek asylum somewhere else?	Yes ◯ No ◯

INFORMATION ABOUT EDUCATION AND PROFESSION

Years of formal education	______ Years
University degree	Yes ◯ No ◯
Do you have a job (incl. housewife)?	Yes ◯ No ◯
Current occupation:	
First occupation:	
Have you ever performed surgery (incl. circumcision)?	Yes ◯ No ◯
Did you ever serve in a (para-)military unit or as a reservist?	Yes ◯ No ◯
Were you ever actively involved in a military mission?	Yes ◯ No ◯
If yes, how old were you then?	
Have you ever been involved in the torture of other people (carried out by self or/and fellow soldiers)?	Yes ◯ No ◯

Contact: anke.koebach@uni-konstanz.de

This page may be reproduced by the purchaser for personal/clinical use.
From: M. Schauer, T. Elbert, & F. Neuner: *Narrative Exposure Therapy (NET) for Survivors of Traumatic Stress* (3rd ed.) (ISBN 9780889375956)
© 2025 Hogrefe Publishing

INFORMATION ABOUT RECREATIONAL ACTIVITIES

Do you hunt? (in leisure time or professionally)	Yes ◯ No ◯
Do you practice martial arts?	Yes ◯ No ◯
Do you have a pet?	Yes ◯ No ◯
If yes, which pet (if dog, ask for its breed):	*Attack dog? Yes* ◯ *No* ◯
Do you possess firearms such as a pistol, gun, grenades, etc.?	Yes ◯ No ◯
Do you possess other weapons such as a knife, nightstick, etc.?	Yes ◯ No ◯

INFORMATION ABOUT THE FAMILY SITUATION

Are you in a long-term relationship?	Yes ◯ No ◯ Widowed ◯	
Do you have children (only biological offspring)?	Yes ◯ No ◯	
If yes, how many daughters and sons?	______ daughters ______ sons	
If yes, do you feel that your children are happy and able to successfully manage their lives?		
Successful in career or at school:	1 ◯ 2 ◯ 3 ◯ 4 ◯ 5 ◯ n.a. ◯	**Scaling information:** 1 = Not at all 2 = Not really 3 = Neutral 4 = Somewhat true 5 = Very true
Successful in finding (a) romantic partner(s):	1 ◯ 2 ◯ 3 ◯ 4 ◯ 5 ◯ n.a. ◯	
Popular within their social environment:	1 ◯ 2 ◯ 3 ◯ 4 ◯ 5 ◯ n.a. ◯	
Good physical and mental health:	1 ◯ 2 ◯ 3 ◯ 4 ◯ 5 ◯ n.a. ◯	
Do you perceive the support within your family as strong?	1 ◯ 2 ◯ 3 ◯ 4 ◯ 5 ◯	

PHYSICAL HEALTH

Have you suffered from one or more of the following health problems within the last 4 weeks:

Headache	Yes ◯ No ◯	Pyrosis	Yes ◯ No ◯
Sniffles	Yes ◯ No ◯	Stomach-ache	Yes ◯ No ◯
Cold	Yes ◯ No ◯	Gastro-intestinal disease	Yes ◯ No ◯
Flu	Yes ◯ No ◯	Skin rash	Yes ◯ No ◯
Fever or chills	Yes ◯ No ◯	Back pain	Yes ◯ No ◯
Pain in the limbs	Yes ◯ No ◯	Joint and muscle pain	Yes ◯ No ◯

Have you ever been diagnosed with a chronic and impairing, or life-threatening disease?	Yes ◯ No ◯
If yes, which disease?	Age:
Did you ever undergo surgery under general anesthetic?	Yes ◯ No ◯
If yes, which type of surgery?	Age:
Have you ever had psychotherapeutic treatment? Which diagnosis? Yes ◯ No ◯	

Have you ingested one or more of the following medications within the last week?

Pain killers	Yes ◯ No ◯	Anxiolytics/Benzodiazepines	Yes ◯ No ◯
Sleeping pills (Hypnotics)	Yes ◯ No ◯	Neuroleptics	Yes ◯ No ◯

Were one or more of your family members ever diagnosed with a chronic and imparing, or life-threatening disease? How old were you at that time?

Father (incl. primary male attachment figure):	Yes ◯ No ◯	Age:
Mother (incl. primary female attachment figure):	Yes ◯ No ◯	Age:
Own child/ren:	Yes ◯ No ◯	Age:
Siblings:	Yes ◯ No ◯	Age:
Spouse:	Yes ◯ No ◯	Age:

Contact: anke.koebach@uni-konstanz.de

This page may be reproduced by the purchaser for personal/clinical use.
From: M. Schauer, T. Elbert, & F. Neuner: *Narrative Exposure Therapy (NET) for Survivors of Traumatic Stress* (3rd ed.) (ISBN 9780889375956)
© 2025 Hogrefe Publishing

Have one or more of your family members died unexpectedly (incident, war, etc.)? How old were you at that time?		
Father (incl. primary male attachment figure):	Yes ◯ No ◯	Age:
Mother (incl. primary female attachment figure):	Yes ◯ No ◯	Age:
Own child/ren:	Yes ◯ No ◯	Age:
Siblings:	Yes ◯ No ◯	Age:
Spouse:	Yes ◯ No ◯	Age:
Does one of your relatives suffer from a hereditary disease (grandparents, parents, siblings, aunts, uncles, own children)?		Yes ◯ No ◯
Is one of your relatives (siblings, aunts, uncles, own children) not able to have children?		Yes ◯ No ◯

EVENT LIST

"In the following part, I will describe a number of different experiences and would like to know if you have encountered any such events in your life. We will not go into details of any specific event, but I will ask you how old you were when it happened, in which context it happened, and whether it happened regularly."

For the interviewer only: *Then ask about the events one after another (main question) and explain them with the help of the examples given on the right-hand side. If your interviewee experienced one or more events of one item, ask for the age at which the event occured, the person or the circumstances responsible for it and the regularity with which the event occured. Note this as follows:*

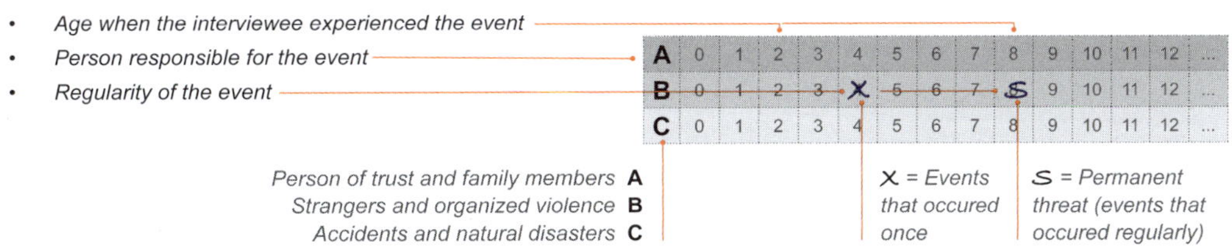

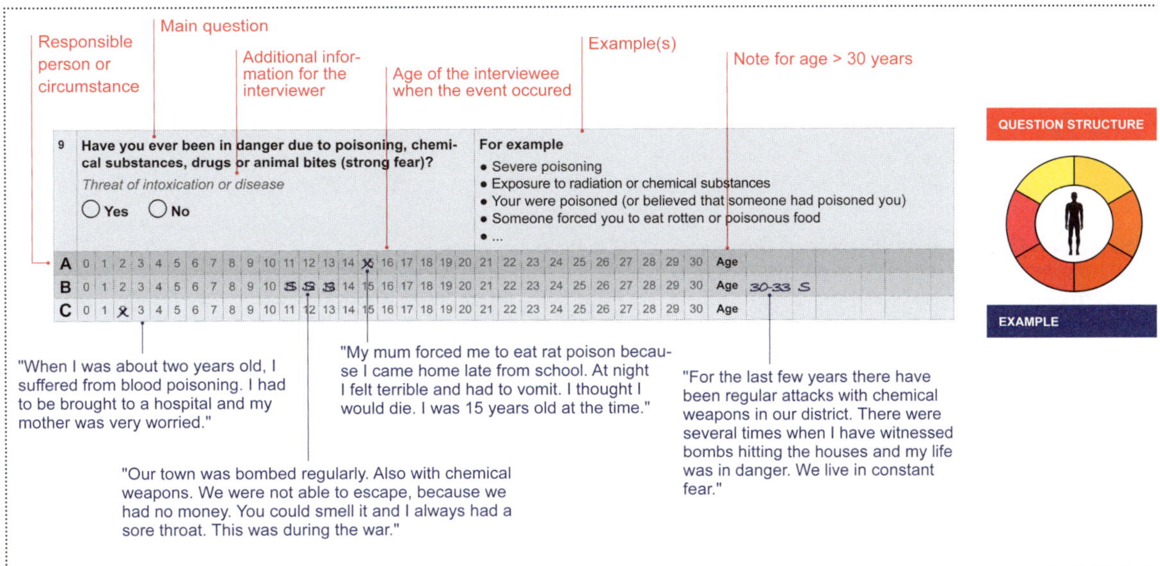

This page may be reproduced by the purchaser for personal/clinical use.
From: M. Schauer, T. Elbert, & F. Neuner: *Narrative Exposure Therapy (NET) for Survivors of Traumatic Stress* (3rd ed.) (ISBN 9780889375956)
© 2025 Hogrefe Publishing

A Person of trust or family member
B Strangers and organized violence
C Accidents and natural disasters

x/s Isolated events versus permanent threats

THREATS TO PHYSICAL INTEGRITY

1 Have you ever been in danger due to extreme height or speed (strong anxiety)?

Threat of fall or high speed

○ Yes ○ No

For example
- Exposure or fall from great height
- Life-threatening, high-speed driving against your will

A	0	1	2	3	4	5	6	7	8	9	10	11	12	13	14	15	16	17	18	19	20	21	22	23	24	25	26	27	28	29	30	Age
B	0	1	2	3	4	5	6	7	8	9	10	11	12	13	14	15	16	17	18	19	20	21	22	23	24	25	26	27	28	29	30	Age
C	0	1	2	3	4	5	6	7	8	9	10	11	12	13	14	15	16	17	18	19	20	21	22	23	24	25	26	27	28	29	30	Age

2 Have you ever thought you would die from hunger or thirst?

○ Yes ○ No

For example
- Famine in times of war
- Extreme poverty
- Deprived of food by caregiver

A	0	1	2	3	4	5	6	7	8	9	10	11	12	13	14	15	16	17	18	19	20	21	22	23	24	25	26	27	28	29	30	Age
B	0	1	2	3	4	5	6	7	8	9	10	11	12	13	14	15	16	17	18	19	20	21	22	23	24	25	26	27	28	29	30	Age
C	0	1	2	3	4	5	6	7	8	9	10	11	12	13	14	15	16	17	18	19	20	21	22	23	24	25	26	27	28	29	30	Age

3 Did you have to escape from a sudden danger?

Escape or run from a sudden life threat (no planned escape or migration)

○ Yes ○ No

For example
- Run away from an aggressive person (offender, robber, hooligan, etc.)
- Escape from police or (para)military violence
- Run away from a dangerous animal
- You had to run away from a dangerous natural force such as an earthquake, tsunami, hurricane, volcanic eruption, etc.

A	0	1	2	3	4	5	6	7	8	9	10	11	12	13	14	15	16	17	18	19	20	21	22	23	24	25	26	27	28	29	30	Age
B	0	1	2	3	4	5	6	7	8	9	10	11	12	13	14	15	16	17	18	19	20	21	22	23	24	25	26	27	28	29	30	Age
C	0	1	2	3	4	5	6	7	8	9	10	11	12	13	14	15	16	17	18	19	20	21	22	23	24	25	26	27	28	29	30	Age

4 Have you ever been injured or endangered by fire or extreme heat (strong fear)?

○ Yes ○ No

For example
- Someone held your hand or another part of your body to a flame
- Someone stubbed out a cigarette on your skin
- Your life was in danger due to a sudden fire in close proximity
- You experienced a volcanic eruption without means of escape
- Someone tortured you with electric shocks
- Someone burnt you with chemicals
- Someone scalded you with hot liquids

A	0	1	2	3	4	5	6	7	8	9	10	11	12	13	14	15	16	17	18	19	20	21	22	23	24	25	26	27	28	29	30	Age
B	0	1	2	3	4	5	6	7	8	9	10	11	12	13	14	15	16	17	18	19	20	21	22	23	24	25	26	27	28	29	30	Age
C	0	1	2	3	4	5	6	7	8	9	10	11	12	13	14	15	16	17	18	19	20	21	22	23	24	25	26	27	28	29	30	Age

5 Have you ever <u>witnessed</u> another person being injured or endangered by fire or extreme heat (strong fear)?

○ Yes ○ No

For example, someone...
- Held hand(s) or another part of a person's body to a flame
- Stubbed out a cigarette on a person's skin
- Was tortured with electric shocks
- Was burnt with chemicals
- Was scalded with hot liquids

A	0	1	2	3	4	5	6	7	8	9	10	11	12	13	14	15	16	17	18	19	20	21	22	23	24	25	26	27	28	29	30	Age
B	0	1	2	3	4	5	6	7	8	9	10	11	12	13	14	15	16	17	18	19	20	21	22	23	24	25	26	27	28	29	30	Age
C	0	1	2	3	4	5	6	7	8	9	10	11	12	13	14	15	16	17	18	19	20	21	22	23	24	25	26	27	28	29	30	Age

6 Has your life ever been in danger due to extreme cold (strong fear)?

Acute threat of freezing to death

○ Yes ○ No

A	0	1	2	3	4	5	6	7	8	9	10	11	12	13	14	15	16	17	18	19	20	21	22	23	24	25	26	27	28	29	30	Age

Contact: anke.koebach@uni-konstanz.de

This page may be reproduced by the purchaser for personal/clinical use.
From: M. Schauer, T. Elbert, & F. Neuner: *Narrative Exposure Therapy (NET) for Survivors of Traumatic Stress* (3rd ed.) (ISBN 9780889375956)
© 2025 Hogrefe Publishing

A Person of trust or family member
B Strangers and organized violence
C Accidents and natural disasters

x/s Isolated events versus permanent threats

7 **Have you ever been afraid of suffocation?**

○ Yes ○ No

For example

- Someone choked you
- You were in acute danger of drowning
- Someone poured water over your head, so you couldn't breathe (waterboarding)
- You did not get enough oxygen due to fire or other gas in a closed room
- Anaphylactic shock

A	0	1	2	3	4	5	6	7	8	9	10	11	12	13	14	15	16	17	18	19	20	21	22	23	24	25	26	27	28	29	30	Age
B	0	1	2	3	4	5	6	7	8	9	10	11	12	13	14	15	16	17	18	19	20	21	22	23	24	25	26	27	28	29	30	Age
C	0	1	2	3	4	5	6	7	8	9	10	11	12	13	14	15	16	17	18	19	20	21	22	23	24	25	26	27	28	29	30	Age

8 **Have you ever <u>witnessed</u> another person in danger of suffocation?**

○ Yes ○ No

For example

- Someone being choked
- Someone was struggling and in danger of drowning
- Water being poured over the person's mouth (waterboarding)
- Someone (almost) died due to fire or other gas in a closed room
- Someone suffered from an acute anaphylactic shock

A	0	1	2	3	4	5	6	7	8	9	10	11	12	13	14	15	16	17	18	19	20	21	22	23	24	25	26	27	28	29	30	Age
B	0	1	2	3	4	5	6	7	8	9	10	11	12	13	14	15	16	17	18	19	20	21	22	23	24	25	26	27	28	29	30	Age
C	0	1	2	3	4	5	6	7	8	9	10	11	12	13	14	15	16	17	18	19	20	21	22	23	24	25	26	27	28	29	30	Age

9 **Have you ever been in danger due to poisoning, chemical substances, drugs or animal bites (strong fear)?**

Threat of intoxication or disease

○ Yes ○ No

For example

- Severe blood poisoning
- Exposure to radiation or chemical substances
- You were poisoned (or believed that someone had poisoned you)
- Someone forced you to eat rotten or poisonous food
- Life-threatening bite from venomous or sick animal (i.e., snake, spider, fox)
- You experienced an attack with a chemical weapon (incl. teargas)
- You had surgery under unhygienic conditions

A	0	1	2	3	4	5	6	7	8	9	10	11	12	13	14	15	16	17	18	19	20	21	22	23	24	25	26	27	28	29	30	Age
B	0	1	2	3	4	5	6	7	8	9	10	11	12	13	14	15	16	17	18	19	20	21	22	23	24	25	26	27	28	29	30	Age
C	0	1	2	3	4	5	6	7	8	9	10	11	12	13	14	15	16	17	18	19	20	21	22	23	24	25	26	27	28	29	30	Age

10 **Have you ever experienced any type of sexual violence (without sexual intercourse)?**

Sexual abuse, assault

○ Yes ○ No

For example

- You were sexually touched against your will
- You were forced to sexually touch or satisfy another person sexually

A	0	1	2	3	4	5	6	7	8	9	10	11	12	13	14	15	16	17	18	19	20	21	22	23	24	25	26	27	28	29	30	Age
B	0	1	2	3	4	5	6	7	8	9	10	11	12	13	14	15	16	17	18	19	20	21	22	23	24	25	26	27	28	29	30	Age
C	0	1	2	3	4	5	6	7	8	9	10	11	12	13	14	15	16	17	18	19	20	21	22	23	24	25	26	27	28	29	30	Age

11 **Have you ever been forced to have sexual intercourse with someone?**

Rape

○ Yes ○ No

For example

- You were (violently) forced to have sexual intercourse with another person against your will, or at a time when you were mentally incapacitated

A	0	1	2	3	4	5	6	7	8	9	10	11	12	13	14	15	16	17	18	19	20	21	22	23	24	25	26	27	28	29	30	Age
B	0	1	2	3	4	5	6	7	8	9	10	11	12	13	14	15	16	17	18	19	20	21	22	23	24	25	26	27	28	29	30	Age
C	0	1	2	3	4	5	6	7	8	9	10	11	12	13	14	15	16	17	18	19	20	21	22	23	24	25	26	27	28	29	30	Age

12 **Have you ever <u>witnessed</u> any type of sexual violence?**

Witnessed sexual abuse or rape

○ Yes ○ No

For example

- You were forced to watch others having sexual intercourse or another person being touched sexually against his/her will

A	0	1	2	3	4	5	6	7	8	9	10	11	12	13	14	15	16	17	18	19	20	21	22	23	24	25	26	27	28	29	30	Age
B	0	1	2	3	4	5	6	7	8	9	10	11	12	13	14	15	16	17	18	19	20	21	22	23	24	25	26	27	28	29	30	Age
C	0	1	2	3	4	5	6	7	8	9	10	11	12	13	14	15	16	17	18	19	20	21	22	23	24	25	26	27	28	29	30	Age

Contact: anke.koebach@uni-konstanz.de

This page may be reproduced by the purchaser for personal/clinical use.
From: M. Schauer, T. Elbert, & F. Neuner: *Narrative Exposure Therapy (NET) for Survivors of Traumatic Stress* (3rd ed.) (ISBN 9780889375956)
© 2025 Hogrefe Publishing

A *Person of trust or family member*
B *Strangers and organized violence*
C *Accidents and natural disasters*

x/s Isolated events versus permanent threats

13 Have you ever been threatened with death?

This item is only applicable if the person really believed that he/she could be murdered or injured

○ Yes ○ No

For example
- Someone threatened verbally and/or with gestures to hurt or kill you (i.e., domestic or organized violence)
- You received threats of death because of something you have done or because of who you are (i.e., ethnicity, race, political activities, etc.)?
- Pseudo-execution
- Someone threatened you with torture (i.e., police, military)
- Someone threatened you with a gun

A	0	1	2	3	4	5	6	7	8	9	10	11	12	13	14	15	16	17	18	19	20	21	22	23	24	25	26	27	28	29	30	Age
B	0	1	2	3	4	5	6	7	8	9	10	11	12	13	14	15	16	17	18	19	20	21	22	23	24	25	26	27	28	29	30	Age

14 Have you ever been physically assaulted by another person (without an object or weapon) or did you have an accident?

Physical abuse

○ Yes ○ No

For example
- Being beaten, restrained, kicked, punched, slapped, etc.
- You were hit by a falling object (constuction work, etc.)
- You had a traffic accident (moderately severe)

! *This may have occurred as a disciplinary measure, e.g., at school, home, etc., in a physical argument with peers, for some other reason or for no reason.*

A	0	1	2	3	4	5	6	7	8	9	10	11	12	13	14	15	16	17	18	19	20	21	22	23	24	25	26	27	28	29	30	Age
B	0	1	2	3	4	5	6	7	8	9	10	11	12	13	14	15	16	17	18	19	20	21	22	23	24	25	26	27	28	29	30	Age
C	0	1	2	3	4	5	6	7	8	9	10	11	12	13	14	15	16	17	18	19	20	21	22	23	24	25	26	27	28	29	30	Age

15 Have you ever witnessed someone else being-physically assaulted by another person (without an object or weapon) or have an accident?

Witnessed physical abuse

○ Yes ○ No

For example, someone...
- Was beaten, restrained, kicked, punched, slapped, etc.
- Was hit by a falling object (construction work, etc.)
- Had a traffic accident (moderately, partly experiences consciously)

! *This may have occurred as a disciplinary measure, e.g., at school, home, etc., in a physical argument with peers, for some other reason or for no reason.*

A	0	1	2	3	4	5	6	7	8	9	10	11	12	13	14	15	16	17	18	19	20	21	22	23	24	25	26	27	28	29	30	Age
B	0	1	2	3	4	5	6	7	8	9	10	11	12	13	14	15	16	17	18	19	20	21	22	23	24	25	26	27	28	29	30	Age
C	0	1	2	3	4	5	6	7	8	9	10	11	12	13	14	15	16	17	18	19	20	21	22	23	24	25	26	27	28	29	30	Age

16 Have you ever been severely physically assaulted by another person (including violence with blunt objects) or did you have a severe accident?

Severe physical abuse

○ Yes ○ No

For example
- You were beaten or kicked so heavily that you thought you would die or be permanently disabled
- You were beaten with a belt, stick, etc.
- Traffic accident (severe, at least partially consciously experienced)
- Other severe accidents with inner tissue damage (amongst other injuries)

A	0	1	2	3	4	5	6	7	8	9	10	11	12	13	14	15	16	17	18	19	20	21	22	23	24	25	26	27	28	29	30	Age
B	0	1	2	3	4	5	6	7	8	9	10	11	12	13	14	15	16	17	18	19	20	21	22	23	24	25	26	27	28	29	30	Age
C	0	1	2	3	4	5	6	7	8	9	10	11	12	13	14	15	16	17	18	19	20	21	22	23	24	25	26	27	28	29	30	Age

17 Have you ever witnessed a severe physical assault (including violence with blunt objects) or a severe accident?

Witnessed severe physical abuse

○ Yes ○ No

For example, someone...
- Being beaten or kicked so heavily that you thought the person would die or be permanently disabled
- Has been beaten with a belt, stick, etc.
- Had a severe traffic accident
- Had another severe accident causing inner tissue damage (amongst other injuries)

A	0	1	2	3	4	5	6	7	8	9	10	11	12	13	14	15	16	17	18	19	20	21	22	23	24	25	26	27	28	29	30	Age
B	0	1	2	3	4	5	6	7	8	9	10	11	12	13	14	15	16	17	18	19	20	21	22	23	24	25	26	27	28	29	30	Age
C	0	1	2	3	4	5	6	7	8	9	10	11	12	13	14	15	16	17	18	19	20	21	22	23	24	25	26	27	28	29	30	Age

18 Have you ever been injured with a firearm?

○ Yes ○ No

For example
- You were shot
- You experienced a bomb attack in very close proximity

A	0	1	2	3	4	5	6	7	8	9	10	11	12	13	14	15	16	17	18	19	20	21	22	23	24	25	26	27	28	29	30	Age
B	0	1	2	3	4	5	6	7	8	9	10	11	12	13	14	15	16	17	18	19	20	21	22	23	24	25	26	27	28	29	30	Age
C	0	1	2	3	4	5	6	7	8	9	10	11	12	13	14	15	16	17	18	19	20	21	22	23	24	25	26	27	28	29	30	Age

Contact: anke.koebach@uni-konstanz.de

This page may be reproduced by the purchaser for personal/clinical use.
From: M. Schauer, T. Elbert, & F. Neuner: *Narrative Exposure Therapy (NET) for Survivors of Traumatic Stress* (3rd ed.) (ISBN 9780889375956)
© 2025 Hogrefe Publishing

A Person of trust or family member
B Strangers and organized violence
C Accidents and natural disasters
x/s Isolated events versus permanent threats

19 Have you ever witnessed another person being injured with a firearm?
○ Yes ○ No

For example
- Someone was shot
- You witnessed a bomb attack or explosion from a distance, without being in serious danger

A	0	1	2	3	4	5	6	7	8	9	10	11	12	13	14	15	16	17	18	19	20	21	22	23	24	25	26	27	28	29	30	Age
B	0	1	2	3	4	5	6	7	8	9	10	11	12	13	14	15	16	17	18	19	20	21	22	23	24	25	26	27	28	29	30	Age
C	0	1	2	3	4	5	6	7	8	9	10	11	12	13	14	15	16	17	18	19	20	21	22	23	24	25	26	27	28	29	30	Age

20 Have you ever been injured or threatened with a sharp object?
○ Yes ○ No

For example
- With a knife, razor blade, machete, teeth, etc.
- Operation without anesthesia

! *No vaccinations or skin surgeries*

A	0	1	2	3	4	5	6	7	8	9	10	11	12	13	14	15	16	17	18	19	20	21	22	23	24	25	26	27	28	29	30	Age
B	0	1	2	3	4	5	6	7	8	9	10	11	12	13	14	15	16	17	18	19	20	21	22	23	24	25	26	27	28	29	30	Age
C	0	1	2	3	4	5	6	7	8	9	10	11	12	13	14	15	16	17	18	19	20	21	22	23	24	25	26	27	28	29	30	Age

21 Have you ever witnessed someone being injured or threatened with a sharp object?
○ Yes ○ No

For example
- Someone being injured with a knife, razor blade, machete, teeth, etc.
- Operation without anesthesia

A	0	1	2	3	4	5	6	7	8	9	10	11	12	13	14	15	16	17	18	19	20	21	22	23	24	25	26	27	28	29	30	Age
B	0	1	2	3	4	5	6	7	8	9	10	11	12	13	14	15	16	17	18	19	20	21	22	23	24	25	26	27	28	29	30	Age
C	0	1	2	3	4	5	6	7	8	9	10	11	12	13	14	15	16	17	18	19	20	21	22	23	24	25	26	27	28	29	30	Age

22 Have you been circumcised?
All types of female genital mutilation or circumcision of the male foreskin
○ Yes ○ No

0	1	2	3	4	5	6	7	8	9	10	11	12	13	14	15	16	17	18	19	20	21	22	23	24	25	26	27	28	29	30	Age

23 a Have you ever witnessed someone dying?
○ Yes ○ No

If yes, who? ______________________

For example
- Someone died because of a severe sickness
- People were shot, stabbed, etc. in a fighting or a physical argument
- Forced killing of family member(s)
- Natural death

C: *Natural death, sickness, fatal accident, death caused by natural disasters, etc.*
B: *Witnessed death, murder, killing, or homicide executed by a (para-)military group, criminals, strangers, etc.*
A: *Witnessed death, murder, killing, homicide executed by a trusted person or family member*

A	0	1	2	3	4	5	6	7	8	9	10	11	12	13	14	15	16	17	18	19	20	21	22	23	24	25	26	27	28	29	30	Age
B	0	1	2	3	4	5	6	7	8	9	10	11	12	13	14	15	16	17	18	19	20	21	22	23	24	25	26	27	28	29	30	Age
C	0	1	2	3	4	5	6	7	8	9	10	11	12	13	14	15	16	17	18	19	20	21	22	23	24	25	26	27	28	29	30	Age

23 b Have you ever seen mutilated dead bodies?
○ Yes ○ No

To the interviewer:
Ask openly and evaluate the physical reaction during the event.
○ *Fear, apparently 'frozen' with fear, palpitation, tension, impulse to run off or fight, tonic immobility (fright)*
○ *Disgust, sickness, weakness, numbness, sudden warmth, unconsciousness (shutdown, dissociative)*
○ *Strength, excitement, palpitation, affirmation, superiority (fight, flight)*

For example
- Beaten to death, shot, burned, mutilated
- Dead bodies disfigured through accident
- Heavily decomposed corpse

! *The person is not present at the moment of the event.*

0	1	2	3	4	5	6	7	8	9	10	11	12	13	14	15	16	17	18	19	20	21	22	23	24	25	26	27	28	29	30	Age

24 Have you ever experienced another life-threatening event?
○ Yes ○ No

Descripion: ____
____
____
____

A	0	1	2	3	4	5	6	7	8	9	10	11	12	13	14	15	16	17	18	19	20	21	22	23	24	25	26	27	28	29	30	Age
B	0	1	2	3	4	5	6	7	8	9	10	11	12	13	14	15	16	17	18	19	20	21	22	23	24	25	26	27	28	29	30	Age
C	0	1	2	3	4	5	6	7	8	9	10	11	12	13	14	15	16	17	18	19	20	21	22	23	24	25	26	27	28	29	30	Age

Contact: anke.koebach@uni-konstanz.de

This page may be reproduced by the purchaser for personal/clinical use.
From: M. Schauer, T. Elbert, & F. Neuner: *Narrative Exposure Therapy (NET) for Survivors of Traumatic Stress* (3rd ed.) (ISBN 9780889375956)
© 2025 Hogrefe Publishing

A Person of trust or family member
B Strangers and organized violence
C Accidents and natural disasters

x/s Isolated events versus permanent threats

25 Do you know if your mother experienced such an event while she was pregnant with you?

Threat to physical integrity

Important: In case of loss of an affiliated person through disease or accident or violent crime, which was not witnessed directly: this has to be noted under threat of question 34 in the following paragraph.

◯ **Yes** ◯ **No**

Item number: ________

For example

- Physical injury (experienced or observed)
- Contamination
- Sexual abuse or rape (experienced or observed)

If yes:

◯ **1. Trimester**
◯ **2. Trimester**
◯ **3. Trimester**
◯ **I don't know**

26 Have you heard of one of these events happening to a person close to you?

◯ **Yes** ◯ **No**

Life threat because of...

- Any type of physical injury
- Contamination
- Sexual abuse or rape (experienced only)

A	0	1	2	3	4	5	6	7	8	9	10	11	12	13	14	15	16	17	18	19	20	21	22	23	24	25	26	27	28	29	30	**Age**
B	0	1	2	3	4	5	6	7	8	9	10	11	12	13	14	15	16	17	18	19	20	21	22	23	24	25	26	27	28	29	30	**Age**
C	0	1	2	3	4	5	6	7	8	9	10	11	12	13	14	15	16	17	18	19	20	21	22	23	24	25	26	27	28	29	30	**Age**

A Person of trust or family member
B Strangers and organized violence

x/s Rather single versus permanent threat

THREATS TO SOCIAL INTEGRITY

27 Was there ever a period in your life, when you had no home or place to live?

◯ **Yes** ◯ **No**

For example

- Eviction from apartment
- Apartment is destroyed
- Escape from home

0	1	2	3	4	5	6	7	8	9	10	11	12	13	14	15	16	17	18	19	20	21	22	23	24	25	26	27	28	29	30	**Age**

28 During your <u>childhood</u>, was there a period when your need for care was not fulfilled?

◯ **Yes** ◯ **No**

For example

- You did not know where to go when you were sick
- Nobody cared whether you had enough to eat or drink
- Nobody took care that you wore clean and tidy clothes
- One of your caregivers threatened to leave you or to go away

A	0	1	2	3	4	5	6	7	8	9	10	11	12	13	14	15	16	17
B	0	1	2	3	4	5	6	7	8	9	10	11	12	13	14	15	16	17

29 Over the course of your whole <u>life</u>, was there a period when your need for care was not fulfilled?

Denial of help in one/several situations where the person depended on care

◯ **Yes** ◯ **No**

For example

- You suffered a prolonged period of loneliness
- You felt alone
- A person you were dependent on because of disease threatened to go away or to leave you
- There was nobody you could contact when you were sad

A	18	19	20	21	22	23	24	25	26	27	28	29	30	**Age**
B	18	19	20	21	22	23	24	25	26	27	28	29	30	**Age**

30 Have you ever been locked in against your will or held in a confined place?

Social isolation

◯ **Yes** ◯ **No**

For example

- You were locked-in alone (solitary confinement, kidnapping, or punishment)
- You were intentionally kept in darkness (i.e., locked in the basement, stranded and lost in a forest, in torture arrest, etc.)

A	0	1	2	3	4	5	6	7	8	9	10	11	12	13	14	15	16	17	18	19	20	21	22	23	24	25	26	27	28	29	30	**Age**
B	0	1	2	3	4	5	6	7	8	9	10	11	12	13	14	15	16	17	18	19	20	21	22	23	24	25	26	27	28	29	30	**Age**

31 Have you ever been excluded intentionally from a group or has somebody said mean things to you and/or about you?

◯ **Yes** ◯ **No**

For example

- You were cursed, insulted, shouted at, or people said mean things to you or about you, e.g., that you were fat, ugly, stupid, etc.
- Mobbing/bullying at school or at work
- Mobbing/bullying via the internet, telephone, etc.

A	0	1	2	3	4	5	6	7	8	9	10	11	12	13	14	15	16	17	18	19	20	21	22	23	24	25	26	27	28	29	30	**Age**
B	0	1	2	3	4	5	6	7	8	9	10	11	12	13	14	15	16	17	18	19	20	21	22	23	24	25	26	27	28	29	30	**Age**

Contact: anke.koebach@uni-konstanz.de

This page may be reproduced by the purchaser for personal/clinical use.
From: M. Schauer, T. Elbert, & F. Neuner: *Narrative Exposure Therapy (NET) for Survivors of Traumatic Stress* (3rd ed.) (ISBN 9780889375956)
© 2025 Hogrefe Publishing

A *Person of trust or family member*
B *Strangers and organized violence*

X/S Isolated events versus permanent threats

32 Have you ever been betrayed or left alone by a partner or close friend suddenly and unexpectedly?

Sudden loss of social cooperation

◯ Yes ◯ No

For example
- Your spouse/partner left or betrayed you unexpectedly
- You were betrayed or dropped by a longstanding friend

A	0	1	2	3	4	5	6	7	8	9	10	11	12	13	14	15	16	17	18	19	20	21	22	23	24	25	26	27	28	29	30	**Age**

33 Have you ever lost status in your community?

◯ Yes ◯ No

For example
- You heard about a major defeat, which damaged your reputation
- You unexpectedly lost your job and with it your position and reputation

A	0	1	2	3	4	5	6	7	8	9	10	11	12	13	14	15	16	17	18	19	20	21	22	23	24	25	26	27	28	29	30	**Age**
B	0	1	2	3	4	5	6	7	8	9	10	11	12	13	14	15	16	17	18	19	20	21	22	23	24	25	26	27	28	29	30	**Age**

34 Have you experienced any other social event that was stressful for you?

◯ Yes ◯ No

Description: ______________________________

____

____

____

A	0	1	2	3	4	5	6	7	8	9	10	11	12	13	14	15	16	17	18	19	20	21	22	23	24	25	26	27	28	29	30	**Age**
B	0	1	2	3	4	5	6	7	8	9	10	11	12	13	14	15	16	17	18	19	20	21	22	23	24	25	26	27	28	29	30	**Age**

35 Do you know if your mother experienced such an event while she was pregnant with you?

Threats to social integrity

◯ Yes ◯ No

Item number: ___________

For example
- Poverty
- Lack of care
- Social isolation
- Loss of status
- Unexpected loss of social cooperation
- Unexpected death of a family member (partner, parents, siblings, child)

If yes:

◯ **1. Trimester**
◯ **2. Trimester**
◯ **3. Trimester**
◯ **I don't know**

X/S Isolated events versus permanent threats

SOCIAL AND PHYSICAL DOMINANCE BEHAVIOR

Consider information from the first part: Information about education and profession and recreational activities

36 Can you remember one or more moments, when you sought out exciting dangerous situations (heart rate and respiration increase, etc)?

Confrontation with exciting threats

◯ Yes ◯ No

For example
- Seeking life-threatening heights (i.e., highway bridges, climbing at extreme hights, etc.), fast and risky driving with car or motor bike, skydiving, bungee-jumping
- Playing with fire, fireworks, explosives
- Cut off oxygen supply (i.e., by strangulation or holding breath)
- Provocation of physical argument(s)

0	1	2	3	4	5	6	7	8	9	10	11	12	13	14	15	16	17	18	19	20	21	22	23	24	25	26	27	28	29	30	**Age**

37 Can you remember one or more moments, when you sought out numbing threatening situations (heart rate decreases, arms and legs become heavy and warm, etc)?

Confrontation with numbing threats

◯ Yes ◯ No

For example
- Injury with sharp objects (i.e., knife, razor blades, syringes, etc.)
- Sexual penetration
- Insertion of objects into orifices (i.e., vagina, anus)
- Injection without medical indication

0	1	2	3	4	5	6	7	8	9	10	11	12	13	14	15	16	17	18	19	20	21	22	23	24	25	26	27	28	29	30	**Age**

38 Have you ever destroyed things intentionally, e.g., to vent your anger or because the situation allowed it?

Violence against things

◯ Yes ◯ No

For example
- Throwing furniture
- Damaging cars or cutting car wheels
- Violent destruction of other things

0	1	2	3	4	5	6	7	8	9	10	11	12	13	14	15	16	17	18	19	20	21	22	23	24	25	26	27	28	29	30	**Age**

Contact: anke.koebach@uni-konstanz.de

This page may be reproduced by the purchaser for personal/clinical use.
From: M. Schauer, T. Elbert, & F. Neuner: *Narrative Exposure Therapy (NET) for Survivors of Traumatic Stress* (3rd ed.) (ISBN 9780889375956)
© 2025 Hogrefe Publishing

SOCIAL AND PHYSICAL DOMINANCE BEHAVIOR

39 Have you ever killed or otherwise inflicted harm to an animal?

Violence against animals

◯ **Yes** ◯ **No**

For example
- Strangled or prevented an animal from breathing
- Burnt or applied electric shocks
- Beaten, kicked, cut open, or caused another injury
- Penetrated with an object, sexually abused or raped
- Deprived from vital warmth, nutrition or water or poisoned

0 1 2 3 4 5 6 7 8 9 10 11 12 13 14 15 16 17 18 19 20 21 22 23 24 25 26 27 28 29 30 **Age**

40 Have you ever intentionally insulted someone or excluded them from a group?

◯ **Yes** ◯ **No**

For example
- Cursed someone
- Called them names or insults such as fat, ugly, stupid, etc.
- Locked someone in a room
- Betrayed someone in order to hurt that person

0 1 2 3 4 5 6 7 8 9 10 11 12 13 14 15 16 17 18 19 20 21 22 23 24 25 26 27 28 29 30 **Age**

41 Have you ever pursued or hunted someone in order to inflict harm upon that person?

◯ **Yes** ◯ **No**

0 1 2 3 4 5 6 7 8 9 10 11 12 13 14 15 16 17 18 19 20 21 22 23 24 25 26 27 28 29 30 **Age**

42 Have you ever been involved in a physical fight?

Physical abuse (causing at worst bruising as a physical injury)

◯ **Yes** ◯ **No**

For example
- Beaten
- Restrained
- Kicked
- Punched
- Slapped someone
- etc.

! *This may have occurred as a disciplinary measure, e.g., at school, home, etc., in a physical argument with peers, for some other reason, or for no reason.*

0 1 2 3 4 5 6 7 8 9 10 11 12 13 14 15 16 17 18 19 20 21 22 23 24 25 26 27 28 29 30 **Age**

43 Have you ever injured someone so badly, that this person presented with visible physical damage and/or had to be provided with medical aid?

Severe physical abuse (also with object; more severe injury than bruises)

◯ **Yes** ◯ **No**

For example
- Severely beaten someone
- You inflicted serious harm upon someone
- You have beaten someone with a stick, belt or another object

! *This may have occurred as a disciplinary measure, e.g., at school, home, etc., in a physical argument with peers, for some other reason, or for no reason.*

0 1 2 3 4 5 6 7 8 9 10 11 12 13 14 15 16 17 18 19 20 21 22 23 24 25 26 27 28 29 30 **Age**

44 Have you ever injured someone with a sharp object, so that you made the person bleed (excluding medical treatment)?

◯ **Yes** ◯ **No**

For example
- You injured a person with a knife or razor blade
- With pieces of (broken) glass
- Or another sharp object

0 1 2 3 4 5 6 7 8 9 10 11 12 13 14 15 16 17 18 19 20 21 22 23 24 25 26 27 28 29 30 **Age**

45 Have you ever injured another person with a firearm or bomb?

◯ **Yes** ◯ **No**

For example
- You shot someone with a gun
- You launched one or more bomb attack(s)

0 1 2 3 4 5 6 7 8 9 10 11 12 13 14 15 16 17 18 19 20 21 22 23 24 25 26 27 28 29 30 **Age**

46 Have you ever intentionally burnt parts of another person's body?

◯ **Yes** ◯ **No**

For example
- You held someone's hand or another body part in a flame or against hot coals
- You crushed a cigarette on someone's skin
- Burnt someone with chemicals
- You tortured someone with electric shocks
- Scald someone with hot liquids

0 1 2 3 4 5 6 7 8 9 10 11 12 13 14 15 16 17 18 19 20 21 22 23 24 25 26 27 28 29 30 **Age**

47 Have you ever intentionally obstructed another person's breathing?

◯ **Yes** ◯ **No**

For example
- You held someone under water until you felt the person struggling for air
- You suffocated or choked a person
- You poured water over someone's mouth, so that the person could no longer breathe (waterboarding)

0 1 2 3 4 5 6 7 8 9 10 11 12 13 14 15 16 17 18 19 20 21 22 23 24 25 26 27 28 29 30 **Age**

Contact: anke.koebach@uni-konstanz.de

This page may be reproduced by the purchaser for personal/clinical use.
From: M. Schauer, T. Elbert, & F. Neuner: *Narrative Exposure Therapy (NET) for Survivors of Traumatic Stress* (3rd ed.) (ISBN 9780889375956)
© 2025 Hogrefe Publishing

SOCIAL AND PHYSICAL DOMINANCE BEHAVIOR

48 Have you ever injected someone or given someone something to eat or drink with the intention to harm that person?

◯ **Yes** ◯ **No**

For example

- (Try to) Poison someone
- Allow or force someone to eat something that you knew or thought would harm them

0 | 1 | 2 | 3 | 4 | 5 | 6 | 7 | 8 | 9 | 10 | 11 | 12 | 13 | 14 | 15 | 16 | 17 | 18 | 19 | 20 | 21 | 22 | 23 | 24 | 25 | 26 | 27 | 28 | 29 | 30 | **Age**

49 Have you ever denied essential care to another person?

◯ **Yes** ◯ **No**

For example

- You deprived someone of food or water for several days
- You prevented someone from sleeping
- Intentionally let someone freeze (to death)

0 | 1 | 2 | 3 | 4 | 5 | 6 | 7 | 8 | 9 | 10 | 11 | 12 | 13 | 14 | 15 | 16 | 17 | 18 | 19 | 20 | 21 | 22 | 23 | 24 | 25 | 26 | 27 | 28 | 29 | 30 | **Age**

50 Do you know if there was someone in your mother's environment, while she was pregnant with you, against whom she committed the acts mentioned before?

Social and physical dominance behavior of the mother

◯ **Yes** ◯ **No** ◯ **I don't know** **Item:**__________

For example

- Ostracize someone
- Physical injury
- Poison someone

If yes:

◯ **1. Trimester**
◯ **2. Trimester**
◯ **3. Trimester**
◯ **I don't know**

51 Do you remember a time in your life when you had sexual intercourse with random partners?

◯ **Yes** ◯ **No**

For example

- Partners you barely knew and with whom you never had contact again
- Ca ≥3 different partners per month, some months in a row

0 | 1 | 2 | 3 | 4 | 5 | 6 | 7 | 8 | 9 | 10 | 11 | 12 | 13 | 14 | 15 | 16 | 17 | 18 | 19 | 20 | 21 | 22 | 23 | 24 | 25 | 26 | 27 | 28 | 29 | 30 | **Age**

52 Do you remember a time in your life, when you had violent sexual intercourse with the consent of your partner?

Intentional stimulation of sexual and aggressive arousal in combination

◯ **Yes** ◯ **No**

0 | 1 | 2 | 3 | 4 | 5 | 6 | 7 | 8 | 9 | 10 | 11 | 12 | 13 | 14 | 15 | 16 | 17 | 18 | 19 | 20 | 21 | 22 | 23 | 24 | 25 | 26 | 27 | 28 | 29 | 30 | **Age**

53 Have ever exposed yourself in front of others in a situation, in which it was not appropriate?

◯ **Yes** ◯ **No**

For example

- Expose genitals in public such as parks, public transportation,...
- Sending picture of your genitals to other persons without their consent

0 | 1 | 2 | 3 | 4 | 5 | 6 | 7 | 8 | 9 | 10 | 11 | 12 | 13 | 14 | 15 | 16 | 17 | 18 | 19 | 20 | 21 | 22 | 23 | 24 | 25 | 26 | 27 | 28 | 29 | 30 | **Age**

54 Have you ever forcibly touched someone's body or forced someone to touch your private body parts?

Sexual abuse

◯ **Yes** ◯ **No**

For example

- You forced someone to touch their genitals
- You kissed a person against his/her will
- You hugged or restrained somebody against his/her consent

0 | 1 | 2 | 3 | 4 | 5 | 6 | 7 | 8 | 9 | 10 | 11 | 12 | 13 | 14 | 15 | 16 | 17 | 18 | 19 | 20 | 21 | 22 | 23 | 24 | 25 | 26 | 27 | 28 | 29 | 30 | **Age**

55 Have you ever forced someone to have sexual intercourse of any type (oral, anal or vaginal) with you or with another person?

Rape (any type of sexual penetration or invasion)

◯ **Yes** ◯ **No**

0 | 1 | 2 | 3 | 4 | 5 | 6 | 7 | 8 | 9 | 10 | 11 | 12 | 13 | 14 | 15 | 16 | 17 | 18 | 19 | 20 | 21 | 22 | 23 | 24 | 25 | 26 | 27 | 28 | 29 | 30 | **Age**

56 Was there another event in your life when you intentionally harmed or injured someone?

◯ **Yes** ◯ **No**

Description:____

____

____

____

0 | 1 | 2 | 3 | 4 | 5 | 6 | 7 | 8 | 9 | 10 | 11 | 12 | 13 | 14 | 15 | 16 | 17 | 18 | 19 | 20 | 21 | 22 | 23 | 24 | 25 | 26 | 27 | 28 | 29 | 30 | **Age**

This page may be reproduced by the purchaser for personal/clinical use.
From: M. Schauer, T. Elbert, & F. Neuner: *Narrative Exposure Therapy (NET) for Survivors of Traumatic Stress* (3rd ed.) (ISBN 9780889375956)
© 2025 Hogrefe Publishing

ADDITIONAL QUESTIONS TO THE INTERVIEWEE

EVALUATION OF THE QUESTIONNAIRE

Have you answered the questions according to the best of your knowledge?

Part 1: Sociodemographic data	1◯ 2◯ 3◯ 4◯ 5◯	**Scaling information:**
Part 2 - Section 1: Threat to physical integrity	1◯ 2◯ 3◯ 4◯ 5◯	1 = Not at all 2 = Not really
Part 2 - Section 2: Threat to social integrity	1◯ 2◯ 3◯ 4◯ 5◯	3 = Neutral 4 = Somewhat true
Part 2 - Section 3: Social and physical dominance behavior	1◯ 2◯ 3◯ 4◯ 5◯	5 = Very true

Did you perceive the interviewee responding to the questions as being aroused and stressed?

Part 1: Sociodemographic data	1◯ 2◯ 3◯ 4◯ 5◯	**Scaling information:**
Part 2 - Section 1: Threat to physical integrity	1◯ 2◯ 3◯ 4◯ 5◯	1 = Not at all 2 = Not really
Part 2 - Section 2: Threat to social integrity	1◯ 2◯ 3◯ 4◯ 5◯	3 = Neutral 4 = Somewhat true
Part 2 - Section 3: Social and physical dominance behavior	1◯ 2◯ 3◯ 4◯ 5◯	5 = Very true

ADDITIONAL QUESTIONS FOR THE INTERVIEWER

GENERAL VALIDITY OF THE ANSWERS

The interviewee answered all questions without hesitation and honestly.

Part 1: Sociodemographic data	1◯ 2◯ 3◯ 4◯ 5◯	**Scaling information:**
Part 2 - Section 1: Threat to physical integrity	1◯ 2◯ 3◯ 4◯ 5◯	1 = Not at all 2 = Not really
Part 2 - Section 2: Threat to social integrity	1◯ 2◯ 3◯ 4◯ 5◯	3 = Neutral 4 = Somewhat true
Part 2 - Section 3: Social and physical dominance behavior	1◯ 2◯ 3◯ 4◯ 5◯	5 = Very true

VALIDITY OF THE AGE

The interviewee had a good understanding of the chronology of his/her life events and could easily tell at what age s/he experienced a certain event.

Part 1: Sociodemographic data	1◯ 2◯ 3◯ 4◯ 5◯	**Scaling information:**
Part 2 - Section 1: Threat to physical integrity	1◯ 2◯ 3◯ 4◯ 5◯	1 = Not at all 2 = Not really
Part 2 - Section 2: Threat to social integrity	1◯ 2◯ 3◯ 4◯ 5◯	3 = Neutral 4 = Somewhat true
Part 2 - Section 3: Social and physical dominance behavior	1◯ 2◯ 3◯ 4◯ 5◯	5 = Very true

The participant tried to remember the most probable age of his/her life events.

Part 1: Sociodemographic data	1◯ 2◯ 3◯ 4◯ 5◯	**Scaling information:**
Part 2 - Section 1: Threat to physical integrity	1◯ 2◯ 3◯ 4◯ 5◯	1 = Not at all 2 = Not really
Part 2 - Section 2: Threat to social integrity	1◯ 2◯ 3◯ 4◯ 5◯	3 = Neutral 4 = Somewhat true
Part 2 - Section 3: Social and physical dominance behavior	1◯ 2◯ 3◯ 4◯ 5◯	5 = Very true

Contact: anke.koebach@uni-konstanz.de

This page may be reproduced by the purchaser for personal/clinical use.
From: M. Schauer, T. Elbert, & F. Neuner: *Narrative Exposure Therapy (NET) for Survivors of Traumatic Stress* (3rd ed.) (ISBN 9780889375956)
© 2025 Hogrefe Publishing

Examples of Narrations of Life Experiences Resulting From NET

All original names and places have been changed.

Excerpt From Testimony 1

I was born on March 23, 1976, in Southwest Region, Mundemba, Cameroon. My family is originally from Kribi, South Cameroon; however, my dad established his business in Mundemba. There were four children in my family: I have three younger brothers. We were a very good and happy family. I was the oldest son, so I had many rights and could get whatever I wanted from my father. I started school and completed primary school in the Southwest Region. I did well in secondary school and intended to study politics.

While in school, I started having problems with my chemistry teacher, Fanzo. He was a member of CPDM, the ruling party, which had been in power since February 2, 1982. During the parliamentary elections we were to have a chemistry test. Fanzo promised that if the ruling party were to win the election, there would be an extra percentage mark in the test for every student. However, the opposition party won the election; and yet power was given to the ruling party. I would have passed my chemistry test, but Fanzo failed me because I stood up against the ruling party. I didn't take it too hard. After failing the test, I was affirmed in my political beliefs.

At that time, I used to show off a lot in school because my dad was a member of the opposition party. I would get punished in school – for example, by being given a large area to clean or by being suspended. Suspension from school used to hurt me the most.

When I was 18 years old, I organized a rally with other children that went on for 2 weeks. After school, I put my school uniform in my backpack and headed to the rally with my gang. In those days if they found you demonstrating in uniform they would make you clean the streets. We were made to remove old cars and other obstacles that the demonstrators had used to block the street to cut off the police. The street was full of policemen and opposition party members. The rally went well, and I came back home safely.

I formed another gang of children and demonstrated against the illegitimate elections. We used to make petrol bombs in response to them shooting and killing my friends. These bombs could not kill – only injure. This was one of the ideas I came up with. Many times they also shot at me but missed.

I was 18 years old when I started politics. My father told me that no matter how I did at school, if I stood up for my rights, I would be a great man in the future. So I became more active. My father was an important member of the Social Democratic Front (SDF) party in the Southwest. While my father was still alive, I used to go to demonstrations with other students. I was always on the front line. Sometimes I was taken to prison for a couple of hours and beaten. They would tell me to quit my political activities. During some of these incidents, I thought that I was going to die. This happened a few times before my father died.

During one incident I was taken to prison for hours and beaten. This happened as follows: After a demonstration, I was driving in a car. At a checkpoint, the police asked for my driver's license. After recognizing my name, they ordered me to turn on my lights. They ordered me to do other things and asked me questions that annoyed me, and I became angry. They asked me to give them my identity card but I refused. We had a verbal quarrel. One of them slapped me. I told him not to slap me again, or I would slap him back. (In my country, we do not talk back to officers.) We began to fight. They started beating me with their batons. I kept quiet, and they stopped beating me and handcuffed me. They drove to the police station with my car. They took me straight to a room and chained me to a chair, without even writing a statement or anything. They put

This page may be reproduced by the purchaser for personal/clinical use.
From: M. Schauer, T. Elbert, & F. Neuner: *Narrative Exposure Therapy (NET) for Survivors of Traumatic Stress* (3rd ed.) (ISBN 9780889375956)
© 2025 Hogrefe Publishing

electrodes to my temples for about 1 second. I screamed. They put them on again. They tortured me for a couple of seconds and let me go only after several hours. I felt okay the next day and went on with my work. I still feel pain in my head sometimes, though. My father brought this case to court, but it was not taken seriously.

The worst case before my father died happened in 1995. I still have a mark on my body – it's a long mark on my back. We used to make campaigns before the elections. During one demonstration, I was together with very good political friends of mine. As students, we used to sing in the streets. I was the leader of the group. My friends and I were caught together as we were running away. We tried to escape into the adjacent streets, but we were surrounded. We ran into the policemen that were ahead of us. They scattered the group with tear gas. When I was caught I was beaten. I saw what they did to a friend of mine. His feet were swept out from underneath him. He fell down. Then they kicked him with their boots. It was very sunny and hot on that day. They turned his face and smashed it into the hot concrete. When he lifted his head, it looked like his face was burnt. I was still being beaten. I cried as I watched him, because I was afraid the same thing would happen to me. I was very afraid that I would be the next. (I have a headache now as I talk about it, my hands are cold, my veins stand out, and my is heart beating fast right now.) We were taken to the police station separately. I was released the next day. This was the worst case before my father died because of what they did to my friend, which also could have happened to me. Sometimes I imagine what I would look like now, if the same thing had happened to me.

One day, life became very hard. They burnt down my father's shop. I saw it; I was at home. It was 6:00 a.m., and we were sleeping. We heard people shouting: "Fire!" and I could smell it because the fire was very big; the sky was red everywhere. I jumped out of my bed and ran outside. My dad, mom, and younger brothers followed. There were a lot of people outside. I discovered that it was my father's shop that was on fire. I was struggling with an axe to break the wall with the valuable things behind it, but it was too late. I went inside the building. I was very nervous and angry during the incident. I was in the very middle of it. I could have even burnt to death in there. I did not think of anything while I was inside, or that I could die; I just thought of saving everything. There was a tarpaulin high up that came down and fell behind me. That is how I hurt my thumbnail. It was all black. (I even showed it to the people in Genf. This one here is a new nail, which has just grown.) We did not manage to save anything from the fire. Apart from the goods, my father had also kept some money in the store. Luckily, no one was hurt in the fire. The ruling party had started the fire. My father had no other investments. Life became a little bit harder for us, but I continued going to school.

When I think about it now I become nervous immediately. Not fearful, but angry. I feel like fighting or harming someone, the bad people or the ruling party. I am afraid only when there are many of them, and I am alone. I feel very bad – angry and sad about the fire and because of what we lost.

One day, my father left the house to meet some friends to discuss political issues. It was at around 5:30 or 6:00 in the evening. Our house was very big, so either my father or I could leave the house without the other noticing. But, in this case I knew he had left the house. On his way back, he was killed. I was at home. I received a phone call 3 hrs after he had left saying that he had died. The caller simply said: "Your father's body is lying in the street beside his car." I went there in one of our other cars. I was not driving; someone else drove. All I saw was my dad's body lying by his car. One side of the car door was open, as if he had been struggling to get out of the car. He had been shot in the heart. Blood was coming out. I rushed to him to see if I could save him. When I reached him I touched him, but his body was already cold. I saw the blood and the bullet in his chest. The bullet was still in his body. Some other people, friends and Party members, came and helped me to bring him to the mortuary because there was nothing else to do. His body stayed in the mortuary for 2 weeks. Then he was given a burial.

Just after my dad died, I could not hold myself back anymore, and I truly went crazy. My family members locked me up to try to calm me down. One friend took me to his own family, 10 kilometers away. He kept me there for some days. A lot of people came to see me there and to arrange the burial because back then I was not able to do anything. The opposition members helped me to arrange the burial. They did most of the organizing and consulted me because I was the oldest son.

This page may be reproduced by the purchaser for personal/clinical use.
From: M. Schauer, T. Elbert, & F. Neuner: *Narrative Exposure Therapy (NET) for Survivors of Traumatic Stress* (3rd ed.) (ISBN 9780889375956)
© 2025 Hogrefe Publishing

It was a big burial because my dad was well known in Cameroon. Even some ministers attended it. He was buried in Kribi. He had only been a visitor in Mundemba. We kept awake till 11 p.m., then we traveled all the way to Kribi from 11 p.m. till 6 a.m. the next day. The roads were bad, and we were very tired. The chiefs were informed, and they all came to the burial. He was buried the next day at 4:00 p.m.

I stayed in Kribi for a week after that; then I went back to Mundemba. My mother came with me, and then she returned to Kribi after a few weeks. She had to go back to the village to mourn her husband, and only came home during the weekends. We mourned my father wearing only white. I was ill after the death of my father. I had a fever for a couple of weeks, and I had a lot of headaches. (I have a headache now as I talk about it. I started having these headaches – not when I saw his dead body – but at the moment I got the news of his death.) I was on relaxants for some time in order to recover quickly. Some friends came to keep us company in our house in Mundemba.

Life became very tough, and still is today, because now I was the head of the family. The day my father died, I did not really feel in danger because I knew they had got what they wanted. Actually, I was in more danger before he died because I had been the son of an important opposition party member, and they could get to him by getting me. After his death, I actually became an active member of the Party and that put my life in danger again.

I feel angry because of the death of my dad. He was not sick. We never got to say goodbye. I lost more than a father; I also lost a leader and an ideal. I remember all the good things he did for me. After his death, I no longer felt safe. I knew that I could be killed as well. Others had been killed before my father – he was not the first. I knew some of them, and there were others I had not known.

Sometimes I see my dad in my dreams. I see him how he was when things were still good and he was still alive. I never see him dead; I only see how he was when life was good. When I see other people's parents of the same caliber as my dad, I feel bad because I have no one to call my own daddy or mum. No one can feel good in such a situation. I shed a lot of tears.

Nobody could help me now with school, and I had to stop my education. I feel angry because my father's good friends, people he used to eat and drink with and discuss issues with (e.g., the assistant inspector of police and the general manager of the CDC), did not show up to help us after he died.

When I dropped out of school, I became a full-fledged member of the SDF. They gave me a post as a propaganda secretary. I used to publish and distribute fliers whenever there was a rally or a meeting. One day, when I was doing this, a policeman came up to me and asked me why I chose to do these things. He said that maybe this was why my life would end. He talked to me politely while I was putting up the fliers. I said that until the president stepped down, I would continue my political work.

Some time after my father died, presidential elections were held. The president went around campaigning. We were demonstrating in the streets. Schools were closed. We began making petrol bombs again.

One day, when we went out to demonstrate, we were on our way to meet another group in order to attack the military together. There were over 150,000 demonstrators. My best friend was next to me on the front line. Some of the demonstrators had bombs and flags. Even important party members were there. The policemen were in front of us, facing us. They commanded us to stop and disperse, but we continued to march. They shot tear gas at us. They shot it inside the group. We started to fight against them; we threw petrol bombs and stones and anything that could hurt them. They shot real bullets at us – real bullets, not rubber ones. We were shocked. These people were so evil, so evil. My friend and I were carrying a lot of bombs, which we distributed to others to fire them. Suddenly we saw a helicopter. It started to throw tear gas at us. We started running, each one for himself. Ahead of us the policemen were already waiting. Gendarmes, policemen, and the military surrounded us. We were running to a hospital that was 1 kilometer away; we wanted to hide there. We found the military already there. We were shocked to see that they were beating people who were inside the hospital. (I feel very angry as I remember this.) My friends and I turned around. The helicopter, which was not just from Mundemba or Duala but had come all the way from Yaounde, had landed and dropped off some soldiers. My friend was shot in the foot by one of them. He fell down. I shouted his name. He shouted back. I tried to help him but I couldn't. There was a crowd of soldiers coming toward us. They were still shooting, and the tear gas was too much: I had to run to save my own life. My friend was killed and his corpse was

This page may be reproduced by the purchaser for personal/clinical use.
From: M. Schauer, T. Elbert, & F. Neuner: *Narrative Exposure Therapy (NET) for Survivors of Traumatic Stress* (3rd ed.) (ISBN 9780889375956)
© 2025 Hogrefe Publishing

left there. I did not actually see how he died. (It was very painful for me, I feel very angry. I do not feel guilty because I did all I could and I had to save my own life.)

I was not at home for 3 days, because I was well-known. I knew one of the men who had shot at us. We went to his house when nobody was there. We broke the door open. We set a fire and burnt his military uniform, his video machine, and all the important things that he had. Then we ran away. I felt happy and satisfied that we did this, because it paid for my friend's death. I was happy to do even more. This incident happened about 1 month after the death of my dad.

There was a military celebration on the 1st of June 2000, about 3 months after the death of my dad. After my dad had been killed, I was the next target. On the night of the 31st of May, I was assigned to distribute pamphlets. These pamphlets said that we needed freedom of speech and human rights in our country. I finished the job before midnight and returned home. The rally was to be in Bertoua, in the morning of June 1st, though it would be celebrated in all of Cameroon. But the president would be in Bertoua in the East. We planned to block the streets.

At midnight, there was a knock on my door. At that time, I used to have my own room, away from my family's house, for security. Sometimes I would sleep in my room, and sometimes I slept at home. I was surprised to hear the knock. I went to open the door, but it was broken in before I reached it. When I was still about 3 meters away from the door, I was confronted with about six policemen. The policemen came in and started to hit me everywhere on my body. They wore blue uniforms with black berets. I struggled and fought with them. They hit me on the forehead with the butt of a gun, and my forehead broke open. Blood started running down my face, and into my mouth and eyes. They dislocated my arm and knocked out one of my teeth with the butt of a gun. They made a hole in my arm and blood ran out. I still struggled and fought with them, but they were too many for me. They beat me severely until I was unconscious. I was unconscious for 3 days. After a few days, I realized that I was in a cell. There was blood all around me. Even the other prisoners asked the police why they did not take me to a hospital first before taking me to the prison.

In the prison, they fed us beans that were only have cooked once a day. The toilet was in the cell. Everything was being done in there. We were undressed before we entered the cell. They had caught me as the leader of my group in order to disband my group. Nobody knew that I was there. While in the cell, a policeman told me that many prisoners had passed through their hands and died, and so would I. I replied that I would die fighting for my rights and for human rights.

I could not stand up. My whole body was injured. They did not beat me again, because I had so many injuries; I had wounds all over. I couldn't sleep, and I had no appetite. They did not clean me, and I received no medical care. I was never washed for the whole time that I was in the cell. I had no power left even after I had recovered.

I was in the cell until the 17th of July. On that day a policeman asked me where my family lived so that they could be informed where I was. I replied that I would rather die alone than together with my family. He left and only came back on the night of the 18th, because they were working in shifts. He was a just man, but he was working for the government and had to obey their rules. He came to my cell at midnight and removed the chain from my feet. I did not know what was happening. I had had no contact with my family. No one knew where I was, so no one had visited me. The policeman asked me to walk out into the night. That's what they usually did to get rid of people: They asked you to walk into the forest or an open place and shot you from behind. He told me to go and not look behind. I knew this was the end of my life. I thought of my mum and my younger brothers. I started thinking about dead people and where they were, and what the place was like where they were. There was a car ahead of me with four people in it, blinking its lights at me. Two of the people were in uniform, and the other two weren't. When I tried to pass the car, they said, "Come here!" I was shocked. The policeman was now no longer behind me. They handed me a pair of trousers and put me into the car. I sat in the back, in the middle seat. I recognized one man from my village Kribi. The commissioner, with four stars, sat in the front. They drove me from Limbe to Duala. That is a 2-hr drive. When we arrived, they cleaned all the blood off my body. I did not know what was happening. I was surprised to see a policeman being nice to me. In the morning they gave me bread and tea.

This page may be reproduced by the purchaser for personal/clinical use.
From: M. Schauer, T. Elbert, & F. Neuner: *Narrative Exposure Therapy (NET) for Survivors of Traumatic Stress* (3rd ed.) (ISBN 9780889375956)
© 2025 Hogrefe Publishing

At night I was taken to the international airport. The man from my community told me that I had to leave the country for my own safety. If I were to remain in Cameroon, I would die. He told me that they had planned to put me in raw acid the next week. No one checked me at Duala Airport, because the commissioner was ahead of me escorting me. I didn't have a passport. At the entrance of the plane, a man beside me gave me a passport with my photograph on it but not my name. It was checked at the airport under a mercury bulb, but it was okay. I was checked normally as I boarded the plane. I asked the man if he could tell me who he was, but he said that I had no right to know. I came into Switzerland wearing the slippers I had been wearing in the cell. I had been tortured in them, and I had to hold them together with a pin now.

We left the country at 11:55 and the plane landed in Vienna at 6:30. There we transferred and took a Swiss airplane to Zürich. This was the last time I saw the man. He took the passport off me. He gave me 40 DM, shook my hand, and said that he had hereby completed his job. He told me to go a human rights organization. He advised me to go to Genf.

It was my first time in Europe. I was afraid of the police, even though they were White. I took the next train to Genf, where I was interviewed 3 days later. Since then, I have had no contact with my family. Sometimes when I see Black people I become suspicious of them. I know I am not safe yet. I saw my name on the Internet, declared "wanted." I never went online again. I believe that even now there are still people looking for me. If the opposition party comes into power, I might go back to Cameroon. But if I go back to Cameroon now, it will be the end of my life.

This page may be reproduced by the purchaser for personal/clinical use.
From: M. Schauer, T. Elbert, & F. Neuner: *Narrative Exposure Therapy (NET) for Survivors of Traumatic Stress* (3rd ed.) (ISBN 9780889375956)
© 2025 Hogrefe Publishing

Lifeline and Excerpt From Testimony 2

I was born on June 28, 1956. We were living in a village in Kazakhstan.

I was born into a good family. I had three sisters and five brothers.

I had a good time at school. I had a math teacher who had a big influence on me, and a couple of good friends.

I had an accident and injured my spine.

After having finished 10th grade (in Russia, schooling ends after 10th grade) we moved to Grozny. In Grozny, I started studying educational science and went to a teacher training college for 4 years. At the college, I met my former boyfriend who was studying with me. He was the love of my life, and the time with him was the happiest time period of my life.

When I was 21 years old and in the last year of my studies, my boyfriend died in a car accident.

I started an apprenticeship as a commercial assistant. I liked the training very much and when I started to work in this field I enjoyed it a lot.

My wedding and happiness with my husband, Ali.

Birth of my first son (1985), Alex.

Birth of my second son (1987), Umar. I had a normal life until the war started in 1990.

From 1990 until 2000, we went through a very hard time. The riots in Grozny started in 1990. My grandmother on my mother's side died.

In 1993, they threw a hand grenade in the house of my mother's brother, and his wife died immediately while he died from his injuries a bit later. That year, I witnessed the death of a young man, and one day our car was shot at while we were driving.

First Chechen War 1994–1995. We were evacuated and our family was separated. Later I learned that my husband had died. I never found out what happened to my son. For 4 or 5 years we were constantly on the run.

April 1996 (Grozny): At the beginning of the war, I was beaten and sexually abused. Umar was not with me when it happened. Later we fled to another town.

Early 1998: I witnessed a massacre: About 200 women who had gone to fetch water were shot.

Winter 1999: We made an attempt to escape to Ingushetia, but the car that was supposed to pick us up never arrived. In the same year, they found my mother-in-law, but she was so confused that she was not able to tell me what had happened with my son.

In 2001: Umar and I arrived in Germany.

2004: Officials wanted to deport us: The police came for us at night, and we had to spend one night in prison.

2006: Death of my father: A grenade exploded while he was praying.

2007: Death of my mother: She had a heart attack when she heard that I had been raped. At first she was paralyzed and then she died.

September 2006: My son qualifies for university admission. We are happy in Germany for now, but I am still afraid that we will be deported.

My wishes for the future:

- I would like Umar to obtain a university degree
- I hope that Alex will be found
- I wish for my son and myself that we can stay here until the end of our life, that we can feel safe and that my son will find his future here
- For myself, I am wishing for health

This page may be reproduced by the purchaser for personal/clinical use.
From: M. Schauer, T. Elbert, & F. Neuner: *Narrative Exposure Therapy (NET) for Survivors of Traumatic Stress* (3rd ed.) (ISBN 9780889375956)
© 2025 Hogrefe Publishing

Revisiting Some Key Events

My name is Roza Magomadov and I was born on June 28, 1956, into a good family; unlike most other men, my father neither drank nor smoked. We were living in a village in Kazakhstan. I had three sisters and five brothers, and I was the third child of our parents. Altogether, my mother gave birth to twelve children, but three of them died.

When I was a child, we had a happy life in our village. We did not have a lot of money since my father was the only one in our family who was working, but we were a happy family *(it makes me smile, when I think back, it is a nice feeling to remember this)*. My brother Malik and I used to play a lot together. For him I was the older sister who was looking after him, particularly at school. Malik was a very good-natured child; he never had any problems with our parents or with other children. *(These memories make me sad and make me cry as he's dead. At home I can't grieve because my son Umar doesn't know that he is dead).*

[...]

After having finished 10th grade (in Russia, schooling ends with 10th grade), we moved to Grozny.

[...]

One day, something terrible happened: It was in Grozny, around the end of April or the beginning of May in 1996. The snow had already melted, but it was not warm yet. We lived in a half-destroyed house in the city of Grozny. Once again, this was a temporary solution. It was very cold; I remember that we stacked pieces of wood for making fire on the concrete floor. There were some mattresses and a couple of blankets, and there were many other women with their children. Plastic bags, not window grates, were covering the windows. These bags were white. One could constantly hear shots from the street; sporadically during the day and a lot during the night. Actually, at that time there was a ceasefire, but nevertheless there were shootings; we could hear the gunshots and see the flashes. I was scared and there was a constant feeling of unrest inside me, the feeling that I should run away. *(Right now I can see the whitish light shine through the bags into the room from the right.)* There was a room that was a bit warmer for the children. We were about 15 women while the men were in another part of the house. We used to cook for them, and some Chechen men provided us with food and water. The constant threat of war had been around for a long time now, and for a long time we had not had a home. Our mood was accordingly, we felt depressed. In Chechnya we say: "Moving house three times is almost as bad as a house burning down," and all we did in this war was move around. Our life was a catastrophe: It was very very hard, and we all had been tired and demoralized for a long time.

It was always dusky in these ruins, and on the day that I am going to talk about it was almost dark outside. It was after lunch, and the children were in the adjoining room which could be heated, when a couple of Russian soldiers arrived. We could not lock the door because they had broken the lock and used to come and go as they pleased. They entered the house without knocking. They came in order to "check." We did not know any of these men, but I realized at once that they were drunk as they had a smelly alcohol breath; they were cursing a lot. They knew what they wanted; the one who had come in first said straightaway: "Our boss said that we are supposed to have fun here." I assumed that they were hungry and wanted us to make them some food, as we would usually make food for these Russian fools. But they did not want to eat, they said: "We are all now going to chose one of you and fuck you *(trachat)!"* We women were actually not that young anymore as the youngest among us were 35 years old. I was around 40. These soldiers were younger than us! They all had weapons: Each of them had a Kalashnikov. All of the women were together in one room, and a lot of men entered. We were sitting on the floor and leaning against the wall. After they had announced what they wanted, we got scared and starting talking to each other. One of them grabbed a woman called Mila. I was still hoping that the men had meant that she was supposed to work for them, like cook for them or do the washing. We were screaming and wanted to do something! But then one man said to another man: "Akhmed, this one's yours." When I heard that, I understood. He added: "When you're finished with her, it will be my turn."

With this sentence, all my hope was gone, and I was overwhelmed by great weakness. I could not sit up any longer; I was like a wash rag. It was so humiliating *(strong feeling of helplessness)*. The woman was next to

This page may be reproduced by the purchaser for personal/clinical use.
From: M. Schauer, T. Elbert, & F. Neuner: *Narrative Exposure Therapy (NET) for Survivors of Traumatic Stress* (3rd ed.) (ISBN 9780889375956)
© 2025 Hogrefe Publishing

me on a mattress on the floor. She did not start screaming straight away since she first tried to defend herself. He pushed her with his hand, and she fell. When we saw this crudeness, our apprehension became inescapable certainty. *(Pain in the neck; touches her neck with her hand.)* The men surrounded the screaming women while I and a couple of other women went to Mila in order to help her. I wanted to release her from the grip of this man. While I was fighting, I felt strong rage, and I felt the urge to hit him with something, like a stone. I looked around but there was nothing I could have used. *(I can see his pig-face right now!)* It is hard to believe but he even looked quite nice and harmless, around 22 years old and well-built.... This contradiction was sickening somehow. We could have been his mother. I kept looking for an object but could not find anything when suddenly I was hit from behind: A man hit me with his gun on the right shoulder. I started panicking! He pulled my hands back, held my wrists behind my back and twisted them. Now I was completely helpless and in terrible pain. He dragged me out of the room. There were no doors to the main room, just a blanket that was hanging in the door frame.

He pushed me to the room where Mila was and then they dragged us through several rooms till we reached the back part of the ruin. It was dark and wet. He ripped off my clothes; I was wearing a light coat and its buttons came open straightaway. I felt terribly ashamed and was in a state of total panic. He was very brutal and greedy: He wanted to have me straight away! At once! He was already half-undressed and became angry when it took a while until he managed to pull down my nylon tights. He cursed and threatened me and swore in Russian: "You battered whore!" *(disgust and anger)*. He tried to kiss me, but I squirmed and turned my head away. His hands were everywhere: On my breasts and then also in my vagina. *(Hears her own screams.)* He looked "evil." He had light hair and blue eyes. He said: "You are not the first, you Chechen women all have to go 'through us.'" He was very close to me, and I could feel his body heat. I hated his hands on my body, and I hated having to feel his body. Everything inside me was struggling. He smelt of alcohol and sweat, like a man smells when he has not taken care of himself for a while. His sour bad breath like cold smoke was mixed with his body odor. *(Waves of revulsion go through my body, I am literally shaking with disgust.)* He threw me on a wooden pallet, as if I was just an object. He was brutal like an animal, as if he wanted to destroy me. I was lying on my back, and he forcibly penetrated my vagina with his penis. Straightaway I felt a strong pain *(hate and desperation)*. He pushed his penis hard inside me several times, and then he came on me, on my face. He was kneeling next to my head and wanted to push his penis into my mouth while I was fighting; trying to press my mouth shut and turn my head away as much as possible *(strong disgust)*. There was such a bad smell. *(Turns her head away and shivers.)* And then suddenly I scratched his face in blind fury: I wanted to rip out his eye and I wanted him to be blind on this eye! I wanted him to remember! He kept trying to push his penis into my mouth while shouting at me angrily. Then I opened my mouth a bit and bit into his penis as strongly as I could. I do not know how badly I managed to hurt him, but he went crazy: He screamed with pain and hit me in the face so brutally that I blacked out and fainted.

When I regained consciousness, I was in a "med-point" in a dilapidated house which served as a kind of military hospital. I do not remember how I got there, but when I woke up I immediately remembered what had happened, and I was very ashamed....

This page may be reproduced by the purchaser for personal/clinical use.
From: M. Schauer, T. Elbert, & F. Neuner: *Narrative Exposure Therapy (NET) for Survivors of Traumatic Stress* (3rd ed.) (ISBN 9780889375956)
© 2025 Hogrefe Publishing

Excerpt From a KIDNET, Testimony 3

I was born in M., Somalia, in 1990. I have no brothers and sisters. The house of my family was a few miles outside of town. It was a big house, and we had a good life. My father was a businessman; he owned a shop. My mother stayed at home. Later I was told that both parents were very happy to have me, since they had waited a long time for a child. I didn't know that. I only felt their love. There are some occasions that I remember clearly: When I was 5 years old, we celebrated my birthday with a party at our home. I was very happy then. Later, when I was 6 years old, I was taken to school. I was very good at school. I remember that I got a special degree. I was the best in my class. My family and I were very happy and proud because of that. I even remember the date of this special day; it was the 15th of August.

During the coming school break, my father took me on a trip around the country to reward me. When we came back, we met my mother again at home. My mother bought new clothes for me, and I got many presents, like video games. It was the time of the Eid festival. I had my friends at school. I invited them home. We played together. My father took us out to nice places, like the beach. When I remember this, I wished this life would come back, I was very happy then.

When I was 9, my father took me to a city called N. for the first time. We were staying in my aunt's home; she used to live there. My aunt was "cool as ice"; she liked to be with kids a lot. She also introduced me to other relatives there. She held a big party for me at her place. However, I remember missing my mother a lot. At least we had phone contact during our trip. I was looking forward to going back home to M. But when we came back, the city was in chaos. Fighting was going on. We heard that my mother had had to flee the town. I was crying heavily and regretting having left. But my father calmed me down and assured me that we would be together with my mother soon. I did not know at the time that I would never see my mother again. We have not found her until today.

Shortly after our return then, I went to the market with the house girl. We wanted to buy some new shoes for me. She was inside a shop. I stood in the street, attracted by shoes in a shop window. Suddenly I heard bullets; there was shooting and panic in the street everywhere around me. People were shouting and running. I can hear the sound of the bullets right now when I remember this, some people were shouting: "Allah Aq'bar," and there was the sound of bullets: "drrrrumm, drrrumm, drrrrumm." I fell down and was crouching close to the ground in the street with my hands over my head to protect myself. A moment later I could feel people running over me. I can feel the pain of their feet on my back right now, how they were stepping on me. My heart is beating fast when I remember this, there is a pain in my back and chest. My head is hurting so much right now. I was injured and in that moment, I thought I would die. I started crying. The house girl must have recognized my voice; she heard me crying. She had been hiding under a roof, and when she heard me, she ran toward me. She was injured too and crying. She wore only one shoe and was bleeding from her head and mouth. She picked me up from the ground and carried me in her arms. I felt I was safe with her. Her name was Amina, she was about 19 or 20 years old then and very beautiful. She called a taxi, we sat inside and drove away. We were safe in this car, and we held each other tightly. I had slung my arms around her, and she had her arms closely around me. We were both crying. There was still shooting, running, and people crying around us in the street, but I felt safe. As we went out of the city, the bullets became fewer. We reached home. My father was there. He held me and hugged me. In that moment all pain was gone, I forgot about all my injuries. All I felt was "I am safe now."

My father took Amina and me to the hospital. We were treated in the same room, lying on beds next to each other. People were there with aid kits. I had terrible pain in my chest. I was bleeding a lot from the nose. I was coughing blood. I still get the nose bleed now when I remember this day. I also get the pain in my chest, and my heart beats fast whenever I remember. I stayed in the hospital for 2 weeks. Then it was time to say goodbye to Amina, I thought we would part only for a few weeks. We sat together for about 30 minutes and said goodbye to each other. When I remember that moment, I feel happy and sad at the same time. Happy because she was the best housekeeper I ever had. She was like a sister to me; she cared for me so much. She saved me, even though she had been scared and injured herself. Since that day I have never seen her again. That makes me very sad every time I think of it.

This page may be reproduced by the purchaser for personal/clinical use.
From: M. Schauer, T. Elbert, & F. Neuner: *Narrative Exposure Therapy (NET) for Survivors of Traumatic Stress* (3rd ed.) (ISBN 9780889375956)
© 2025 Hogrefe Publishing

When I came out of hospital, I was somehow ok, but still feeling very low. My father took me to my grandma. She was living in a village further away from M. He thought it would be safer for us there. The village was called K. and was not far from the ocean. In K., I made several good friends after some time. I went to Madrasah Qu'ran school again.

About 1 month after I had moved to the village, I walked around with some friends. By that time the war had nearly reached the village. I wanted to look at the ocean because I liked looking at the water a lot. It always made me calm and happy. My friends went into the forest, so we separated. I went to the ocean alone. When I got to the shore, I stood on a rock and looked down over the water. What I saw was horrible. The water was full of dead bodies up to my feet. At first, I had thought people were out swimming. But I realized that there were about 20 floating bodies. They were black, there was blood, most of them were children, about 8 or 9 years old, some women, even pregnant ones with big bellies, and a few men. The bodies were floating there with their faces up and the eyes wide open. Their stomachs were already swelling. The moment I saw all these dead bodies I got a shock. I started shouting and crying: "Woowooowoo..!" I was shaking all over, I was frozen there on the rock although all I wanted to do was to run away. I felt intense fear, my heart was racing. I even feel it now, when I talk about this moment.

My friends heard me and came. They took me home. The memory of the street shooting in M. had also come back strongly. My nose started bleeding, I had a terrible headache, and the pain in my back where people had stepped on me came back badly. At home, I got first aid, my father put a piece of cloth on my head and neck. For 1 week I could not talk, I could not eat, I was in a state of total shock. Then my grandmother managed to calm me down, she explained about life and death to me, she said: "We all have to die one day; when the time comes that God has decided for you, you will die, no matter if there is war or not, that will be your day...." Slowly the confusion in my head cleared up. I became clearer in my thoughts. I started eating and talking again and felt ok. I woke up from that stage, walked around with my friends again and went to school.

At that time, I met Halimo; she was a friend of some of my friends. She had heard about what had happened to me. One day she asked me how I was doing now. This was the first time we talked to each other. She was my age and very beautiful; her skin was dark brown. We liked each other instantly. Soon we were spending most of our time together. We were walking around the neighborhood and talking a lot. When I wanted to go running, she went with me. We went to the shops together, and she helped me with the housework. She taught me a lot of things, and I taught her other things that she did not know. She was like Amina, she cared for me and was kind. We were having a great time. She was so cool. We started giving little gifts to each other. One of them was a postcard that she gave me one day. It read: "Love with all my friendship and all my heart." Halimo was always there for me whatever I wanted to do. She went with me and helped me forget all the bad things that had happened to me. We shared the root of our hearts. Can you ever forget such a beautiful friend?

One day we came back from the Madrasah school together. We were a group of about 20 girls and boys. It was about 1:30 in the afternoon. We separated because everybody had to walk in different directions to get home. Soon only Halimo and I were left. We decided to use a shortcut. It was a narrow path, bushland with some trees. We were talking. Suddenly there were three grown-up men in front of us. They had guns. Four others showed up behind us. Halimo was the one who realized first that they were killers. She took my left hand, pulled me, and we ran sideways into the bushes. One of them started shooting. It was rapid fire, one bullet hit my buttock, on the left side. At first, I didn't feel the pain, then I noticed that my left leg was failing to function. It became awfully heavy. Then the pain came. It was a strong pumping kind of pain. I wanted to get away, so I grabbed my trousers with my hands and tried to pull the leg forward. I had worn white trousers that day. My left side was already full of blood. It was running down my leg, soaking the white cloth. My hands were full of blood, too. Then my leg became too weak. I fell down. Halimo was still pulling my hand. She tried to get me back up, so we could continue running. She was crying and shouting: "Get up, let's run, please! Abdul, let's run!" Her face was full of fear, her eyes were wide open, looking terrified. I couldn't talk; I was just looking at her. One of the men had already reached us and hit me with the back of

This page may be reproduced by the purchaser for personal/clinical use.
From: M. Schauer, T. Elbert, & F. Neuner: *Narrative Exposure Therapy (NET) for Survivors of Traumatic Stress* (3rd ed.) (ISBN 9780889375956)
© 2025 Hogrefe Publishing

his gun on the left side of my head from behind. I fainted. I must have been unconscious for about 1 minute. When I woke up, I was lying on my stomach, bleeding. I felt the pain in my injured leg. I couldn't see properly. I touched and rubbed my eyes. I thought I would go blind. Everything I saw was red and flickering or flashing, like a red curtain in front of me. And then I saw Halimo, she was about 5 meters away, lying on her back. Two men were holding her arms. All seven men were there. They were looking ugly; their cloths were dirty and torn. Halimo's clothes were torn, and she was naked. One of the men had pulled down his trousers to his knees. I saw him penetrating her, moving up and down. One side of his face was very damaged. There was hardly any skin, and the left eye was like pushed inside the skull. It was so ugly and disgusting, I was horrified. When I remember this, I start seeing everything red, like in that very moment. When I look at the faces of men in such a state of memory and fear, any face in front of me can turn into the face of that rapist. That's when I lose control. All I want is try to beat and chase the person. I can get very angry and aggressive. It sometimes happens even when it is the face of my father, or other people who I like and admire. Then I feel like as if there are two people inside me. While the deformed man was raping Halimo, the others were standing there watching, laughing, and constantly shooting into the air. These are the only sounds I could hear, and they are ringing in my ear whenever I think of that day. Halimo's lips were swollen and bleeding. She was injured on her right cheek near the eye. Her eyes were open and dark. She seemed to be unconscious. I felt terrible pain. But I tried to move, shout, do anything, throw a stone at least, to make them stop, but I was frozen, paralyzed. I could not move. I was annoyed and very angry. My body failed me completely; I could not move at all. I was trapped. I felt so helpless and guilty. Since then I blame myself for not helping her, whereas she was always helping me so much. This guilt and sadness has weighed very heavy on me ever since. When the first man had finished, the next one was raping her. He was the one with the scar. He pulled off his clothes in a hurry. He wore a long shirt. He was penetrating her, too. When I saw him moving up and down, I fainted again. It was just too much; it was too terrible to bear. The next thing I remember was that I woke up seeing white things. There were voices talking. First I thought I was in another world, or dead, or something like that. I was in hospital. I saw blood dripping from a bottle on the right side of my bed. It was an infusion. My dad was there beside me. He was holding my hand. I was still fearing a lot. Then a doctor came and for the first time the face of an ordinary man turned into the disgusting face of the rapist. I was terrified and screamed: "This is the guy I saw and I know what he did!" I was furious and angry, full of tension. My dad tried to calm me down, but I shouted: "I will kill you!" My dad explained to me that it was just the doctor, and that he wanted to help me. My father also tried to find out what had happened to me, but I could not tell him.

After that incident I got a single room for a period of time. The nights in the hospital were horrible. I couldn't sleep. I saw the face of the rapist. I saw everything red when I remembered. I could not eat. I was blaming myself for what had happened. I was feeling guilty. I was terribly angry. A very deep feeling of darkness came into my heart and has never left me up to today. I had no future, no hope. After some time, when I seemed to have become more normal, it was decided that I should share a room again. But it didn't take long, and I attacked my roommate. I shouted at him and pulled at his infusion because I thought he, too, was one of the rapists. So I was moved to a solitary room again. I was having nightmares about the rape scene and the dead bodies floating at the shore all the time. When I saw children playing and being happy, I had to cry because I thought I could never do something like that again. I was in hospital for 3 months. In the end I was somehow okay again. Then the day I left the hospital, at the gate my dad and I met a stranger and again everything turned red, and I saw the rapist in that innocent man. I ran after him, shouted at him, and wanted to hurt him. My father got me and held me tight. He said: "What is wrong with you? What's wrong?" I have never told him or anybody else what had happened to me exactly during that day of the rape, and he also doesn't know what goes on in my mind and body when I get out of control. This is why I felt and still feel a certain distance to everybody around me. People don't understand why I act strange sometimes, and I cannot tell them.

Some time later Halimo's parents visited me at my home. They had brought gifts and wanted to see how I was doing. I could not face them. I could not open the door. I felt so bad and guilty. How could she ever forgive me for not having helped her when she needed me most? Sometimes she comes to me in my dreams, even now, and she looks beautiful and kind, just like she used to. But I cannot forgive myself. I don't even

This page may be reproduced by the purchaser for personal/clinical use.
From: M. Schauer, T. Elbert, & F. Neuner: *Narrative Exposure Therapy (NET) for Survivors of Traumatic Stress* (3rd ed.) (ISBN 9780889375956)
© 2025 Hogrefe Publishing

know whether she is still alive. I can't get myself to find out. I can't imagine how it would be to see her again. I only know I would run away.

After my days in the hospital, my father took me to a friend of his. He lived in a small and quiet village. There were a lot of children in the village, playing football. I spend most of the time inside, just watching them, doing nothing. I was completely absent, far away, dealing with the darkness in my heart. After 3 weeks in the village, I started to relax a bit. I ate more and slept a bit. Then fighting reached even this little remote village. One day at 12 noon, there was a heavy attack. There were explosions, fire, and the sounds of bullets all over the place. First, I was inside the house alone. People ran around and fled toward the forest. I was full of fear, shocked and paralyzed, but I ran behind the house. From there I could not move, I just stood there, my heart was racing and my whole body was shaking. Many people were passing by, some were injured, some shot, some were running although they were lacking an arm. One man lying very near to me on the ground was torn into two parts. A shell must have hit him. His upper part was lying far from his lower part, yet he was still crying and screaming. There was a lot of blood. The sight of him was horrible, it just looked so awful. All I did was close my eyes, I could not move. I don't know how long I was frozen there in terror and fear, crying until my dad came and carried me into a pickup. He was holding me as I was shaking and crying. I sat beside my dad and the driver in the front seat. Suddenly, as we were already heading out of the village, a bullet hit our driver through the front window. The glass shattered. The bullet went into the front of his head and something came out of his neck. The driver fell backwards and blood spilled over my eye. The vehicle lost control, and we went into a ditch with great speed. When the pickup crashed, I was catapulted out through the window and fainted. When I woke up, I was lying halfway on the front of the car, halfway on the ground. I was more or less ok and immediately checked on my dad. He was unconscious, blood was coming out of his mouth, and his shoulder and chest were injured. By that time people had come, and they helped us on a truck to get to the nearby hospital. My father was unconscious for a long time. I kept sitting by his bedside, holding his hand and talking to him. I was scared he would not come back. I told him: "Don't worry. I'm ok. Please wake up, wake up!" I stayed in the hospital with my dad for 2 weeks, for there was no other place I could have gone to. Sometimes a guy came and gave me some fruit to eat.

When my dad was feeling better, we went to friends and they brought us to G. There we met my aunt. We stayed there for a while. My dad had no job. He was just there with me thinking about what should happen to us in the future. I was feeling safer in G. but I had still problems with sleeping. After a while my aunty married, and I was somehow happy, but there was nothing I could enjoy any more, even the marriage party was not enjoyable for me.

Then we decided to move on to U. In U., I made new friends, and one day we met at a friend's place to watch the movie *Black Hawk Down.* It is a film about the war in Somalia. At first it was okay, but when the shooting in the film started, and a lot of blood was shown I got out of control. I started to see everything red, I was breathing fast, my heart was racing. I got scared, furious, angry. I started shaking and then I took a chair and threw it into the TV screen. The television exploded and everybody screamed and shouted. I didn't realize the panic and chaos around me. It was like I was not in my world anymore. I was full of panic, I ran out of the room and down the stairs. I fell and cut my tongue badly, blood was dripping out of my mouth and on my trousers. I was still in total shock and panic when they found me. I was taken to hospital and treated for about 1 month. I could not talk properly for some time because my tongue was swollen and stitched together. My dad did not understand what had happened. He just said he had to pay a lot of money for the damage that I had done.

In those days we were living with another aunt, actually it was not my aunt, it was the wife of one of my dad's friends. Altogether we spent about 1 year in U. My dad was unemployed during that time, but he was helping the friends we stayed with.

Then in 1999 my dad got to know a woman from Tanzania in U. They decided to get married, and we moved to the refugee camp in 2000. The woman is okay, although I don't talk to her too much. She also doesn't know anything about my past, and I don't know what she thinks is wrong with me when I get out of control. Sometimes she makes an effort and tries to talk to me. She asks me questions about my experiences in the past, but I cannot tell her. She tries, but still I do not feel very close to her.

This page may be reproduced by the purchaser for personal/clinical use.
From: M. Schauer, T. Elbert, & F. Neuner: *Narrative Exposure Therapy (NET) for Survivors of Traumatic Stress* (3rd ed.) (ISBN 9780889375956)
© 2025 Hogrefe Publishing

Even now, many years later, the pictures of the day when Halimo got raped keep coming back to my mind. I look at normal people, like a teacher or a friend, and suddenly the face of the rapist appears. Then I get angry and aggressive and try to hurt the person. I throw things and get violent. Sometimes I find myself sitting in strange places, like on top of the roof, crying, and I have no idea how I got there. It is as if there are two personalities living inside me. One is smart and kind and normal, the other one is crazy and violent. I try so hard to control this other side of me. But I fail. Sometimes I feel tears running down my cheek, and I wonder why. Sometimes I walk down the street, and suddenly I see the path in the bush of that day in front of me, and I feel Halimo's hand pulling my hand, trying to make me run and escape together. Since that day I can't walk shortcuts anymore. Even a normal bush can bring back all these memories. And when the memory of the rape comes, all the other pictures are in my mind as well, like the dead bodies in the ocean. Since we are in the camp, it is especially bad, since there is so much bushland around.

Now that I have talked about all that has happened to me, I would also like my father to know. I want him to read my story. I also want to register now with the Red Cross Tracing Service, to find Halimo. Maybe she is still in Somalia or lives as a refugee in Nairobi. Wherever she is now, I want to find out how her life is today. Maybe she will write to me, or we can even meet? Until today, I have never started a friendship with a girl again. I didn't want to get close to them anymore. They remind me of what happened to Halimo and me. In the future I wish I can live like a normal person, get married, and have children. I would like to be a doctor or a lawyer. I would love to help people.

Date and Place:

________________ ________________ ________________

Signature Survivor | Signature Therapist | Signature Interpreter

This page may be reproduced by the purchaser for personal/clinical use.
From: M. Schauer, T. Elbert, & F. Neuner: *Narrative Exposure Therapy (NET) for Survivors of Traumatic Stress* (3rd ed.) (ISBN 9780889375956)
© 2025 Hogrefe Publishing

Peer Commentaries

In this superb presentation by the developers of an exceptional and invaluable psychotherapy for trauma survivors, Narrative Exposure Therapy (NET), the authors have succeeded in exemplifying the essence of the intervention by putting into words *NET's rigorous and fundamentally humane rationale and its wonderfully creative therapeutic process. NET stands out among the many other trauma-focused psychotherapies by providing a unique approach to memory processing that embeds this crucial therapeutic work in the survivor's autobiographical lifeline, connecting and re-integrating fragmented memories, and also extending the healing process to the entire community. This book is essential reading for all psychotherapists who work with trauma survivors as it provides a framework and specific interventions that will extend and enhance the ability of practitioners, trainers, and trainees from every theoretical orientation and across all therapeutic allegiances.*

Julian D. Ford, PhD, ABPP, Director of the Center for the Treatment of Developmental Trauma Disorders at the University of Connecticut Health School of Medicine; Past President of the International Society for Traumatic Stress Studies; Editor of the *Journal of Trauma and Dissociation*

In my opinion, there can be no text on trauma and narrative more authoritative than this one. The authors have expertly crafted a manual that provides the perfect marriage of theoretical foundation, scientific evidence, practical step-by-step guidance, and authentic case study discussion, simplifying the heavy lifting of working with traumatised individuals, groups, and communities in different violence-ridden contexts. The suite of interventions (e.g., KIDNET, eNET, ElderNET, FORNET), addressing life course needs, is unique and demonstrates an unwavering commitment on the part of the authors to give voice, across the lifespan, to "victims," and truly relieve suffering and promote sustainable healing.

Soraya Seedat, MD, PhD, Distinguished Professor of Psychiatry, Faculty of Medicine and Health Science, Stellenbosch University, Cape Town, South Africa

Since its creation, Narrative Exposure Therapy has become a highly respected and increasingly used evidence-based treatment for people with posttraumatic stress disorder, especially those with more complex presentations. The authors are to be commended on this excellent update of the NET handbook. The detailed explanation of NET's theoretical basis and step-by-step guidance on the delivery of NET and its adaptations for specific populations will be invaluable to therapists. I have no doubt that the updated handbook will help further establish NET as an effective treatment for traumatised people.

Jonathan I. Bisson, DM FRCPsych, Clinical Professor in Psychiatry, Cardiff University, UK; Director of Traumatic Stress Wales

This manual is an invaluable resource for clinicians working with survivors of organized violence. Clear step-by-step instructions, diagrams, bullet-point summaries and example transcripts provide practical guidance for novice and expert clinicians alike. Beyond the outstanding clinical content, this manual is imbued with a strong social justice perspective. It emphasizes the clinician's role as a healer and advocate, recognizing the systemic forces that contribute to the suffering of violence-affected communities and encouraging a compassionate, community-centered approach to healing. Overall, this manual combines rigorously researched evidence-based methodologies with an unwavering commitment to safeguarding the rights and dignity of those affected by violence, making it an indispensable tool for those working with traumatized individuals and communities.

Angela Nickerson, Professor and Director of the Refugee Trauma and Recovery Program, School of Psychology, UNSW Sydney, Australia

New edition of this effective toolbox for treating trauma survivors is even more comprehensive

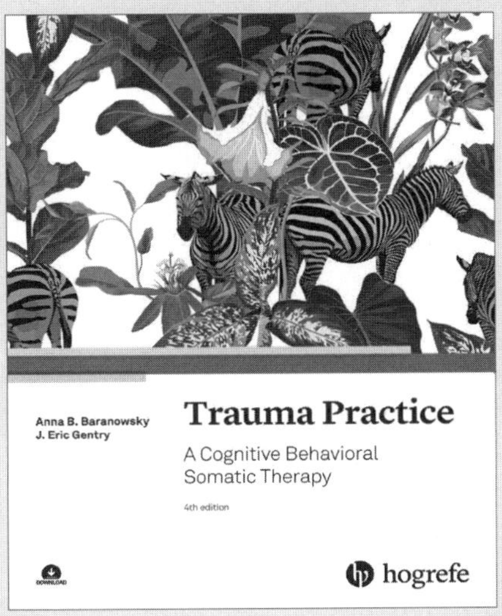

4th ed. 2023, xii + 226 pp.,
$59.00/€ 50.95
ISBN 978-0-88937-592-5
Also available as eBook

Anna B. Baranowsky/J. Eric Gentry

Trauma Practice

A Cognitive Behavioral Somatic Therapy

This popular, practical resource for clinicians caring for trauma survivors has been fully updated and expanded. It remains a key toolkit of cognitive behavioral somatic therapy (CBST) techniques for clinicians who want to enhance their skills in treating trauma. Baranowsky and Gentry help practitioners find the right tools to guide trauma survivors toward growth and healing. Reinforcing this powerful intervention is the addition of a deeper emphasis on the preparatory phase for therapists, including the therapists' own ability to self-regulate their autonomic system during client encounters.

Throughout the acclaimed book, an effective tri-phasic model for trauma treatment is constructed (safety and stabilization; working through trauma; reconnection with a meaningful life) as guiding principle, enabling a phased delivery that is fitted to the survivor's relational and processing style. The authors present, clearly and in detail, an array of techniques, protocols, and interventions for treating trauma survivors (cognitive, behavioral, somatic, and emotional/relational). These include popular and effective CBST techniques, approaches inspired by research on neuroplasticity, and interventions informed by polyvagal theory. Many techniques include links to video or audio material demonstrating how to carry-out the intervention. Further sections are devoted to forward-facing trauma therapy, a safe, effective, and accelerated method of treating trauma, and to clinician self-care.

Over 40 video and audio demonstrations of many of the techniques are available for download. There are also 36 handouts for clients that can be downloaded and printed for clinical use.

"Carefully researched, theoretically grounded, and beautifully written, [this book] is a must-read for any clinician who treats interpersonal trauma. Highly recommended."

Robert T. Muller, PhD, Professor, Faculty of Health, York University, Toronto, ON, Canada; Fellow of the International Society for the Study of Trauma & Dissociation(from the Foreword of the 1st ed.)

www.hogrefe.com

hogrefe

Don’t miss a thing with this excellent guide to diagnosing the impact of trauma

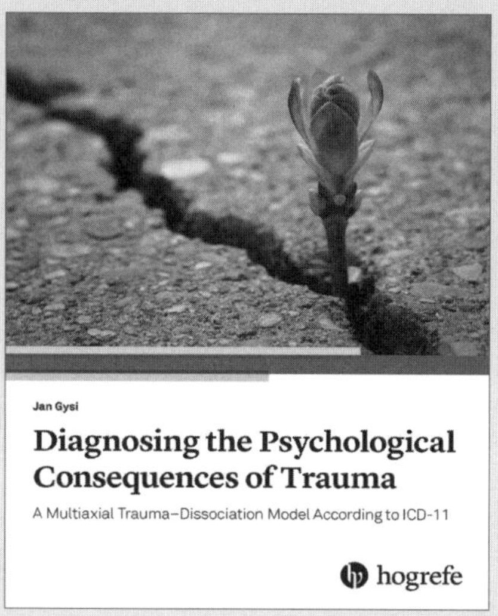

Due April 2025, approx. xiv + 250 pp.,
Approx. $86.00/74.95
ISBN 978-0-88937-636-6
Also available as eBook

Jan Gysi

Diagnosing the Psychological Consequences of Trauma

A Multiaxial Trauma–Dissociation Model According to ICD-11

Tremendous progress has been made in the diagnosis and treatment of the consequences of trauma over the past two decades, which has led to significant changes being introduced in the ICD-11 and the DSM-5. Navigating this wealth of new knowledge in psychotraumatology, as well as keeping track of the various posttraumatic symptoms and disorders that can present in clients, can be challenging.

The brilliantly structured, full-color navigation charts in this volume help both early career and experienced professionals to keep track of the variety of diagnostic options to be considered or excluded while not overlooking anything. After an introduction to the trauma–dissociation axis model, the five axes are then presented in detail, including case examples, differential diagnoses, recommendations, decision paths, and questionnaires:

- Axis I: Personality disorders (including, borderline)
- Axis II: Disorders specifically associated with stress (including, PTSD, CPTSD, and prolonged grief disorder)
- Axis III: Structural dissociation of the personality (dissociative and partial dissociative identity disorder)
- Axis IV: Other dissociative disorders (dissociative neurological symptom disorder, depersonalization-derealization disorder, dissociative amnesia)
- Axis V: Comorbid disorders

The last two chapters provide an overview of the special diagnostic aspects of reporting to law enforcement agencies, and a catalog of questions collated by the author to help guide diagnosis and inform treatment. This volume is an exceptional resource for psychiatrists, clinical psychologists, psychotherapists, and other mental health professionals who work with traumatized individuals.

www.hogrefe.com

hogrefe